STUDY GUIDE FOR THE

Core Curriculum
for Oncology
Nursing

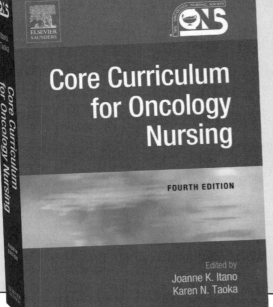

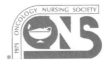

STUDY GUIDE FOR THE
Core Curriculum
for Oncology
Nursing

FOURTH EDITION

Suzanne M. Mahon, RN, DNSc, AOCN®, APNG
Assistant Clinical Professor
Division of Hematology/Oncology
Department of Internal Medicine
Saint Louis University Cancer Center
St. Louis, Missouri

ELSEVIER
SAUNDERS

ELSEVIER
SAUNDERS

11830 Westline Industrial Drive
St. Louis, Missouri 63146

NOTICE

Oncology Nursing is an ever-changing field. Standard safety precautions must be followed, but as new research and clinical experience broaden our knowledge, changes in treatment and drug therapy may become necessary or appropriate. Readers are advised to check the most current product information provided by the manufacturer of each drug to be administered to verify the recommended dose, the method and duration of administration, and contraindications. It is the responsibility of the licensed prescriber, relying on experience and knowledge of the patient, to determine dosages and the best treatment for each individual patient. Neither the publisher nor the author assumes any liability for any injury and/or damage to persons or property arising from this publication.

The use of brand names in this text is not an assertion of trademark ownership or an endorsement of any product. The brand names cited are not comprehensive; more than one company may manufacture or market a product known by the same brand name. Every effort was made to ensure the accuracy of this information at press time. However, trademark ownership often changes, as do the names and locations of companies; therefore, the publisher and contributors take no responsibility for the accuracy of the brand names cited. Do not use this information without verifying it to ensure that the brand names are up-to-date.

ISBN-13: 978-0-7216-0359-9
ISBN-10: 0-7216-0359-9

Executive Publisher: Barbara Nelson Cullen
Acquisitions Editor: Sandra Clark Brown
Senior Developmental Editor: Cindi Anderson
Publishing Services Manager: Catherine Jackson
Senior Project Manager: Anne Konopka
Designer: Teresa McBryan

Printed in the United States of America.

Last digit is the print number: 9   8   7   6   5   4

Working together to grow
libraries in developing countries

www.elsevier.com | www.bookaid.org | www.sabre.org

ELSEVIER   BOOK AID International   Sabre Foundation

Contributors

Carol S. Blecher, RN, MS, AOCN®, APN, C
Advanced Practice Nurse, Clinical Manager
Hematology & Oncology Associates of
    New Jersey, LLC
Union, New Jersey
The Education Process

Patricia C. Buchsel, RN, MSN, FAAN
Adjuvant Faculty
College of Nursing
Seattle University
Seattle, Washington
*Nursing Implications of Hematopoietic Stem Cell
    Transplantation*

Joe Burrage, Jr., PhD, RN
Associate Professor
School of Nursing
University of Alabama–Birmingham
Birmingham, Alabama
Nursing Care of the Client with HIV-Related Cancers

Jeannine M. Brant, RN, MS, AOCN®
Oncology Clinical Nurse Specialist
Pain Consultant
St. Vincent Healthcare
Billings, Montana
Comfort

Kathleen A. Calzone, RN, MSN, APNG
Senior Nurse Specialist (Research)
Center for Cancer Research, Genetics Branch
National Cancer Institute
Bethesda, Maryland
Genetics

Dawn Camp-Sorrell, MSN, FNP, AOCN®
Oncology Nurse Practitioner
Central Alabama Oncology, LLC
Alabaster, Alabama
Myelosuppression

Ellen Carr, RN, MSN, AOCN®
Case Manager
Head/Neck Oncology
Rebecca and John Moores Cancer Center
University of California, San Diego
San Diego, California
*Nursing Care of the Client with Head and Neck
    Cancer*
*Nursing Care of the Client with Bone and Soft Tissue
    Cancers*

Cindy Catlin-Huth, RN, MSN, OCN®, ANP-C
Nurse Practitioner
Department of Hematology Oncology
Duke University Adult Bone Marrow
    Transplant Program
Durham, North Carolina
Nursing Implications of Radiation Therapy

Cynthia Chernecky, PhD, RN, CNS, AOCN®
Professor
School of Nursing
Medical College of Georgia
Augusta, Georgia
Alterations in Ventilation

Diane G. Cope, PhD, ARNP, BC, AOCN®
Nurse Practitioner
Florida Cancer Specialists
Fort Meyers, Florida
Nursing Care of the Client with Breast Cancer

Robin L. Coyne, RN, MSN, FNP
Family Nurse Practitioner
Cancer Prevention Center
The University of Texas MD Anderson Cancer
    Center
Houston, Texas
Early Detection of Cancer

Denise Murray Edwards, CS, ARNP, MA, MEd, MTS

Mental Health Nurse Practitioner
The Center for Health and Well-Being
Iowa Health Systems
West Des Moines, Iowa
  Supportive Care: Nonpharmacologic Interventions

Constance B. Ellis, MN, RNC, CWOCN, OCN®

Director, Wound, Ostomy, Continence Nurse
  Education Program
The University of Texas MD Anderson Cancer
  Center
Houston, Texas
  Professional Issues in Cancer Care

Jean M. Ellsworth-Wolk, RN, MS, AOCN®

Oncology Clinical Nurse Specialist
Lakewood Hospital
Lakewood, Ohio
  *Principles of Preparation, Administration, and
    Disposal of Hazardous Drugs*

Peg Esper, MSN, RN, CS, AOCN®

Nurse Practitioner
Department of Medical Oncology
University of Michigan
Ann Arbor, Michigan
  *Nursing Implications of Biotherapy and Molecular
    Targeted Therapy*

Susan Ezzone, MS, RN, CNP

Nurse Practitioner
Bone & Marrow Transplant Program
Arthur G. James Cancer Hospital and Richard
  Solove Institute
The Ohio State University Medical Center
Columbus, Ohio
  *Nursing Care of the Client with Lymphoma or
    Multiple Myeloma*

Marie Flannery, RN, PhD, AOCN®

Senior Nurse Practitioner
James P. Wilmot Cancer Center
Assistant Professor
University of Rochester School of Nursing
Rochester, New York
  Nursing Care of the Client with Lung Cancer

Jo Ann A. Flounders, MSN, CRNP, APRN, BC, AOCN®, CHPN

Nurse Practitioner
Consultants in Medical Oncology and
  Hematology
Drexel Hill, Pennsylvania
  Structural Emergencies

Paula Forest, MSN, OCN®, GNP, CHPN, ARNP

Medicine Cancer Service
Mercy Medical Center
Cedar Rapids, Iowa
  *Nursing Care of the Client with Cancers of the
    Reproductive System*
  *Nursing Care of the Client with Cancers of the
    Urinary System*

Beth A. Freitas, RN, MN, OCN®

Clinical Nurse Specialist
Pain and Palliative Care Department
The Queen's Medical Center
Honolulu, Hawaii
  Coping: Altered Body Image and Alopecia

Sue L. Frymark, RN, BS

Executive Director
Cancer Care Resources/Northwest Cancer
  Specialists Foundation
Portland, Oregon
  Supportive Care: Rehabilitation and Resources

Barbara Holmes Gobel, RN, MS, AOCN®

Oncology Clinical Nurse Specialist
Northwestern Memorial Hospital
Chicago, Illinois
  Metabolic Emergencies

Patricia M. Grimm, PhD, RN, APRN, BC

Clinical Staff
HopeWELL Cancer Support
Baltimore, Maryland
  Coping: Psychosocial Issues

Robert J. Ignoffo, PharmD, FASHP, FCSHP

Clinical Professor
Department of Clinical Pharmacy
University of California, San Francisco
San Francisco, California
  Supportive Care: Pharmacologic Interventions

Gabriela Kaplan RN, MSN, AOCN®

Oncology Education Specialist
The Cancer Institute of New Jersey
New Brunswick, New Jersey
  Selected Ethical Issues in Cancer Care

Shirley J. Kern, RN, MSN, AOCN®, APRN-BC

Oncology Clinical Nurse Specialist
Lung Cancer Program
North Memorial Medical Center
Minneapolis, Minnesota
Nursing Care of the Client with Cancers of the Neurologic System

Valerie Kogut, MA, RD, LDN

Nutrition Coordinator
Department of Otolaryngology
University of Pittsburgh Physicians
Pittsburgh, Pennsylvania
Alterations in Nutrition

Linda U. Krebs, RN, PhD, AOCN®

Associate Professor
School of Nursing
University of Colorado at Denver and Health Sciences Center
Denver, Colorado
Application of the Statement on the Scope and Standards of Oncology Nursing Practice *and Evidence-Based Practice*

Kim K. Kuebler, MN, RN, ANP, CS

Adjuvant Therapies Inc.
Private Practice
  Primary/Oncology/Palliative Care
Atlanta, Georgia
Legal Issues Influencing Cancer Care

Evelyn H. Larrison, RN, BSN

Gynecologic Oncology Nurse Consultant
DeForest, Wisconsin
Sexuality

Colleen O. Lee, RN, MS, AOCN®

CDR, US Public Health Service
Practice Assessment Program Manager
Office of Cancer Complementary and Alternative Medicine
National Cancer Institute
Bethesda, Maryland
Complementary and Alternative Medicines

Susan Leigh, BSN, RN

Cancer Survivorship Consultant
Tucson, Arizona
Coping: Survivorship Issues and Financial Concerns

Molly Loney, RN, MSN, AOCN®

Clinical Nurse Specialist
Hillcrest Hospital
The Cleveland Clinic Health System
Cleveland, Ohio
Supportive Care: Dying and Death
Cancer Economics and Health Care Reform

Alice J. Longman, RN, EdD, FAAN

Professor Emeritus
The University of Arizona College of Nursing
Tucson, Arizona
Nursing Care of the Client with Skin Cancer

Suzanne M. Mahon RN, DNSc, AOCN®, APNG

Assistant Clinical Professor
Division of Hematology/Oncology
Department of Internal Medicine
Saint Louis University Cancer Center
St. Louis, Missouri
Epidemiology and Prevention of Cancer

Jan Hawthorne Maxson, RN, MSN, AOCN®

Nurse Practitioner
Division of Gynecologic Oncology
University Hospitals of Cleveland
Cleveland, Ohio
Principles of Preparation, Administration, and Disposal of Hazardous Drugs

Molly J. Moran, MS, APRN, BC

Clinical Nurse Specialist
Department of Oncology Nursing
James Cancer Hospital and Solove Research Institute
Columbus, Ohio
Nursing Care of the Client with Leukemia

Zoe Ngo, PharmD

Oncology Pharmacist
Assistant Clinical Professor
Department of Clinical Pharmacy
UCSF Comprehensive Cancer Center
San Francisco, California
Supportive Care: Pharmacologic Interventions

Bridget O'Brien, ND, RN, CS-FNP, OCN®

Gastrointestinal Oncology Nurse Practitioner
Department of Hematology/Oncology
Northwestern Medical Faculty Foundation
Robert H. Lurie Comprehensive Cancer Center
Chicago, Illinois
Nursing Care of the Client with Cancers of the Gastrointestinal Tract

James C. Pace, DSN, RN, MDiv, ANP-BC
Professor of Nursing
Adult Nurse Practitioner
Program/Palliative Care Focus
Vanderbilt University School of Nursing
Nashville, Tennessee
Immunology

Jennifer Douglas Pearce, RN, MSN, CNS
Associate Professor
Department of Nursing
University of Cincinnati
Raymond Walters College
Cincinnati, Ohio
*Alterations in Mobility, Skin Integrity, and
Neurologic Status*

Janice Phillips, PhD, RN, FAAN
Nurse Researcher
University of Chicago Hospitals and Clinics
Chicago, Illinois
Coping: Cultural Issues

Barbara C. Poniatowski, MS, RN,C, AOCN®
Senior Clinical Nurse Educator
Oncology Division
GlaxoSmithKline
Philadelphia, Pennsylvania
Nursing Implications of Antineoplastic Therapy

Elisa Ricciardi, BA, MS
Patient Care Manager
Wound, Ostomy, Continence Nurse
Department of Hematology/Oncology, Inpatient
Unit
Childrens Hospitals and Clinics
Minneapolis, Minnesota
Alterations in Elimination

Kristine Turner Story, RN, MSN, APRN
Nurse Practitioner
Department of Internal Medicine
Physicians Clinic, Internal Medicine Health
West
Omaha, Nebraska
Alterations in Circulation

Lisa Stucky-Marshall, RN, MS, AOCN®
Oncology Advanced Practice Nurse
Oncology Services
Elmhurst Memorial Hospital
Elmhurst, Illinois
*Nursing Care of the Client with Cancers of the
Gastrointestinal Tract*

Thomas J. Szopa, RN, MS, WOCN
Clinical Nurse Specialist
Oncology and Ostomy/Wound Management
Elliot Hospital
Manchester, New Hampshire
Nursing Implications of Surgical Treatment

Susan Vogt Temple, RN, MSN, ETN, AOCN®
Senior Clinical Educator
GlaxoSmithKline Oncology
Seale, Alabama
*Nursing Care of the Client with Cancers of the
Reproductive System
Nursing Implications of Antineoplastic Therapy*

Cynthia H. Umstead, RN, MSN, OCN®
Senior Clinical Educator
GlaxoSmithKline Pharmaceuticals
Philadelphia, Pennsylvania
*Nursing Care of the Client with Cancers of the
Reproductive System*

Carol S. Viele, RN, MS
Clinical Nurse Specialist
Department of Hematology-Oncology-Bone
Marrow Transplant
Assistant Clinical Professor
Department of Physiological Nursing
School of Nursing
University of California, San Francisco
San Francisco, California
Supportive Care: Pharmacologic Interventions

Deborah L. Volker, RN, PhD, AOCN®
Assistant Professor
School of Nursing
The University of Texas at Austin
Austin, Texas
Biology of Cancer and Carcinogenesis

Marjorie Whitman, RN, MS(N), AOCN®
Clinical Instructor of Nursing
Sinclair School of Nursing
University of Missouri–Columbia
Columbia, Missouri
Supportive Care: Support Therapies and Procedures

Reviewers

Elaine S. DeMeyer RN, MSN, AOCN®

Independent Oncology Nurse Consultant
President and CEO
Creative Cancer Concepts, Inc.
Rockwall, Texas

Pat Gillett, RN, MSN, ACNP

Clinical Instructor
College of Nursing
The University of New Mexico
Albuquerque, New Mexico

Jeanne Held-Warmkessel, MSN, RN, AOCN®, APRN, BC

Clinical Nurse Specialist
Fox Chase Cancer Center
Philadelphia, Pennsylvania

Bernadette M. Lombardi, RN, MSN, MA, MS, PhD(c)

Assistant Director
Northeast Health Albany and Samaritan
  Hospitals School of Nursing
Albany, New York

Julie D. Painter, RNC, MSN, OCN®

Clinical Nurse Specialist
Community Health Network
Indianapolis, Indiana

Phyllis G. Peterson, RN, MN, AOCN®

Assistant Professor
Division of Nursing
Our Lady of Holy Cross College
New Orleans, Louisiana

Carmencita M. Poe, RN, EdD, CD, OCN®, CHPN

Clinical Nurse Manager
Department of Oncology/Medical-Surgical
  Nursing
Bon Secours DePaul Medical Center
Norfolk, Virginia

Cheryl Reggio, RN, OCN®

Clinical Staff Nurse
Department of Hematology/Oncology
Children's National Medical Center
Silver Spring, Maryland

Noemi Salcido, RN, BSN

El Paso Cancer Treatment Center
El Paso, Texas

Patti C. Simmons, RN, MN

Assistant Professor of Nursing
Department of Nursing
North Georgia College and State University
Dahlonega, Georgia

Miriam E. Sleven, RN, MS, OCN®

Oncology Nurse Consultant
Clovis, California

Susan K. Steele, DNS, RN, AOCN®

Assistant Professor of Nursing
School of Nursing
Louisiana State University Health Sciences
  Center
New Orleans, Louisiana

Scott Carter Thigpen, RN, MSN, CCRN, CEN

Assistant Professor of Nursing
Division of Nursing
South Georgia College
Douglas, Georgia

Constance Visovsky PhD, RN, ACNP

Assistant Professor of Nursing
Case Western Reserve University
Cleveland, Ohio

M. Linda Workman, RN, PhD, FAAN

The Gertrude Perkins Olivia Professor of
  Oncology Nursing
Case Western Reserve University
Cleveland, Ohio

Preface

The *Study Guide for the Core Curriculum for Oncology Nursing,* fourth edition, is a companion text to the *Core Curriculum for Oncology Nursing,* fourth edition, and a resource for oncology nursing. Clinical nurses, educators, and managers will find this book a useful source of questions to guide the development of oncology-related classes.

The questions for the fourth edition are based on the *Core Curriculum for Oncology Nursing* and present a question followed by multiple-choice answers. The rationales for not only the correct answer but also the incorrect options are provided in the Answer sections. The manuscripts have undergone peer review by clinical oncology nurses and oncology nurse educators for completeness, clinical relevance, accuracy, and clarity. Answers were chosen to reflect national practice trends at the time the text was written and may not reflect some regional clinical practices.

The resources for the questions and the rationale for the answers are based on the *Core Curriculum for Oncology Nursing,* fourth edition, and other current references that support the answers. All of these references can be used for further study of the content area.

The number of questions on each topic was derived from the percent of questions for that content area established by the Oncology Nursing Certification Corporation (ONCC) in the OCN® Test Blueprint provided to applicants for the certification examination. The OCN® Test Blueprint can be found in the *Oncology Nursing Certification Bulletin* (2005). The subjects covered in both this study guide and in the *Core Curriculum for Oncology Nursing* go beyond those known to be included in the certification exam.

I would like to dedicate this book to my family. My gratitude goes to my parents, Ted and Jackie Dubuque, who provided the foundation and education that initiated my career and who have always encouraged me to pursue my dreams. I thank my husband, Jerry, who continues to be a source of support. I am grateful for my three beautiful daughters, Emily, Maureen, and Elaine, who each through her own special gifts, have provided me with constant joy and hope for the future.

This book would not have been possible without the contributions of the many authors. I appreciate their willingness to share their expertise with other oncology nurses.

In a special way I want to acknowledge and thank Barbara Sigler, RN, MNEd, who is Director of Commercial Publishing and Technical Editor for the Oncology Nursing Society Publishing Division. Barb has been a constant source of assistance, guidance, and encouragement. She helps me keep things in perspective. She has taught me much about the publication process, for which I am most grateful. Barb paid great attention to detail during every phase of the project and provided much insight into ways to improve the book. Without her, the book would not have been possible.

Suzanne M. Mahon

REFERENCE

Oncology Nursing Certification Corporation. (2005). *Oncology Nursing Certification Bulletin.* Pittsburgh: Author.

Contents

PART SIX

Scientific Basis for Practice, 171

PART SEVEN

Health Promotion, 279

PART EIGHT

Professional Performance, 295

PART ONE

QUALITY OF LIFE

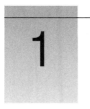

1 Comfort

JEANNINE M. BRANT

Select the best answer for each of the following questions:

1. Pain is defined as an unpleasant sensory and emotional experience associated with
   A. actual tissue damage.
   B. actual or potential tissue damage.
   C. observable pain behaviors.
   D. physiologic signs and symptoms that the pain exists.

2. Neuropathic pain characteristics include
   A. well-localized syndrome with aching and gnawing sensations.
   B. the activation of nociceptors in deep and cutaneous tissue.
   C. peripheral or central mediation of pain.
   D. cramping and poorly localized sensations.

3. After experiencing nausea and vomiting for 48 hours, a client is unable to take the scheduled opioids for cancer pain and begins to withdraw. The withdrawal is due to
   A. physical dependence.
   B. drug tolerance.
   C. addiction.
   D. equianalgesia.

4. The pain physiology step that includes neurons descending from the brainstem to the dorsal horn of the spinal cord to release neuromediators is called

   A. transduction.
   B. transmission.
   C. perception.
   D. modulation.

5. The most common source of cancer pain is
   A. bone metastases.
   B. liver metastases.
   C. pancreatic involvement.
   D. nerve compression or injury.

6. When assessing for pain in the pediatric population,
   A. ask the parent about the child's level of pain.
   B. use the "0-10" scale to assess pain intensity for children aged 7 and older.
   C. encourage children to use the pain faces to describe pain.
   D. use a pain scale that is appropriate to the developmental level of the child.

7. Mrs. J. recently was given the diagnosis of multiple myeloma and is undergoing her first cycle of chemotherapy. While her pain is rated as "2" on a scale of "0-10" when she is at rest and not moving, the pain increases to "8" with any type of movement or activity. She is taking 30 mg of controlled-release oxycodone every 12 hours and 5 to 10 mg of immediate-release oxycodone every 4 hours as needed. The nurse's best recommendation for the management plan would be to

A. add a nonsteroidal antiinflammatory medication for the bone pain.

B. increase the dose and frequency of the breakthrough opioid medication and administer before anticipated activity.

C. encourage Mrs. J. to use a bedside table to keep items near her to prevent movement.

D. encourage her that the pain will decrease once the chemotherapy begins to work.

8. Mrs. Q. has a history of rheumatoid arthritis and has been taking pentazocine (Talwin) for the last 2 years. She was recently given the diagnosis of metastatic breast cancer and has been experiencing low back pain related to bone metastases of "8" intensity. She is given a fentanyl (Duragesic) patch. What should be considered with this client?

A. The pentazocine and Duragesic will work synergistically to provide more optimal pain relief.

B. Mrs. Q. will have an exacerbation of side effects related to the two opioids she is taking.

C. The pentazocine, an agonist-antagonist, should be discontinued, because the Duragesic will not work effectively in combination with an agonist-antagonist.

D. An alternative agent to pentazocine, such as nalbuphine (Nubain), should be substituted for the arthritic pain.

9. Bisphosphonates such as pamidronate (Aredia) and zoledronic acid (Zometa) are used for relief of pain associated with

A. visceral metastases.

B. neuropathic pain.

C. osteolytic bone metastases.

D. headache associated with increased intracranial pressure.

10. One type of autonomic nervous system block used to prevent pain from pancreatic cancer is the

A. peripheral nervous system block.

B. celiac plexus block.

C. dorsal rhizotomy.

D. commissural myelotomy.

11. Drug tolerance is which type of phenomenon?

A. Physiologic.

B. Psychologic.

C. Addictive.

D. Obsessive-compulsive.

12. Which class of analgesic adjuvants is helpful for peripherally mediated neuropathic pain?

A. Analeptics.

B. Tricyclic antidepressants.

C. Serotonin-specific reuptake inhibitor antidepressants.

D. Benzodiazepines.

13. A client with cancer has a pain score of "2" on a "0-10" scale but complains of "always being sleepy." An appropriate intervention would be to recommend the addition of

A. amitriptyline (Elavil).

B. phenytoin (Dilantin).

C. methylphenidate (Ritalin).

D. a nonsteroidal antiinflammatory drug.

14. The most common side effect of cancer therapy is

A. pain.

B. nausea and vomiting.

C. mucositis.

D. fatigue.

15. Chemotherapy-related fatigue generally peaks

A. on the day of the chemotherapy administration.

B. on the third day after the chemotherapy administration.

C. 3 to 4 days after the nadir.

D. throughout the course of chemotherapy.

16. A potential laboratory finding in anemia-related fatigue includes a(n)

A. decreased white blood cell count.

B. decreased red blood cell count.

C. increased hemoglobin.

D. increased P_{O_2}.

17. Red blood cell growth factors used in the management of anemia include

A. erythropoietin (rHuEPO) (Epogen, Procrit) and oprelvekin (Neumega).

B. darbepoetin alfa (Aranesp) and erythropoietin.

C. oprelvekin and pegfilgrastim (Neulasta).

D. erythropoietin and sargramostim (Leukine).

18. Mary is a 42-year-old client with lymphoma who is undergoing chemotherapy. She has completed two of six cycles of therapy and is complaining of fatigue level "8" on a "0-10" scale. What suggestions would help Mary with her fatigue?
  A. Maintain a vegetarian diet to increase the vitamin stores in her body.
  B. Sleep during the day when fatigued and get up only as needed.
  C. Engage in some activity as tolerated during the day to maintain energy stores.
  D. Continue the regular schedule that was used before the illness.

19. Which of the following should be included in the assessment of fatigue?
  A. Blood urea nitrogen (BUN) and creatinine.
  B. Platelet count.
  C. Family perception of the client's fatigue.
  D. Depression scales.

20. To assess the effect of fatigue on a client's cognitive or mental function, ask the client
  A. about the ability to concentrate on the family finances and paperwork.
  B. to count backwards by 3s beginning at 100.
  C. to read a paragraph in a book.
  D. about the ability to organize and perform activities of daily living (ADLs).

21. Which statement is true about the physiology of pruritus?
  A. The physiology of pruritus is closely linked to the physiology of pain.
  B. Delta fibers are the neurons responsible for itch.
  C. The initiating stimulus occurs external to the body.
  D. Serotonin is the neurotransmitter responsible for the transmission of pruritus.

22. Which of the following is a risk factor for pruritus?
  A. History of alcohol abuse.
  B. Male gender.
  C. History of cardiac disease.
  D. Age older than 70.

23. One malignancy that typically causes pruritus is
  A. Hodgkin's disease.
  B. breast cancer.
  C. bladder cancer.
  D. melanoma.

24. Mr. O. returned from colon resection surgery 2 hours ago. Client-controlled analgesia morphine was begun in the postanesthesia recovery unit, and he is now complaining of pruritus. The nurse phones the physician to recommend the best intervention, which is to
  A. administer an opioid antagonist to block the pruritic influence.
  B. administer diphenhydramine, an H_1-receptor antagonist.
  C. change the opioid to meperidine.
  D. place a fan in the room to control the pruritus.

25. Which malignancy can cause facial and nasal itching?
  A. Lymphomas.
  B. Prostate cancer.
  C. Leukemia.
  D. Gliomas.

26. Which of the following is an appropriate nursing intervention for pruritus?
  A. Keep the room humidity at 30% to 40%.
  B. Keep the room temperature warm to prevent vasoconstriction.
  C. Encourage fluid intake of 1000 ml/day.
  D. Wear tight clothing that will rub on the pruritic skin.

27. The nurse makes a home visit to a client with end-stage pancreatic cancer. Upon assessment, the nurse discovers scratch marks and scabs on the trunk and upper extremities. The client reports that she has been itching in the evenings before bedtime, and the itching is "driving her crazy." In addition to managing the underlying cause, an appropriate nursing intervention to prevent further scratching would be to
  A. encourage the family member to scratch the affected area to prevent skin irritation.
  B. encourage a warm bath in the evening when the pruritus is most likely to occur.

C. drink a glass of wine each evening before bedtime for relaxation.
D. encourage television, reading, and crafts in the evening to distract from the pruritus.

28. Which of the following is true about rapid eye movement (REM) sleep?
   A. It is the transition between wakefulness and sleep.
   B. It is also called quiet sleep.
   C. The cycle of REM sleep is approximately 30 minutes.
   D. REM sleep cycles occur approximately four to five times per night in clients with optimal sleep patterns.

29. Approximately how many clients with a new diagnosis of cancer or who have recently been treated for cancer experience sleep disorder?
   A. 100%.
   B. 60%-80%.
   C. 30%-50%.
   D. <25%.

30. Melatonin is a hormone released by the pineal gland that
   A. mediates night and day rhythms.
   B. increases with age.
   C. increases during the daylight hours.
   D. increases with menopause.

31. Which category of sleep medications has more selective hypnotic properties with fewer residual side effects the next day?
   A. Benzodiazepines.
   B. Nonbenzodiazepine hypnotics.
   C. Tricyclic antidepressants.
   D. Anxiolytics.

32. Nonpharmacologic interventions for sleep include
   A. going to bed at a scheduled time whether sleepy or not.
   B. arising at the same time each morning.
   C. exercising 1 hour before retiring for bed.
   D. staying in bed upon awakening at night until sleep resumes.

33. Which of the following characteristics or lifestyle factors may interfere with sleep?

   A. Male gender.
   B. Younger age.
   C. Regular, physical activity.
   D. Alcohol intake.

34. Physical signs of sleep deprivation include
   A. dark circles under the eyes, nystagmus, incorrect word use.
   B. dark circles under the eyes, overpronunciation of words, and a loud voice.
   C. stuttering, nystagmus, and loss of balance.
   D. slurred speech, a loud voice, and an impaired gait.

35. The respiratory center that controls breathing lies within
   A. the medulla.
   B. the bronchus.
   C. the carotid receptors.
   D. the chemoreceptors.

36. Examples of mechanoreceptors that may provide input into the respiratory center to create dyspnea include
   A. pulmonary edema and pleural effusion.
   B. poor nutritional status.
   C. changes in oxygenation.
   D. input from the cerebral cortex.

37. Which of the following is a disease-related risk factor for dyspnea?
   A. Peripheral edema.
   B. Syndrome of inappropriate antidiuretic hormone.
   C. Hepatomegaly.
   D. Hypercalcemia.

38. To assess the intensity of the dyspnea that a client is experiencing,
   A. ask the client to describe how the dyspnea feels.
   B. ask the client what makes the dyspnea worse.
   C. ask the client about a smoking history that may affect the dyspnea.
   D. ask the client to rate the dyspnea on a "0-10" scale.

39. Mr. W. is a 79-year-old man with mantle cell lymphoma. He recently completed two cycles of chemotherapy that included

cyclophosphamide (Cytoxan), doxorubicin (Adriamycin), vincristine (Oncovin), and prednisone. He arrives at the clinic for his third cycle of chemotherapy with complaints of dyspnea. His lungs have a few rales bilaterally on auscultation. Before chemotherapy, his pulmonary function and cardiac ejection fraction were within normal limits. The two most likely differential diagnoses of the dyspnea include
   A. anemia and congestive heart failure.
   B. anemia and pleural effusion.
   C. superior vena cava syndrome and congestive heart failure.
   D. pulmonary embolus and anemia.

40. The most reliable way to assess dyspnea is to
   A. monitor the O_2 saturation.
   B. monitor the hemoglobin and hematocrit for anemia.
   C. ask the client about the intensity of dyspnea.
   D. ask the family members about how the dyspnea interferes with the client's activities of daily living.

41. Ms. A. has lung cancer with superior vena cava syndrome. A chest x-ray film shows that a tumor is compressing the vena cava. One strategy used to manage the underlying cause of the dyspnea would be to
   A. administer a respiratory sedative to slow the respiratory rate.
   B. administer supplemental oxygen.
   C. begin nebulized morphine.
   D. begin radiation therapy.

42. Respiratory sedatives such as phenothiazines and benzodiazepines are given to suppress respiratory awareness and
   A. treat the underlying cause of the dyspnea.
   B. decrease the inflammation in the lungs that is causing the dyspnea.
   C. manage anxiety associated with dyspnea.

   D. act as a bronchodilator for airway obstruction.

43. The pharmacologic agents of choice for bronchial airway obstruction include
   A. bronchodilators and corticosteroids.
   B. respiratory sedatives and antidepressants.
   C. opioids and anxiolytics.
   D. antidepressants and anxiolytics.

44. Shivering or chills may occur as a response to
   A. fever.
   B. heat loss.
   C. tumor cells.
   D. paraneoplastic syndromes.

45. The body temperature is regulated by the
   A. medulla.
   B. cerebral cortex.
   C. hypothalamus.
   D. parathyroid.

46. Larry is a 25-year-old client with acute myelocytic leukemia. He is on day 14 after induction therapy. A red blood cell transfusion was completed 1 hour previously when he calls the nurse to the room complaining of fever and chills. The best initial intervention would be to
   A. administer 650 mg acetaminophen.
   B. call the physician and request starting an antibiotic.
   C. collect a urine specimen.
   D. administer intravenous meperidine for the chills.

47. Acetaminophen, often used to treat fever and chills, should be limited to
   A. 2 g/day.
   B. 4 g/day.
   C. 6 g/day.
   D. there is no ceiling dose.

ANSWERS

1. **Answer:** B
   Rationale: Pain is a warning sign of actual or potential tissue damage; thus the damage may not have occurred yet. Although observable signs such as grimacing and splinting may indicate pain, these behaviors are often unreliable and are affected by gender, culture, and familial preferences. In addition, physiologic signs such as tachycardia and hypertension may be associated with acute pain. This is inconsistent; physiologic adaptation occurs over time, and vital signs may or may not be affected.

2. **Answer:** C
   Rationale: Neuropathic pain is the result of compression or injury that is mediated (generated and spread) through the peripheral, central, and/or sympathetic nervous system. Well-localized pain that is aching or gnawing is consistent with somatic pain such as bone metastases. Visceral pain such as pancreatitis can be characterized by cramping and poorly localized pain. Both somatic and visceral pain are nociceptive pains that stimulate deep and cutaneous tissues.

3. **Answer:** A
   Rationale: Withdrawal occurs in clients who are "physically dependent" on an opioid and abrupt cessation occurs. The administration of an antagonist can also precipitate withdrawal. This is a physiologic phenomenon that the client cannot control. Tolerance means that after repeated administration of an opioid, a given dosage begins to lose its effectiveness; it begins to have a shorter duration of action and then less analgesic action. Addiction is a psychologic occurrence when clients have an overwhelming need to obtain and use a drug for a nonmedical purpose.

4. **Answer:** D
   Rationale: In response to the pain stimuli, the brain sends neuromediators to the dorsal horn such as opioids, norepinephrine, and serotonin to modulate the pain experience.

5. **Answer:** A
   Rationale: Bone destruction or compression of the bone on nerves and soft tissue is the most common source of cancer pain. Bone metastases are common in the following malignancies: breast, prostate, lung, and multiple myeloma.

6. **Answer:** D
   Rationale: Biologic age cannot be used when choosing a pain assessment tool for the pediatric population; rather the clinician should choose the tool that the child can developmentally interpret.

7. **Answer:** B
   Rationale: The client is experiencing "incident pain," that is, increased pain with movement or activity. It is important to get on top of the pain quickly and before anticipated activity, and so the best response is to increase the dose and interval of the breakthrough opioid medication. The client should also take the breakthrough medication approximately 30 minutes before activity so that the medication will be most effective while the client is moving, and hence the client can move and complete activities of daily living more easily and comfortably.

8. **Answer:** C
   Rationale: Pentazocine is not an optimal drug of choice for any type of pain because of the psychomimetric effects. When agonist-antagonists are added to pure agonists, the combination can also prevent full receptor binding of the agonist and can precipitate withdrawal in some clients.

9. **Answer:** C
   Rationale: Bisphosphonates are used for the relief of pain in osteolytic bone metastases such as metastatic breast cancer.

10. **Answer:** B
    Rationale: The celiac plexus block is a surgical intervention for pain related to pancreatic cancer that is effective in up to 80% of clients.

11. **Answer:** A
    Rationale: Drug tolerance is a physiologic phenomenon that occurs after repeated

administration of an opioid, and the opioid begins to lose its effectiveness with a shorter duration of action and less analgesic action.

12. *Answer:* B
Rationale: The tricyclic antidepressants block the reuptake of serotonin, norepinephrine, and dopamine in the central nervous system. No research suggests that the serotonin-specific antidepressants are as effective for pain. Analeptics are used to counteract sedation, and benzodiazepines are used for pruritic pain and anxiety associated with pain.

13. *Answer:* C
Rationale: Analeptics such as Ritalin may counteract sedation and may improve quality of life. Another commonly used analeptic is dextroamphetamine.

14. *Answer:* D
Rationale: Fatigue affects approximately 100% of clients undergoing all types of cancer therapy.

15. *Answer:* C
Rationale: Chemotherapy-related fatigue often peaks on the third or fourth day after the nadir, possibly related to the declining red blood cell count.

16. *Answer:* B
Rationale: A decreased red blood cell count often is indicative of anemia and fatigue. The hemoglobin and PO_2 are often decreased, not elevated, in clients with anemia. The low hemoglobin and subsequent low PO_2 result in a decreased oxygen capacity caused by a low number of red blood cells. The white blood count is not a laboratory test for anemia.

17. *Answer:* B
Rationale: Darbepoetin alfa and erythropoietin are both growth factors that stimulate the production of red blood cells in the bone marrow. Oprelvekin is a platelet growth factor, and sargramostim and pegfilgrastim are white blood cell growth factors.

18. *Answer:* C
Rationale: It is important to take part in some type of activity or exercise as tolerated. Studies show that clients who exercise have decreased levels of fatigue. Too much sleep will not assist with the fatigue. A diet should be balanced with adequate amounts of protein, and schedule adjustments with prioritizing needs are important to manage the overwhelming fatigue.

19. *Answer:* D
Rationale: Depression and fatigue often share the same symptoms, and therefore a differential diagnosis is important. Blood urea nitrogen, creatinine, and platelet counts are not reliable tests in the assessment of fatigue. In addition, family perceptions are often inaccurate, and fatigue can only be measured by asking the individual client. Fatigue, like pain, is a subjective symptom.

20. *Answer:* B
Rationale: The cognitive or mental dimension of fatigue involves the assessment of concentration, memory, and alertness; counting backward by 3s is an example. Asking the client about the ability to concentrate or organize and perform ADLs provides a subjective rather than an objective answer. Reading a paragraph does not assess cognitive function but rather reading skills.

21. *Answer:* A
Rationale: Pruritus transmission is closely linked to the transmission of pain and is conducted along polymodal C-nociceptors. The stimuli can originate anywhere along the afferent pathway, and the cause is often linked to an internal cause.

22. *Answer:* D
Rationale: Pruritus increases with age and is especially prevalent in those over the age of 70.

23. *Answer:* A
Rationale: Pruritus is common in hematologic malignancies including Hodgkin's and nonHodgkin's lymphomas.

24. *Answer:* B
Rationale: H_1-receptor antagonists are the first drugs of choice for pruritus. Small doses of opioid antagonists are sometimes used for pruritus caused by intraspinal analgesia. Rotating opioids takes time and interrupts the

pain management plan, and meperidine is not a drug of choice. Placing a fan in the room does not manage the underlying cause of the pruritus.

25. *Answer:* D
Rationale: Gliomas are often associated with facial and nostril itching, and the pruritus may be a presenting sign.

26. *Answer:* A
Rationale: All of the answers are inappropriate interventions for pruritus except for A. Fluid intake should be at least 3000 L/day, and the room should be kept cool to prevent vasodilation. The room humidity should be kept at 30% to 40% to prevent dry skin that can contribute to pruritus.

27. *Answer:* D
Rationale: Scratching should be avoided because it can disrupt the skin integrity. Medicated baths can help with pruritus, but the temperature should be cool to minimize vasodilation. Alcohol can cause vasodilation and contribute to the pruritus. Distraction methods such as television and other activities may be helpful, because pruritus is often exacerbated with stress and anxiety.

28. *Answer:* D
Rationale: REM sleep, also known as paradoxical sleep, is characterized by deep sleep cycles of 90 minutes in duration that occur four to five times per night. Non-REM sleep is the transition between wakefulness and sleep.

29. *Answer:* C
Rationale: Approximately 30% to 50% of clients with a recent diagnosis of cancer or those recently treated experience sleep disorder.

30. *Answer:* A
Rationale: Melatonin mediates or regulates the day and night rhythms. Normally, the levels increase at night during sleep and decrease during the daylight hours. Melatonin decreases with menopause and age, and this is reflective of the fact that as people age, they experience sleep disturbances more often.

31. *Answer:* B
Rationale: The nonbenzodiazepine hypnotics such as zolpidem and zaleplon are more selective for sleep, and clients experience less drowsiness and sedation the next day.

32. *Answer:* B
Rationale: Arising at the same time each morning facilitates a routine that enhances sleep. Going to bed when not sleepy may not be helpful, and although routine exercise often helps with sleep disturbance, exercise should be avoided 2 hours before bedtime. Exercise can stimulate the client and lead to insomnia right before bedtime. If clients awaken at night, it may be helpful to leave the bed and return when sleepy.

33. *Answer:* D
Rationale: Female gender rather than male, increased age rather than younger age, and physical inactivity versus physical activity are all factors that can interfere with sleep. Alcohol intake can also interfere with normal sleep patterns.

34. *Answer:* A
Rationale: Dark circles under the eyes, nystagmus, incorrect word use, slurred speech, frequent yawning, and ptosis of the eyelids are all physical signs of sleep deprivation. Stuttering and a loud voice are not usually associated with sleep disorders.

35. *Answer:* A
Rationale: The respiratory center is the autonomic control of respiration that lies within the medulla.

36. *Answer:* C
Rationale: Mechanoreceptors are sensitive in changes in pressure on the lung. The pressure can be caused by fluid in or around the lung or by compression on the lung such as a tumor.

37. *Answer:* C
Rationale: Coexisting pulmonary disease, superior vena cava syndrome, and hepatomegaly can all interfere with pulmonary function and contribute to dyspnea. Hypercalcemia does not cause dyspnea.

38. *Answer:* D
Rationale: The intensity of dyspnea, like pain, is best rated by the client on a "0-10"

scale, with "0" being no breathlessness and "10" being the worst breathlessness imagined.

39. *Answer:* A

Rationale: Anemia and congestive heart failure should be evaluated first. Anemia likely is due to the chemotherapy. In addition, the client received doxorubicin, a cardiotoxic chemotherapeutic agent that can cause congestive heart failure, and so this needs to be carefully evaluated as well. Pleural effusion is not likely, because the lower lobe breath sounds are not decreased and pleural effusion is not highly associated with lymphoma. Assessment finding with superior vena cava syndrome would also include edema of the upper extremities and possibly jugular vein distention. A pulmonary embolus usually would be accompanied by chest pain.

40. *Answer:* C

Rationale: Dyspnea, like pain, is a subjective phenomenon. The most accurate method to assess dyspnea is to ask the client. Other methods may be unreliable.

41. *Answer:* D

Rationale: Radiation therapy is the only strategy listed that will treat the underlying cause of the dyspnea, a tumor that is pressing on the vena cava. Other interventions are used for symptom management.

42. *Answer:* C

Rationale: Many benzodiazepines and phenothiazines are also anxiolytics and can assist with anxiety that can accompany dyspnea. These agents are not antiinflammatory, and they are not bronchodilators. Strategies used to treat the underlying cause include anticancer therapies.

43. *Answer:* A

Rationale: Bronchodilators act by expanding the ventilatory airway that can be compromised by obstruction, while corticosteroids decrease the inflammation caused by the obstruction.

44. *Answer:* B

Rationale: Chills and shivering often follow fever and are the result of heat loss from the body.

45. *Answer:* C

Rationale: The hypothalamus is the body's thermal regulator.

46. *Answer:* A

Rationale: Providing the client with acetaminophen initially will bring the fever down and make the client more comfortable. Drawing blood cultures would be the second intervention, because the fever and chills likely are due to infection during an immunosuppressive period. Although the client recently had a transfusion, it was completed, and the fever and chills likely are not due to this.

47. *Answer:* B

Rationale: Acetaminophen overdose can lead to hepatotoxicity. The dose should be limited to 4 g (4000 mg)/day.

BIBLIOGRAPHY

American Pain Society. (1999). *Principles of analgesic use in the treatment of acute pain and cancer pain* (4th ed.). Glenview, IL: American Pain Society.

Body, J.J., & Mancini, I. (2002). Bisphosphonates for cancer patients: Why, how, and when? *Supportive Care in Cancer 10,* 399-407.

Brown, K., Esper, P., Kelleher, L., et al. (2001). *Chemotherapy and biotherapy guidelines and recommendations for practice.* Pittsburgh: Oncology Nursing Press.

Davidson, J.R., Waisberg, J.L., Brundage, M.D., & MacLean, W. (2001). Nonpharmacologic group treatment of insomnia: A preliminary study with cancer survivors. *Psycho-Oncology 10,* 389-397.

Dudgeon, D.J. (2002). Managing dyspnea and cough. *Hematology Oncology Clinics of North America 16,* 557-577.

Dworkin, R.H. (2002). An overview of neuropathic pain: Syndromes, symptoms, signs, and several mechanisms. *The Clinical Journal of Pain 18,* 343-349.

Krajnik, M., & Zylicz, Z. (2001). Pruritus in advanced internal diseases: Pathogenesis and treatment. *The Netherlands Journal of Medicine 58,* 27-40.

McCaffery, M., & Pasero, C. (1998). *Pain: Clinical manual for nursing practice* (2nd ed.). St. Louis: Mosby.

McMillan, C. (2001). Breakthrough pain: Assessment and management in cancer patients. *British Journal of Nursing 10,* 860-866.

Redeker, N.S., Lev, E.L., & Ruggiero, J. (2000). Insomnia, fatigue, anxiety, depression, and quality of life of cancer patients undergoing chemotherapy. *Scholarly Inquiry for Nursing Practice: An International Journal 14,* 275-290.

Savard, J., & Morin, C.M. (2001). Insomnia in the context of cancer: A review of a neglected problem. *Journal of Clinical Oncology 19,* 895-908.

Thomas, J.R., & Won Gunten, C.F. (2002). Treatment of dyspnea in cancer patients. *Oncology 16,* 745-760.

NOTES

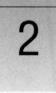

2 Coping: Psychosocial Issues

PATRICIA M. GRIMM

Select the best answer for each of the following questions:

1. In considering what places a client with cancer at risk for emotional distress, which one of the following factors can be influenced by nursing interventions?
   A. Disruption of age-specific developmental-like tasks.
   B. Lack of prognostic certainty.
   C. Knowledge of cancer diagnosis, treatment, and expected outcomes.
   D. Previous life experiences and coping ability.

2. In caring for a client with a diagnosis of ineffective individual coping, which intervention will require the most participation on the part of the client?
   A. Evaluation with the client on the effectiveness of current coping strategies.
   B. Instruction in relaxation, imagery, and other holistic stress reduction techniques.
   C. Providing referrals as needed to the psychiatric liaison nurse, psychologist, or social worker.
   D. Strengthening the client's social support system.

3. Mrs. R. is a 76-year-old retired banker who has done well for 2 years after pelvic exenteration. Recently she experienced a recurrence. She now has multiple draining fistulae and has been told that she is not a candidate for further treatment. Her son said that her response has been complete withdrawal. She has changed from a meticulous dresser and housekeeper to neglecting both. She refuses to eat and blames herself for not going for regular Pap smears. She refuses help from her son, saying he is "wasting his time, I deserve to die." Her responses reflect developmental, situational, and disease-related characteristics most suggestive of
   A. fear of death.
   B. low self-esteem.
   C. neurotic anxiety.
   D. role abandonment.

4. Mrs. R. was hospitalized for management of the fistulae. Once the drainage was managed effectively, Mrs. R. seemed to show more interest in her care. During this phase, the most therapeutic nursing approach to facilitate adaptive behavior would be to
   A. initiate a referral for rehabilitative counseling.
   B. make no demands on Mrs. R. for her own care.
   C. positively reinforce Mrs. R.'s approaches to self-care.
   D. transfer responsibility for Mrs. R.'s care to her family.

5. The nursing plan included a referral to a client support program to assist Mrs. R. in

adapting to the life changes imposed by the progression of her cancer. Which of the following would provide this service?
    A. I Can Cope
    B. National Cancer Institute (NCI)
    C. Reach to Recovery
    D. The Wellness Community

6. Mr. L. is admitted to an oncology unit, and assessment reveals flushed skin, sweating, jerky hand movements, and asking questions repeatedly. The most probable nursing diagnosis would be which of the following?
    A. Anxiety.
    B. Fear.
    C. Low self-esteem.
    D. Phobias.

7. Mr. L. has started taking an antianxiety drug. He tells you that he feels much calmer but that his mouth is so uncomfortably dry that he is thinking about discontinuing the drug. The most therapeutic response would be to
    A. assure him that the dry mouth is not as bad as the anxiety.
    B. call the physician and request an order for another antianxiety drug.
    C. explain that the dryness generally diminishes; increase fluid intake.
    D. support him in his decision and hold the daily dose.

8. Mr. L. returns to the oncology outpatient clinic for his 1-year follow-up appointment. He states that he is having problems with sleeping, flashbacks of his initial treatment, and difficulty concentrating. You refer him for psychiatric evaluation, suspecting that he is experiencing
    A. bipolar disorder.
    B. generalized anxiety stress disorder.
    C. posttraumatic stress disorder.
    D. psychotic disorder.

9. Antianxiety drugs are not discontinued abruptly because a possible withdrawal effect is
    A. hypertensive episodes.
    B. narcolepsy.
    C. seizures.
    D. severe depression.

10. Mrs. S. is admitted to the hospital for the evaluation of metastatic disease related to her diagnosis of breast cancer. Her family is concerned about recent changes in her behavior such as crying, lack of interest in her appearance, and changes in sleeping and eating. In considering a referral for evaluation of depression in this client, it is most important to assess
    A. effect of behavior on family members.
    B. meaning of the illness to the client.
    C. meaning of appearance to patient and family.
    D. mental status as an indicator of delirium.

11. The nurse's assessment of treatment-related risk factors for depression in individuals with cancer should include
    A. chemotherapeutic agents being given.
    B. sleeping and eating patterns.
    C. symptom control, particularly pain.
    D. type of cancer.

12. Which of the following risk factors for development of depressive symptoms is most amenable to direct nursing interventions?
    A. Family developmental and situational crises.
    B. Inadequate social support.
    C. Inadequate symptom control.
    D. Client history of suicidal thoughts.

13. Physical findings most descriptive of a depressed state include
    A. facial pallor, tense posturing, vocal tremors, and diaphoresis.
    B. flat affect, lack of spontaneity, minimal eye contract, and slumped posture.
    C. inappropriate affect, disheveled dress, sweaty hands, and tremors.
    D. labile emotions, hyperactivity, sighing respirations, and overtalkativeness.

14. Which of the following responses by the nurse would be most therapeutic in helping the client deal with the somatic complaints often associated with depression?
    A. Advising the client to minimize these symptoms, thus conserving energy to fight the disease.
    B. Explaining that the symptoms are not "real" and therefore need no treatment.

C. Listening nonjudgmentally and trying diversional techniques as a possible method of alleviation.
D. Validating that symptoms do or do not have a physiologic basis

15. In teaching management of the side effects of antidepressant medication, which of the following would be most important for an elderly client?
    A. Change from a lying to a standing position slowly.
    B. Monitor changes in visual acuity.
    C. Increase fluid intake.
    D. Take medication at bedtime.

16. The most serious potential outcome of depression in cancer clients is
    A. interference with social roles.
    B. lack of compliance with medical treatment.
    C. severe psychologic regression with loss of function.
    D. suicidal ideation and/or attempt.

17. Mr. G. returns to the oncology clinic for treatment of recurrent lymphoma after bone marrow transplant. He tells you that it is hard to believe that there is a purpose to his experience, tearfully stating, "I'm really angry and I don't trust anything anymore." The most probable nursing diagnosis would be
    A. anxiety.
    B. ineffective coping.
    C. self-esteem disturbance.
    D. spiritual distress.

18. Spiritual distress is often misdiagnosed as
    A. cognitive problems.
    B. lack of social support.
    C. noncompliance.
    D. psychologic distress.

19. From your past contact with Mr. G., you know him to be a deeply spiritual person, attending church and using prayer to manage the demands of his illness and treatment. Today he angrily refuses when you volunteer to call his pastor for him. Your best response to this would be:
    A. Getting angry with God isn't going to help.

B. Perhaps you'd like to tell me more about what you're feeling right now.
C. Sounds like you'd like some privacy, I'll be back soon.
D. Would you like me to pray with you?

20. In considering barriers that influence a client's ability to continue his or her spiritual beliefs and practices, the most significant one is
    A. activity and dietary restrictions.
    B. ignorance of health care providers.
    C. lack of privacy.
    D. treatment regimen requirements.

21. Mr. G.'s family can best enhance his spiritual well-being by
    A. avoiding discussion of his spiritual concerns with him.
    B. discussing their opposition to his spiritual beliefs.
    C. participating in his spiritual practices with him.
    D. sharing their perceptions of his spiritual distress.

22. Mr. J., a 48-year-old businessman, has recently been given the diagnosis of lung cancer. His family states that since his diagnosis, he has refused to participate in decision making regarding his treatment, is ignoring postbiopsy instructions, and has become more withdrawn. The most accurate nursing diagnosis would be
    A. anxiety.
    B. ineffective coping.
    C. powerlessness.
    D. spiritual distress.

23. An individual's response to the loss of personal control depends primarily on which of the following:
    A. duration of time since diagnosis.
    B. individual patterns of coping.
    C. meaning of the loss.
    D. response of family and friends.

24. Mr. J. states, "I don't feel like I have any control over what is happening to me." Which of the following is an appropriate statement for the nurse to make?
    A. "Ask your doctor about your care, and he will answer your questions."

B. "Ask your wife to let you do more things for yourself."

C. "Let's spend some time talking about your feelings."

D. "We will develop a routine schedule for your care so you will know what to expect."

25. The most basic nursing intervention designed to facilitate Mr. J.'s sense of personal control would be
   A. asking family to make decisions regarding burdensome areas of treatment and care.
   B. discussing with him his feelings regarding personal control.
   C. encouraging identification of areas over which control can be maintained.
   D. providing successful management of symptoms.

26. Before discharge, the most important nursing intervention for facilitation of a sense of control for both Mr. J. and his family would be:
   A. Make a referral to an appropriate home care agency.
   B. Organize a health team meeting to plan his care.
   C. Provide specific care instructions for family members.
   D. Seek client's and family's opinions and suggestions about his care at home.

27. A behavior that would indicate a need for immediate professional assistance (mental health professional) with Mr. J. is
   A. inability to perform activities of daily living.
   B. noncompliance with treatment regimen.
   C. refusal to discuss personal feelings.
   D. verbalization of self-harm intentions.

28. Grief is defined as changes in thinking, feeling, and behaving that occur in response to
   A. death of a significant other.
   B. disease with an uncertain prognosis.
   C. losses related to the aging process.
   D. loss of a valued object or person.

29. In addition to the developmental and situational factors that most people experience, individuals with cancer may also experience

A. changes in body structure/function.
B. changes in employment, including retirement.
C. multiple losses and unanticipated losses.
D. symbolic losses, including independence.

30. In discussing the process of grief with clients or family members, the most basic point to emphasize is:
   A. One's grief response will be influenced by past experiences with loss and grief.
   B. Each family member will grieve in their own fashion.
   C. Somatic symptoms of grief often occur.
   D. Specific stages of grief exist.

31. Resolution of the grief process may be facilitated by which of the following interventions?
   A. Encouraging discussion of the feelings related to the loss.
   B. Discouraging expression of negative feelings, such as anger.
   C. Providing sedation as suggested by others.
   D. Restricting visitors to family members only.

32. Which of the following client responses is most representative of a dysfunctional grief response?
   A. A 76-year-old man who cared for his wife during the terminal phases of colon cancer reports frequent vivid dreams about his wife and himself.
   B. A mother who cries continuously and keeps saying, "No, he can't die," as she attends her 21-year-old son who is dying of leukemia.
   C. A 35-year-old woman who, at 6 weeks after a mastectomy, avoids hugs and physical contact with family and friends and has not allowed her husband to look at the surgical site.
   D. A 35-year-old widower who prides himself on keeping all of his wife's possessions and visiting her grave daily for the 5 years since her death while neglecting his other responsibilities.

33. Of the following grief responses, which is indicative of the need for mental health intervention?
    A. Crying, angry outbursts.
    B. Preoccupation with lost object/person.
    C. Somatic symptoms.
    D. Withdrawal or social isolation.

34. Ms. P., an 18-year-old with a recent diagnosis of leukemia, comes to the clinic for evaluation and determination of treatment. In your assessment of Ms. P., you determine that she has lived on her own this past year and has a conflictual relationship with her parents. As you continue your assessment, which additional finding might be indicative of a potential for social dysfunction?
    A. Admits she has a temper and has "gotten in trouble before."
    B. Has two roommates who accompany her to the clinic.
    C. Lives in a community with ethnic and cultural characteristics similar to her own.
    D. Seems knowledgeable about her illness and its treatment.

35. Ms. P. is admitted to the hospital for induction chemotherapy. Her parents come to visit regularly, and often their visits end with angry shouting matches. As Ms. P.'s nurse, you schedule a meeting with the family. Given the above, your initial interventions are directed at
    A. assisting family members to discuss their thoughts and feeling about Ms. P.'s illness.
    B. establishing limits on problematic behavior.
    C. instruction regarding the disease and treatment regimen.
    D. referral of family to appropriate resources.

36. The most basic psychologic requirement of social functioning is
    A. ability to problem solve.
    B. effective interaction with others.
    C. effective reality testing.
    D. intact family structure.

37. Ms. P. will be discharged soon and will need to move home with her parents for a period of time. In preparing Ms. P. and her parents for discharge, it is most important to
    A. encourage Ms. P. to participate in self-care.
    B. encourage her parents to limit social contacts.
    C. plan for ongoing evaluation of effects of caring on caregivers.
    D. provide the client and family with skills required for day-to-day care.

38. Mr. O., a 30-year-old unemployed factory worker, is admitted to your unit with a diagnosis of colon cancer. A nursing assessment reveals that he is a recent immigrant who has been living with a cousin since losing his job. Which factor places Mr. O. at most risk for social dysfunction?
    A. Language or cultural differences.
    B. Living situation.
    C. Poor social and interpersonal skills.
    D. Prolonged hospitalization.

39. Mr. O. has surgery for his colon cancer and is scheduled for outpatient chemotherapy treatment. In preparing him for the beginning of this treatment, it is most important to assess his
    A. extent of social support in the community.
    B. problem-solving and decision-making skills.
    C. psychiatric history of antisocial personality.
    D. need for financial assistance.

40. A history of poorly developed social and interpersonal skills, social isolation, and prolonged cancer treatment hospitalization may place a person at risk for the nursing diagnosis:
    A. Ineffective coping.
    B. Powerlessness.
    C. Impaired social interaction.
    D. Spiritual distress.

41. In preparing Mr. O. for discharge, the most important nursing intervention would be
    A. assessing his understanding of his illness and its treatment.
    B. contacting immigration services for support information.
    C. providing him with social and financial services information.
    D. supporting his enrollment in an English as a Second Language course.

ANSWERS

1. *Answer:* C
   Rationale: Client teaching will help with anxiety and fears. Client teaching is a nursing intervention.

2. *Answer:* D
   Rationale: Although the nurse may help the client to identify the current social support system, only the client can determine the need to, or ways in which to, strengthen it.

3. *Answer:* B
   Rationale: Self-negation and self-blame are the defining characteristics that differentiate between low self-esteem and the other mood states.

4. *Answer:* C
   Rationale: Option A is premature, based on the information given. Option B does not facilitate adaptive behavior. Option D fosters dependency. Option C is a behavioral approach that reinforces the desired behavior and is therefore the best response.

5. *Answer:* D
   Rationale: The Wellness Community is the only support program listed. I Can Cope is a group program only. Reach to Recovery is for mastectomy clients. The NCI is for research.

6. *Answer:* A
   Rationale: Option A is correct, and these are classic signs of anxiety. The stimulus is diffuse, thereby ruling out fear and phobias. Self-negation is not included, thus ruling out Option C (low self-esteem).

7. *Answer:* C
   Rationale: Option C represents knowledge of the reactions to the drug and a definitive strategy to alleviate the side effects. Option A negates the feelings of the client. Option B is premature or not indicated. Option D may lead to symptoms of withdrawal.

8. *Answer:* C
   Rationale: Contact with reality is intact, so Option D is not true. No history of mood swings is given, thus eliminating Option A as a possibility. Although Option B may be present, the experience of flashbacks, with the other symptoms, may be indicative of Option C.

9. *Answer:* C
   Rationale: Withdrawal symptoms similar in character to those noted with barbiturates and alcohol, including seizures, have been reported after abrupt discontinuation of antianxiety drugs.

10. *Answer:* D
    Rationale: It is important to assess for delirium with this client, who may be experiencing behavioral changes related to metastatic disease. Options A, B, and C are valid considerations, but organic causes of behavior must be ruled out first.

11. *Answer:* A
    Rationale: Although all of those factors are important to consider, only Option A reflects a treatment-related risk factor.

12. *Answer:* C
    Rationale: Crises and social support can be affected by interventions, but the nurse has limited control of these. Although a history of suicidal thoughts is important to consider, interventions to enhance symptom control, particularly pain, may have a more direct effect on depressive symptoms.

13. *Answer:* B
    Rationale: Questions require differentiation among depression (Option B), anxiety (Option A), psychosis (Option C), and panic (Option D). Depression is a state of feeling sad or discouraged. Anxiety is a state of feeling uneasy and apprehensive in response to a vague, nonspecific threat. Psychosis refers to disintegration of personality and loss of contact with reality. Panic is acute anxiety, terror, or fright.

14. *Answer:* C
    Rationale: When there is no physiologic basis for the symptoms, "treatment" of somatic

aspects of depression is contraindicated, because such actions reinforce these maladaptive behaviors and symptoms. To ask the client to "buck up" is asking the impossible and instilling guilt. The symptoms are "real" to the client, and diversion may help.

15. *Answer:* A

Rationale: Risk for falls is a primary concern with an older client. Option B may or may not be necessary. Option C is recommended for dry mouth associated with most antidepressants. Option D depends on the specific drug being taken.

16. *Answer:* D

Rationale: At one time, it was thought that clients with cancer did not attempt suicide. However, with cancer now being a chronic disease, suicidal thoughts and/or attempts are more common. Therefore, Option D is the most serious potential outcome of depression in clients with cancer.

17. *Answer:* D

Rationale: Loss of purpose, beliefs, and trust is indicative of spiritual distress. Anxiety symptoms are not present, ineffective coping is not specific enough, and the client is not exhibiting any self-negating behavior indicative of self-esteem problems.

18. *Answer:* D

Rationale: Cognitive problems would be indicated by other symptoms. No information is given that would lead to the conclusion that Options B or C exist. Spiritual distress is often confused with psychologic distress because of symptom similarity and comfort with attributing these symptoms to psychologic, rather than spiritual, difficulties.

19. *Answer:* B

Rationale: B is a therapeutic response and acknowledges the client's discomfort. Option A denies his feelings. Option C indicates the nurse's discomfort. Option D is imposing the nurse's beliefs.

20. *Answer:* B

Rationale: The nurse's lack of knowledge can be the most significant barrier. Once we understand beliefs and practices, we can then, it is hoped, consider and explain Options A, C, and D.

21. *Answer:* C

Rationale: Avoiding or challenging spiritual concerns will not provide support and enhancement of spiritual well-being. Although sharing perceptions may be helpful, there is not enough information given to know how supportive this may be. Option C represents a concrete way to enhance spiritual well-being.

22. *Answer:* C

Rationale: Symptoms presented are indicative of powerlessness. Options A and D are not represented by these symptoms. Option B is not specific enough.

23. *Answer:* B

Rationale: Loss of personal control is just that, personal; therefore Option B is the primary influencing factor. Options A and D may be influences. Assessment of Option C is not present.

24. *Answer:* C

Rationale: Use an open-ended statement to elicit individual perceptions of the response without jumping to conclusions of a diagnosis of loss of personal control.

25. *Answer:* D

Rationale: Management of symptoms is a basic nursing intervention in facilitating a client's sense of personal control. Options B and C would be additional interventions once symptom control is accomplished. Option A would not be therapeutic for the client.

26. *Answer:* D

Rationale: Seeking the opinions of both client and family about his care is most facilitative of his sense of control. Options A, B, and C, although important, represent doing something for the client, not facilitating his sense of control.

27. *Answer:* D

Rationale: Statements of suicidal intentions require immediate response for further assessment by a mental health professional. Option A or B requires problem solving by care providers, and Option C may be the client's choice.

28. *Answer:* D
Rationale: All of the situations given may precipitate the grief process, but the best definition of grief is Option D.

29. *Answer:* A
Rationale: Options B, C, and D are factors that all people may experience. Changes in body structure and function are more specific to the experiences of cancer diagnosis and treatment.

30. *Answer:* A
Rationale: One's past experiences are basic to one's grief responses throughout life; therefore Option A is the most basic point. Options B, C, and D are also applicable.

31. *Answer:* A
Rationale: Responses other than Option A represent strategies that block grief work and resolution of loss.

32. *Answer:* D
Rationale: Options A, B, and C represent normal grief responses. Option D is the best answer because of the evidence of a prolonged and unresolved grief process.

33. *Answer:* D
Rationale: Withdrawal or social isolation could be a symptom of clinical depression and deserves further evaluation. Options A, B, and C represent normal grief responses.

34. *Answer:* A
Rationale: A history of violence and possible legal difficulties may place her at risk. Other data indicate social functioning.

35. *Answer:* A
Rationale: Although limit setting (Option B) is appropriate, the first goal would be to better understand this family's emotional issues. Other interventions, although appropriate, do not address the identified problems.

36. *Answer:* C
Rationale: Options A and B would not be possible if the more basic requirement of effec-

tive reality testing were not present. Option D is not a requirement of social functioning.

37. *Answer:* D
Rationale: Providing both client and family with care skills is important to the client's participation and successful self-care (Options A and C). Option B is a nontherapeutic intervention.

38. *Answer:* A
Rationale: Language and cultural difference place individuals at risk for social dysfunction. The nursing assessment does not indicate Options B, C, or D.

39. *Answer:* B
Rationale: Basic to the success of outpatient treatment are the client's problem-solving and decision-making skills. Options A and D are also important factors to consider. No indication of a psychiatric assessment is present.

40. *Answer:* C
Rationale: Factors identified are indicative of the potential for impaired social interaction. Option A is not specific enough. Options B and C are not indicated by factors presented.

41. *Answer:* A
Rationale: Option A is basic to the success of the client's future care. Options B and C are not the responsibility of the nurse, and Option C, although important, would be based on a further assessment of need.

BIBLIOGRAPHY

American Cancer Society. (2000). *Complementary and alternative cancer methods.* Atlanta: American Cancer Society.

American Psychiatric Association. (2000). *Diagnostic and statistical manual of mental disorders* (4th ed., text revision). Washington, DC: American Psychiatric Association.

Brown-Saltzman, K. (1998). Transforming the grief experience. In R.M. Carroll-Johnson, L. Gorman & N.J. Bush (Eds.). *Psychosocial nursing care along the cancer continuum.* Pittsburgh: Oncology Nursing Press, pp. 192-214.

Bush, N.J. (1998a). Anxiety and the cancer experience. In R.M. Carroll-Johnson, L. Gorman & N.J. Bush (Eds.). *Psychosocial nursing care along the cancer continuum.* Pittsburgh: Oncology Nursing Press, pp. 125-138.

Bush, N.J. (1998b). Coping and adaptation. In R.M. Carroll-Johnson, L. Gorman & N.J. Bush (Eds.). *Psychosocial nursing care along the cancer continuum.* Pittsburgh: Oncology Nursing Press, pp. 192-214.

Carpenito, L.J. (Ed.). (2002). *Nursing diagnosis: Application in clinical practice* (9th ed.). Philadelphia: Lippincott Williams & Wilkins.

Carson, V. (1989). *Spiritual dimensions of nursing practice.* Philadelphia: W.B. Saunders.

Grimm, P. (2005). Coping: Psychological issues. In J. Itano & K. Taoka (Eds.) *Core curriculum for oncology nursing* (4th ed.). St. Louis: Elsevier.

NOTES

3 Coping: Altered Body Image and Alopecia

BETH A. FREITAS

Select the best answer for each of the following questions:

1. Persons with body image disturbances may exhibit self-destructive behavior. In dealing with such behavior, the primary goal of the nurse is to assist the client to identify
   A. logical basis for behavior.
   B. adverse effects of behavior.
   C. moral implications of behavior.
   D. psychologic basis for behavior.

2. Which of the following client outcome behaviors represents the highest level of adaptation to body image changes?
   A. Discusses plans to return to previous work role.
   B. Discusses changes in body structure and function.
   C. Serves as a volunteer in a client-to-client visitation program.
   D. Lists emergency resources to deal with self-destructive behavior.

3. The predominant fear for an adolescent female whose treatment plan includes an amputation is
   A. desertion.
   B. loss of status.
   C. disfigurement.
   D. hospitalization.

4. A primary objective of a client visit by a trained volunteer who has adjusted successfully to a similar experience, for example, Reach to Recovery program for mastectomy clients, is to promote adaptation changes in
   A. body structure and functioning by discussing prostheses, clothing, and appearance.
   B. sexual and social functioning by discussing sexual dysfunction.
   C. prognosis and life expectancy by discussing the similarity of the visitor's and the client's disease.
   D. role functioning and lifestyles by discussing a vocational rehabilitation plan for the individual client.

5. A client had a colostomy 48 hours ago. Which of the following demonstrates a concern regarding his body image changes?
   A. Neglect in bathing self.
   B. Refusing to get out of bed.
   C. Not answering the telephone.
   D. Refusal to cough and deep breathe.

6. Nurses can assist clients in the acceptance of a changed body image. Which of the following nursing interventions is the most supportive?
   A. Stressing a time frame to grieve and then quickly moving on.
   B. Facilitating conversations between client and long-lost family.

C. Educating family immediately regarding body image changes.

D. Allowing ventilation of negative emotions, especially anger and guilt.

7. Which of the following strategies is helpful to a 12-year-old daughter's adjustment when her mother has cancer and body image issues?

A. Have another family member inform the child.

B. Keep a structured communication style in place.

C. Inform the child about the specifics of the illness.

D. Inform the child when the disease outcome is known, approximately a year after diagnosis.

8. The most accurate estimate of usual hair regrowth is

A. 1 to 2 weeks after completion of chemotherapy.

B. 1 to 6 months after completion of chemotherapy.

C. 6 to 7 months after completion of chemotherapy.

D. more than 12 months after completion of chemotherapy.

9. Which of the following statements is correct in regard to chemotherapy-induced alopecia?

A. Hair loss is usually permanent.

B. Eyelashes and nasal hair are spared.

C. Type of drug administered affects the severity of alopecia.

D. Administration of multiple drugs decreases the severity of alopecia.

10. Which of the following is considered a common side effect of paclitaxel (Taxol)?

A. Nausea.

B. Fatigue

C. Hair loss.

D. Constipation.

11. Which of the following treatments is most likely to cause permanent hair loss?

A. Cyclophosphamide, methotrexate, 5-FU (CMF) for breast cancer

B. 6000 cGy radiation for brain tumor.

C. High-dose cytarabine (ARA-C) for leukemia.

D. Mechlorethamine, vincristine (Oncovin), procarbazine, prednisone (MOPP) therapy for Hodgkin's disease.

12. Client teaching for individuals receiving high doses of chemotherapy drugs should include which of the following suggestions?

A. Perm or color hair to disguise hair loss.

B. The best client outcome results when a plan is developed before hair loss.

C. Because of the slow rate of hair loss, there is adequate time to plan once hair loss begins.

D. Because hair regrowth will be similar to original hair, wigs should closely resemble original hair.

13. Which of the following is an appropriate method to reduce hair loss?

A. Sleep on a satin pillow.

B. Use a soft-bristled hairbrush.

C. Use a cold scalp cap during chemotherapy treatments.

D. There is no research-based method to reduce hair loss.

14. Body image is defined as

A. how one looks.

B. how one feels about one's body.

C. how others see the client's body.

D. how the client and other's view the client's body.

15. The long-term body image impact on adolescents with a childhood cancer has been shown to result in

A. changes in sexual function.

B. an altered genetic makeup.

C. changes in their treatment protocol.

D. a disturbed body image even with positive coping.

16. As a nurse assists a client to integrate into the workplace related to a body image issue, the nurse should

A. tell the client it is going to be ok and it's time to get back to work.

B. go into the workplace and share all about the client's disease and treatment.

C. have the client take as much medical leave as possible to regain emotional strength to face the coworkers.

D. Assist the client to verbalize specific concerns, identify supports, and dialogue concerning possible responses of coworkers.

17. Body image disturbance ranks behind ____ as an oncology client's primary concern when diagnosed.

A. fear of death
B. role adjustment
C. financial concerns
D. fear of sexual dysfunction

18. A client's body image disturbance may affect which hierarchy of need?

A. Physiologic.
B. Safety and security.
C. Perception of how others look.
D. Feelings of how client will re-enter the work force.

19. Which of the following is a positive coping behavior for families to use to discuss body image issues?

A. Humor.
B. Rigid communication.
C. Ignore the body image change.
D. Spend hours of focus on the body image change.

20. Which statement is true regarding radiation therapy–induced hair loss?

A. It is always permanent.
B. It occurs over the entire body.
C. It depends on the dosage of radiation to the site.
D. If the client puts gel on the hair, it will prevent hair loss.

21. This dosage of radiation therapy will most likely cause permanent hair loss in the treatment field.

A. 10 Gy
B. 50 Gy
C. 50 cGy
D. 100 cGy

22. A positive coping strategy to assist a client with alopecia is

A. staying inside to keep the sun off a bald head.
B. cutting fingernails short to prevent scratching self.
C. trying out new styles on a computer model before purchasing a wig.
D. educating about concerns other clients have experienced.

23. A nursing intervention that may increase the severity of a body image disturbance is to

A. use active listening skills and facilitate discussion of concerns.
B. educate client/family about body image changes after surgery.
C. stress the temporary nature of some side effects and limits in function.
D. allow the client to return to work after head/neck surgery before talking about reactions of coworkers.

24. The client's diagnosis of body image disturbance occurs if the nurse

A. has a full client spiritual history.
B. is able to ask all her clients what their body image score is.
C. identifies a gap between how the client sees himself or herself and is unable to return to school because of this.
D. identifies a gap between how the client sees himself or herself and how the client's significant other sees him or her and is able to talk this through.

25. A client intervention to assist with side effect management of alopecia is

A. keep head bare.
B. wear sunglasses.
C. shave arms and legs.
D. put sunscreen on arms and legs.

ANSWERS

1. *Answer:* B
   Rationale: The adverse effects of body image disturbances have implications for client safety and should be given priority. Attention to adverse effects is a response that can be an independent nursing role. Other responses refer to interventions that are not necessarily appropriate or are representative of the role of other health professionals or an advanced practice nurse.

2. *Answer:* C
   Rational: Option C represents actual, rather than a plan, and reintegration with constructive channeling of energies. Therefore Option C represents a higher level of adaptation than planned activity (Option A), knowledge (Option B), or attention to safety (Option D).

3. *Answer:* C
   Rationale: Although each person is different, body image is crucial in adolescents. Although not identified in this question, fear of death may be the predominant fear.

4. *Answer:* A
   Rationale: Option A delineates the limits of the volunteer's role. Prognosis, personal diseases, and sexual counseling are beyond the scope of responsibility for volunteers.

5. *Answer:* A
   Rationale: Options B, C, and D are more likely related to the client's fear of pain with movement versus body image perception of self. Validation of the client's feelings of motivation regarding these actions is required. Option A is more likely related to client's perception of self.

6. *Answer:* D
   Rationale: Nurses often find it more difficult to allow client's to share negative emotions, but it may be the most supportive role of a nurse. Option A is not accurate because grief has no time frame. Option B is not accurate because body image is not affected by this activity. Option C is not accurate because this is a preoperative role, and knowledge is not congruent with acceptance.

7. *Answer:* C
   Rationale: Option D is not appropriate because the client should communicate with the child. Options A and B are not correct because communication about the effects of the disease should be done within 1 year, and the communication style should be open and age-appropriate.

8. *Answer:* B
   Rationale: Regrowth is rare before 1 month and after 6 months.

9. *Answer:* C
   Rationale: Chemotherapy drugs may affect all hair bulbs. Administration of multiple drugs may increase the severity of hair loss. Hair loss is usually not permanent with chemotherapy but may be permanent with radiation therapy.

10. *Answer:* C
    Rationale: Hair loss is the most common side effect listed. The other responses are not side effects of paclitaxel.

11. *Answer:* B
    Rationale: Chemotherapy generally causes temporary hair loss. Radiation doses above 4500 cGy generally induce permanent loss.

12. *Answer:* B
    Rationale: Options A, C, and D contain incorrect information. Hair loss is generally rapid; hair texture may be different when it grows back, and treating hair may damage it and increase hair loss.

13. *Answer:* D
    Rationale: Although hair loss has a significant impact on the clients' body image, no large-scale research study supports any method of reducing hair loss. In some studies it has been found that scalp-cooling methods have allowed cancer cells to survive.

14. *Answer:* B
    Rationale: Body image is based on how one feels about how one's body looks and functions.

15. *Answer:* D
Rationale: Adolescent females who survived childhood leukemia have shown a severely altered body image even with apparent appropriate coping skills. Their sexual function and genetic makeup have not changed related to their body image.

16. *Answer:* D
Rationale: The nurse's role to assist reintegration is one focused on positive coping strategies of role-play and problem solving versus lack of empathy, improper disclosure, or avoidance.

17. *Answer:* A
Rationale: Fear of death is the number one concern of most cancer survivors. The concerns regarding role adjustment and financial and sexual dysfunction vary in priority depending on the individual.

18. *Answer:* A
Rationale: A body image change may affect one's ability to eat (physiologic). Options C and D are not part of the hierarchy of needs.

19. *Answer:* A
Rationale: Although humor is not always a family's coping pattern, it is used effectively to assist change. Rigid communication, spending hours of focus, or ignoring the body image changes are not effective in problem solving or progressing to acceptance of the changes.

20. *Answer:* C
Rationale: Hair loss occurs only at the site of radiation therapy. A small study has identified using gel to decrease hair loss, but this study was for clients undergoing chemotherapy. The gel may be harmful in clients undergoing radiation therapy.

21. *Answer:* B
Rationale: 100 cGy = 100 rad and 1 Gy = 100 rad. Any dose greater than 45 Gy or 4500 cGy will cause permanent hair loss.

22. *Answer:* C
Rationale: Option A is an avoidance behavior. Option B is not related to hair loss. Option D is an intervention that should be done before hair loss occurs.

23. *Answer:* D
Rationale: Options A, B, and C are positive coping strategies. Option D is avoidance of a possible issue.

24. *Answer:* C
Rationale: The body image change has affected the client's social interaction. Options A and B are assessments but are not specific to an individual client. Option D is an intervention.

25. *Answer:* B
Rationale: Wearing sunglasses will protect eyes because of a lack of eyelashes. The head should be kept covered, at least with sunscreen. Limbs do not need to be shaved, because hair loss will also occur there. Sunscreen should always be worn. This is not dependent on alopecia.

BIBLIOGRAPHY

Alley, E., Green, R., & Schuchter, L. (2002). Cutaneous toxicities of cancer therapy. *Current Opinion in Oncology* 14(2), 212-216.

Batchelor, D. (2001). Hair and cancer chemotherapy: Consequences and nursing care: A literature study. *European Journal of Cancer Care 10*, 147-163.

Cohen, M.Z., Kahn, D.L., & Steeves, R.H. (1998). Beyond body image: The experience of breast cancer. *Oncology Nursing Forum 25*(5), 835-841.

Dropkin, M.J. (1999). Body image and quality of life after head and neck cancer surgery. *Cancer Practice 7*(6), 309-313.

Kraus, P.L. (1999). Body image, decision making, and breast cancer treatment. *Cancer Nursing* 22(6), 421-427.

McGarvey, E.L., Baum, L.D., Pinkerton, R.C., & Rogers, L.M. (2001). Psychological sequela and alopecia among women with cancer. *Cancer Practice 9*(6), 283-289.

Newell, B. (2002). Terminal illness and body image. *Nursing Times 98*(14), 36-37.

Pickard-Holley, S. (1995). The symptom experience of alopecia. *Seminars in Oncology Nursing 11*(4), 235-238, 298.

Price, B. (2000). Altered body image: Managing social encounters. *International Journal of Palliative Nursing 6*(4), 179-185.

Weber, C., Bronner, E., Their, P., et al. (2001). Body experience and mental representation of body image in patients with haematological malignancies and cancer as assessed with the Body Grid. *British Journal of Medical Psychology 74*, 507-521.

4 Coping: Cultural Issues

JANICE PHILLIPS

Select the best answer for each of the following questions:

1. Which of the following groups has the highest incidence of cancer for all sites combined?
   A. Caucasian males.
   B. African American males.
   C. American Indian females.
   D. Native Hawaiian females.

2. African American males have the highest incidence of which of the following cancer(s)?
   A. Colon and rectum.
   B. Lung.
   C. Prostate.
   D. Liver.

3. Which of the following racial and ethnic minority groups has the lowest incidence of cancer?
   A. African Americans
   B. American Indians/Alaskan Natives.
   C. Hispanics.
   D. Chinese Americans.

4. Although African American women have a lower incidence of breast cancer, they are less likely to survive 5 years compared with Caucasian women. This difference in outcome is **least** likely to be due to
   A. family predisposition.
   B. late stage at detection.

   C. more aggressive tumor types.
   D. presence of additional illnesses.

5. Acculturation is best defined as
   A. the process of integrating various world views.
   B. one's country of origin, ethnicity, or culture.
   C. the ways in which individuals and cultural groups adapt and change over time.
   D. the process in which health care providers engage directly in cross-cultural encounters.

6. A 72-year-old American Indian woman with advanced cancer is comatose. She has a small discolored pouch around her neck. While bathing her, the most appropriate action for the nurse is to
   A. discard the pouch as it is a source of infection.
   B. remove it and place it in the drawer as you would with any personal belongings.
   C. leave it on.
   D. remove it and talk with the family when they come.

7. The nurse would be most cautious when entering the personal space of which of the following clients?
   A. A 36-year-old American Indian man.

B. A 40-year-old Hispanic woman.

C. A 52-year-old African American woman.

D. A 62-year-old Vietnamese man.

8. Suggesting whole milk or cheese as a means to improve nutritional status should be used with caution for which of the following racial/ethnic groups?

A. Asian and Pacific Islanders and African Americans.

B. Hispanic Americans.

C. American Indians and Alaskan Natives.

D. Caucasians.

9. A major factor explaining the differences in cancer incidence, mortality, and survival within different racial/ethnic groups is

A. skin color.

B. generation immigrated to the United States.

C. language.

D. poverty.

10. A wife has been at her husband's bedside continually since his admission 3 days ago. She is clearly tired. In considering their Japanese American background, the most appropriate nursing action is to

A. insist that the wife go home at night.

B. talk with the client to have him tell his wife to go home at night.

C. do nothing as it is the wife's duty to be at the bedside at all times.

D. talk with the family about other family members who might help stay with the client.

11. Given the tremendous increase in culturally diverse populations receiving care at your institution, you have been asked to serve on your hospital's cultural competence planning committee. During the initial planning session, which of the following is an appropriate first step?

A. Developing family-focused interventions.

B. Conducting an assessment of one's own cultural beliefs and values.

C. Emphasizing that good health comes from good luck despite cultural heritage.

D. Conducting focus groups with diverse communities.

12. Recent population trends indicate a tremendous increase in minority populations by the year 2020. Which of the following represents the fastest growing racial and ethnic minority populations?

A. African Americans.

B. Hispanics.

C. American Indians/Alaskan Natives.

D. Asian and Pacific Islanders.

13. In addition to the emphasis on cultural competence, there is a requirement for health care organizations to develop standards for linguistically appropriate care. Which of the following is least likely to meet the requirement of linguistically appropriate care?

A. Providing care that is meaningful and fits with cultural beliefs and lifeways.

B. Providing all clients with limited English proficiency with access to bilingual interpretation services.

C. Providing oral and written notices, including translated signage at key points of entry.

D. Ensuring the patient's preferred spoken language is included in the organization's information system.

14. Cultural competence is an ongoing process in which the health care provider strives to effectively work with the client (individual, family, community) within the appropriate cultural context. In the process of pursuing cultural competence, the point in which the provider demonstrates a genuine passion to be open and flexible with others is referred to as

A. cultural desire.

B. cultural knowledge.

C. cultural skill.

D. cultural encounter.

15. Mr. M. is a 40-year-old African American male whose father and grandfather were given the diagnosis of prostate cancer in their fifties. At what age should Mr. Mitchell begin prostate cancer screening?

A. Age 30.

B. Age 40.

C. Age 45.

D. Age 50.

16. As an outreach worker working with an American Indian community, you noted a sudden decrease in mammography participation. This reluctance was particularly noted after several diagnoses of breast cancer. After many unsuccessful attempts to increase mammography participation, what is the most appropriate strategy to pursue?
   A. Continue to explore beliefs and practices with outside consultants.
   B. Extend mammography screening hours.
   C. Prepare more culturally appropriate materials.
   D. Consult with respected American Indian leaders for assistance and suggestions.

17. A description of the health status and related needs of Asian and Pacific Islander communities may be underestimated because of
   A. cultural differences.
   B. degree of acculturation.
   C. higher socioeconomic status.
   D. lack of identification of the many groups and their subpopulations.

18. The belief that one has little control over personal health outcomes and that death is inevitable when cancer is present is referred to as
   A. assimilation.
   B. fatalism.
   C. religiosity.
   D. external control.

19. When planning programs targeting culturally diverse populations, which of the following is **least** likely to facilitate success?
   A. Consulting with key leaders after completing the program.
   B. Creating and sustaining partnerships.
   C. Recognizing intracultural variations.

   D. Incorporating traditional values, beliefs, and traditions.

20. In assessing a client's beliefs about the cause of his cancer, he states that it is caused by an imbalance in nature. This is an example of which health belief system?
   A. Magico-religious.
   B. Biomedical.
   C. Holistic health.
   D. Fatalistic.

21. Talking Circles are particularly helpful when designing health programs targeting which of the following groups?
   A. African American women.
   B. Newly arrived immigrants.
   C. American Indians.
   D. Hispanics.

22. The curandero, a type of folk healer, generally uses which of the following to address health concerns within the Hispanic community?
   A. Applies massage therapy to bones and joints in the absence of a physician.
   B. Practices black magic.
   C. Calls on the assistance of a well-known or deceased healer.
   D. Uses rituals, prayers, pledges, and herbal baths to facilitate healing.

23. Generalizations are best defined as
   A. a projection of one's own values or world views.
   B. starting points that require more assessment of beliefs and practices that are shared by a group.
   C. end points when planning culturally competent care.
   D. a simplified inflexible belief of a population or subgroup.

ANSWERS

1. *Answer:* B
   Rationale: According to the American Cancer Society, African American males have the highest incidence rates for all sites combined at 696.8 per 100,000 population.

2. *Answer:* C
   Rationale: According to the American Cancer Society, African American males have the highest incidence of prostate cancer compared with Caucasians and other racial and ethnic minority populations. The incidence rate for prostate cancer for African American males is 272.1 per 100,000, followed by 164.3 for Caucasians, 137.2 for Hispanics, 106.0 for Asian and Pacific Islanders, and 53.6 for American Indian/Alaskan Native males. The mortality rate for African American males is 73.0 per 100,000, followed by 30.2 for Caucasians, 24.1 for Hispanics, 21.9 for American Indians/Alaskan Natives, and 13.9 for Asian and Pacific Islander males.

3. *Answer:* B
   Rationale: According to the American Cancer Society, American Indians and Alaskan Natives experience lower cancer incidence and death rates for all cancers combined, with an annual incidence of 488.2 per 100,000.

4. *Answer:* A
   Rationale: Family predisposition to cancer has little effect on the survival of these women. Scientists believe that more than half of the difference in survival can be attributed to later stage at detection and tumors that are more aggressive and less responsive to treatment. Additional factors thought to contribute to this difference include the presence of additional illnesses and various sociodemographic factors.

5. *Answer:* C
   Rationale: Acculturation, ways in which individuals and cultural groups change over time, is an important concept when interfacing with various racial and ethnic or culturally diverse groups. Although some acculturation may take place, many groups will maintain traditional cultural traits. Nurses need to understand the degree to which patients and various groups adhere to traditional values. Many factors influence how likely individuals or groups will be to maintain traditional beliefs and practices. These factors can include the length of time a person lives in a new country, the ability to communicate with the majority culture, size of the racial and ethnic or culturally diverse group, rigidity or flexibility of the host country, age, and socioeconomic status.

6. *Answer:* C
   Rationale: American Indians may carry objects believed to guard against witchcraft or have objects that are considered curative, given to the client by the native healers. The latter may be considered sacred. As long as the object does not interfere with the client's care, there is no harm in leaving it on. If for some reason it needs to be removed, consult with the family since the client is comatose.

7. *Answer:* D
   Rationale: In general, Asian and Pacific Islanders are noncontact people compared with the other ethnic groups. They may feel uncomfortable with close, physical contact.

8. *Answer:* A
   Rationale: Lactose intolerance is high in both Asian and Pacific Islanders and African Americans.

9. *Answer:* D
   Rationale: Poverty, not race, accounts for a 10% to 15% lower survival rate from cancer in many ethnic groups. When data are corrected for economic status, African Americans have a slightly lower incidence and mortality for a number of cancers than did Caucasians. The disproportionate number of African Americans in the lower socioeconomic strata accounted for the increased incidence. In another study, when only Caucasians who received the same level of care were included in the study, it was found that indigent clients, regardless of ethnicity, had poorer survival

rates for each cancer type. The impact of poverty on cancer is felt in ethnic minorities because a disproportionate number of ethnic minorities comprise the poor of America.

10. *Answer:* D
Rationale: There is an expectation for the wife to be the primary caretaker in the Japanese culture. Other family members may also share the duties. To "not bother the nurses" is also a common belief. Options A and B do not consider their cultural beliefs, whereas Option C does. However, it does not consider the health of the wife and possible caregiver burnout.

11. *Answer:* B
Rationale: Becoming culturally competent requires an ongoing process that begins with self-awareness. Ideally, one should begin to assess his or her personal cultural beliefs and professional values and identify how these help to shape personal behaviors and attitudes. The process of cultural awareness includes the recognition of one's biases, prejudices, and assumptions about individuals who are different. Without an awareness of the influence of one's own cultural or professional values, the health care provider runs the risk of engaging in cultural imposition: imposing one's beliefs and values on another culture.

12. *Answer:* B
Rationale: In 2000, the American population was 71.4% Caucasian, 11.8% Hispanic, 12.2% African American, 3.9% Asian and Pacific Islander, and 0.7% American Indian. Projections indicate that by 2020, the American population will consist of 63.8% Caucasians, 17% Hispanics, 12.8% African Americans, 5.7% Asian and Pacific Islanders, and 0.8% American Indian/Alaskan Natives.

13. *Answer:* A
Rationale: Linguistic relates to language. The National Standards and Outcomes-Focused Research Agenda calls for the design of culturally and linguistically competent health care services. Linguistically appropriate responses include the use of interpreter staff, translated written materials, and the communication of such services to clients.

14. *Answer:* A
Rationale: Cultural desire is the motivation of the health care provider to want to, rather than have to, engage in the process of becoming culturally aware, culturally knowledgeable, culturally skillful, and familiar with cultural encounters.

15. *Answer:* C
Rationale: According to the American Cancer Society, the prostate specific antigen (PSA) test and the digital rectal examination should be offered annually, beginning at age 50, to men with a life expectancy of 10 years. However, men at high risk, African Americans and those with strong family history (first-degree relatives given the diagnosis of prostate cancer at an early age), should begin testing at age 45. As always, men should confer with their health care provider to gather information and make an informed decision.

16. *Answer:* D
Rationale: Program success is greatly enhanced when respected leaders are involved in all phases of a project, beginning with problem identification to completion of the project. In this instance the health care team can work with a respected American Indian leader to address the low participation. As a result, a respected Indian healer might perform a cleansing ceremony and blessing of the mammography machine. This may help the women to feel more comfortable and willing to participate in mammography screening.

17. *Answer:* D
Rationale: Information regarding the health status of Asian and Pacific Islanders has been inadequate because of the lack of specification and identification of the many groups. When all Asian and Pacific Islanders are aggregated, many inherent differences are not readily apparent. Inadequate classification and reporting contributes to the belief that Asian and Pacific Islanders do not require special care or that they are healthier than the general population.

18. *Answer:* B
Rationale: The concept of fatalism has often been cited in the oncology literature. Some authors have reported fatalism among

African Americans, females, and people with low incomes and low educational levels. Research shows that these populations believe that cancer is a death sentence and that there is little that one could do to prevent cancer and/or to treat cancer. However, fatalism is not limited just to these populations, nor should it be generalized to all segments of these populations.

19. *Answer:* A

Rationale: The community should be involved in all phases of the project, beginning with the needs assessment to the final completion and dissemination of results. Many authors highlight that participation of those affected by the problem might well be the most important aspect of program development.

20. *Answer:* C

Rationale: In the holistic health view, the forces of nature must be in balance or in harmony. Human life is one aspect of nature and must be in harmony with the rest of nature. Native Americans often have this view. That health and illness are controlled by supernatural forces is the belief in the magico-religious view. Some African Americans may believe in voodoo, whereas Hispanic Americans often believe that illness is caused by the evil eye (mal ojo). The biomedical health belief view is that life and life processes are controlled by physical and biochemical processes that can be manipulated by humans. The client will expect medications, a treatment, or surgery to cure the health problem.

21. *Answer:* C

Rationale: Talking circles incorporate American Indian or Alaskan Native culture into story as a means to reinforce traditional roles and values of American Indian and Alaska Native cultures. Talking circles incorporate the tradition of oral storytelling and are facilitated by respected community members. These stories are helpful in forming a foundation for educational messages and may vary from tribe to tribe.

22. *Answer:* D

Rationale: Many culturally diverse groups use folk healers to cure illness. Although the Hispanic community is very diverse, many share a common belief system that consists of a folk medical system called curanderismo. The curandero, or folk healer, generally uses rituals, prayers, pledges, and herbal baths to assist in healing. This is in contrast to a yerbalista, who uses herbal prescription, a sobador/sobadora, who uses massage to manipulate joints and bones in the absences of a doctor, a brujas/brujos and hechiceros, who work with black magic, or an espiritistas/espiritualistas, who may solicit the assistance of a well-known deceased healer to cure illness. The use of folk healers continues to be a very important cultural value for the Hispanic community. The use of folk healers must be assessed and considered when working with this population. The use of traditional healers is also important to other groups (e.g., American Indian/Alaskan Natives) and should be assessed for possible incorporation into health programs.

23. *Answer:* B

Rationale: When working with any population regardless of ethnicity, race, or culture, one must be careful not to make generalizations. Although many culturally diverse groups have shared values, beliefs and practices, one must be careful to avoid a "one size fits all approach." Generalizations are common patterns for beliefs and behaviors that are shared by a group. In some cases the generalizations may be inaccurate when applied to specific individuals of that group. Thus they serve as starting points and serve as a basis for further assessment.

BIBLIOGRAPHY

American Cancer Society. (2001). *Cancer facts and figures for Hispanics 2000-2001*. Atlanta: Author.

American Cancer Society. (2002). *Breast cancer facts and figures 2001-2002*. Atlanta: Author.

American Cancer Society. (2003). *Cancer facts and figures for African Americans 2003-2004*. Atlanta: Author.

American Cancer Society. (2004). *Cancer facts and figures 2004*. Atlanta: Author.

Boyle, J. (2003). Culture, family, and community. In M.M. Andrews & J.S. Boyle (Eds.). *Transcultural concepts in nursing care*. Philadelphia: Lippincott Williams & Wilkins, pp. 335-336.

Burhansstipanov, L., & Olsen, S.J. (2001). Cancer prevention and early detection in American Indian and Alaska Native populations. In

M. Frank-Stromborg & S.J. Olsen (Eds.). *Cancer prevention in diverse populations: Cultural implications for the multidisciplinary team.* Pittsburgh: Oncology Nursing Society, pp. 5-52.

Campinha-Bachote, J. (2002). The process of cultural competence in the delivery of healthcare services: A model of care. *Journal of Transcultural Nursing 13(3)*, 181-184.

Chen, M.S., & Hawks, B.L. (1995). A debunking of the myth of healthy Asian Americans and Pacific Islanders. *American Journal of Health Promotion 9*, 261-268.

Frank-Stromborg, M., & Olsen, S.J. (Eds.). (2001). *Cancer prevention in diverse populations: Cultural implications for the multidisciplinary team* (2nd ed.). Pittsburgh: Oncology Nursing Society, Inc.

Freeman, H. (1989). Cancer in the socioeconomically disadvantaged. *CA: A Cancer Journal for Clinicians 39(5)*, 266-288.

Huff, R.M., & Kline, M.V. (1999). *Promoting health in multicultural populations: A handbook for practitioners.* Thousand Oaks, CA: Sage Publications.

Kline, M.V. (1999). Planning health programs and disease prevention programs in multicultural populations. In R.M. Huff & M.V. Kline (Eds.). *Promoting health in multicultural populations:*

A handbook for practitioners. Thousand Oaks, CA: Sage Publications, p.73-102.

Office of Minority Health. (1999). *Assuring cultural competence in health care: Recommendations for national standards and an outcomes-focused research agenda.* Washington, DC: U.S. Department of Health and Human Services, Washington, DC. www.omhrc.gov/clas/ds.htm.

Oncology Nursing Society. (2000). *Oncology nursing society multicultural outcomes: Guidelines for cultural competence.* Pittsburgh: Oncology Nursing Press, Inc.

Phillips, J., Cohen, M., & Moses, G. (1999). Breast cancer screening and African American Women: Fear, fatalism, and silence. *Oncology Nursing Forum 26*, 561-571.

Powe, B. (1995). Cancer fatalism among elderly Caucasians and African Americans. *Oncology Nursing Forum 22*, 1355-1359.

Powe, B., & Weinrich, S. (1999). An intervention to decrease cancer fatalism. *Oncology Nursing Forum 26(3)*, 583-588.

U.S. Census Bureau. (2003). *Population projections.* Retrieved April 9, 2003 from http://www.census.gov/population/www/projections/natsum-T5.html.

NOTES

5 Coping: Survivorship Issues and Financial Concerns

SUSAN LEIGH

Select the best answer for each of the following questions:

1. In relation to cancer survivorship, the term "secondary survivors" refers to what population?
   A. Anyone who is given the diagnosis of more than one cancer.
   B. Someone who recurs with the original primary disease.
   C. A family member who also has cancer.
   D. Any member of a social network—personal or professional—who is affected by someone's cancer diagnosis.

2. "Seasons of Survival," the survivorship model described by Mullan, illustrates
   A. the extent that disease has progressed.
   B. an estimate of when death will occur.
   C. a continuum of acute, extended, and permanent stages.
   D. a description of cure.

3. If survivorship is viewed as a continuum, what statement best describes the acute stage?
   A. The time when symptoms from treatment are most severe.
   B. The stage when the initial diagnosis is made and treatment begins.
   C. The stage when treatment is no longer effective and the prognosis is terminal.
   D. The period of watchful waiting.

4. During the acute or immediate stage of survival, survivors would rarely encounter
   A. the fear of dying.
   B. nausea and vomiting.
   C. disruption in family and social roles.
   D. delayed effects of treatment.

5. Survivors in the extended or intermediate stage of survival are
   A. finished completely with all medical treatments.
   B. in remission or receiving maintenance therapy.
   C. considered "cured" of their disease.
   D. undergoing initial therapy.

6. Which statement best characterizes someone in the permanent or long-term stage of survival?
   A. The survivor is cancer free.
   B. The survivor is guaranteed a cure.
   C. The survivor's cancer status has gradually evolved to where the probability for disease recurrence is minimal.
   D. The survivor has not responded to multiple courses of therapy and is preparing to die.

7. Which of the following best describes symptoms or effects that persist for months or years after therapy is completed?
   A. Progressive effects.
   B. Iatrogenic effects.

C. Erroneous effects.

D. Long-term effects.

8. Cardiomyopathy, pulmonary fibrosis, and sterility are examples of

A. long-term, late, or delayed effects of cancer therapy.

B. acute toxicity from cancer treatment.

C. inevitable side effects from all radiation therapy.

D. reversible effects once treatment has ended.

9. A 32-year-old woman who had received mantle radiation for Hodgkin's disease at the age of 17 asks the oncology nurse why a baseline mammogram was ordered? Knowing this history, the nurse explains that

A. this is a mistake, because this survivor is too young for a baseline mammogram and her breasts would be too dense for a definitive procedure.

B. she should have had a baseline mammogram before treatment began.

C. the radiation would prevent any cancer from developing.

D. that follow-up guidelines for young women treated for Hodgkin's disease now suggest a baseline mammogram approximately 10 years after initial therapy because of an increased risk of breast cancer after mantle radiation.

10. Which of the following statements accurately describes a psychosocial effect of long-term survival?

A. Most cancer survivors have severe and permanent psychologic impairment.

B. After therapy is completed, there is rarely, if ever, any need for continued psychosocial support.

C. The fear of recurrence may persist for many years after completion of therapy and may range anywhere between a mild or chronic anxiety all the way to disabling fear.

D. The Damocles syndrome refers to a genetic predisposition to cancer.

11. Although employment discrimination continues to haunt some survivors, there are laws that offer protection to most people with histories of cancer. When survivors qualify for new jobs, promotions, or retention of existing jobs, current laws

A. are the same laws that protect the mentally and physically disabled.

B. are legislated only through state government.

C. apply to private employers only.

D. have a statute of limitations.

12. During a follow-up visit, a former client confides that he will soon be laid off from his job and that losing health insurance is his greatest concern. For immediate short-term protection, you inform him that there is a law that mandates certain employers to offer time-limited access to continued insurance coverage. This coverage is available for 18 months for the person losing the job and for 36 months for dependents. This protection is the

A. Social Security Disability Insurance Program.

B. Consolidated Omnibus Budget Reconciliation Act (COBRA).

C. Family and Medical Leave Act (FMLA).

D. Americans with Disabilities Act (ADA).

13. After experiencing cancer, many survivors critically examine their lives, search for meaning, and feel an increased appreciation for life. This can best be described as

A. positive, spiritual transformation or existential effect that is an individual and personal reaction to having cancer.

B. an impossibility, because nothing good can come from a diagnosis of cancer.

C. a warning sign that further psychologic therapy is needed.

D. feelings experienced by all survivors regardless of outcome.

14. Mrs. P. is having a difficult time going to her breast cancer support group. Although she is doing well and is free of disease 2 years after completing treatment, she feels sad and despondent when she sees others suffer or die of the same illness she had. She asks herself why she is alive and doing well when so many others are not. This phenomenon has been described as

A. posttraumatic stress disorder.

B. acute reactive syndrome.

C. bipolar disorder.

D. survivor's guilt.

15. Which statement best describes the current state of long-term follow-up care for adult cancer survivors in the United States?
   A. All long-term survivors are seen in specialty follow-up clinics for the rest of their lives.
   B. Although pediatric survivors undergo follow-up for indefinite periods of time in long-term survivor specialty clinics, adult cancer survivors rarely have access to this type of oncology follow-up.
   C. Adult survivors are eligible to be seen in follow-up clinics after being free of disease for 5 years.
   D. Primary care physicians are best prepared to identify oncology-related follow-up problems.

16. As survivors near the end of their initial treatment, how can the oncology team help the survivor transition to completing therapy and entering the extended stage of survival?
   A. Establish a time for an exit interview so that the health care team can help the survivor and family develop a plan of action for what life will look like after the initial treatment is completed.
   B. Encourage the survivor to try to forget the past painful months and get on with life once therapy is completed.
   C. Discuss the risks of recurrence with the family so that the survivor does not worry.
   D. Have a party or ceremony to celebrate the end of treatment.

17. The Americans with Disabilities Act is one of the first laws to offer protection against discrimination to cancer survivors. Although not perfect, this law best describes protection for which of the following?

   A. Survivors who have noticeable amputations only, such as leg amputations.
   B. Survivors who have disabilities that were identified before the cancer diagnosis.
   C. Survivors with mental health problems.
   D. Survivors who work for employment agencies, labor unions, local and state government offices, or private employers that have 15 or more employees.

18. Assessing the risk or probability for recurrence of disease and long-term and late effects would ideally happen within what context?
   A. At a late effects clinic or long-term follow-up visit, ideally by a health care team that would include the oncology nurse.
   B. At an internal medicine office.
   C. At a family practice office.
   D. No need to assess unless there are symptoms that may be related to the primary disease or treatment.

19. A 52-year-old breast cancer survivor who was treated 12 years ago has moved to your area and comes to your oncology clinic for the first time. With this introductory history, which type of information would be **least** important for you to begin your assessment?
   A. Type and date of surgical procedures, including pathology reports and diagnostic indicators.
   B. Specific therapies, including chemotherapy drugs and radiation fields, doses, and dates.
   C. Her willingness to be a community advocate.
   D. Financial status.

ANSWERS

1. *Answer:* D
   Rationale: Rarely does cancer affect only an individual. Family units, social acquaintances, coworkers, and even health care professionals are affected in multiple ways by someone else's cancer diagnosis. Their issues must also be addressed with appropriate support and resources.

2. *Answer:* C
   Rationale: Introduced by Mullan and embraced by the National Coalition for Cancer Survivorship, the model of seasons—or stages of survival—describe survivorship as a dynamic, evolutionary process that begins at diagnosis and proceeds along a continuum through and beyond treatment, regardless of outcome. This model has helped to identify issues that affect quality of life and longer term survivors and that warrant intervention by the health care community and society at large.

3. *Answer:* B
   Rationale: The acute stage of survival begins at the time cancer is diagnosed and extends through the initial phase of therapy.

4. *Answer:* D
   Rationale: Delayed or late effects of treatment occur months to years after therapy is completed.

5. *Answer:* B
   Rationale: When disease is in remission or survivors have completed the basic, rigorous course of treatment, the extended or intermediate stage begins. They may or may not continue to receive maintenance therapy and will not know for years whether treatment has been successful.

6. *Answer:* C
   Rationale: This stage is roughly equated to "cure," yet there is no such thing as a guarantee. Rather than a guarantee of cure, there is a gradual evolution from the extended stage of survival into a period where the likelihood of the disease recurring is sufficiently small that the cancer can be considered permanently arrested.

7. *Answer:* D
   Rationale: Long-term effects of cancer and cancer therapy begin during the acute stage and continue indefinitely after treatment ends. Many of these effects gradually subside (e.g., hair regrows), whereas others can become chronic conditions (e.g., neuropathies).

8. *Answer:* A
   Rationale: Cardiomyopathy, pulmonary fibrosis, and sterility are late and/or long-term effects of specific cancer therapies that become apparent months to years after therapy completion. These medical problems are due to subclinical tissue or cellular damage during treatment that progress over time. Although these effects are not necessarily inevitable, they are rarely reversible.

9. *Answer:* D
   Rationale: Although the overall risk for second malignancies in general is still relatively low, breast cancer is the most frequently seen second malignancy in young women who were treated with mantle radiation for Hodgkin's disease. Although breast tissue is, in fact, dense in young women, mammography remains the best option for screening at this time. Also, tumors occur as late effects and usually occur more than a decade after initial treatment.

10. *Answer:* C
    Rationale: Although much of the fear associated with cancer gradually subsides over time, an underlying fear of the cancer recurring can remain for the remainder of life. This is often referred to as the Damocles syndrome (story that describes a guest at a mythologic banquet with all the food and drink he can consume, but with a sword attached by a mere thread dangling over his head). This fear can be triggered at the time of medical follow-up visits, during an anniversary of diagnosis or painful procedures, or at any time a suspicious symptom arises. Although survivors

have varying needs for continued psychosocial support after therapy is completed, few are considered to have overt mental illness because of their cancer diagnosis.

11. *Answer:* A

Rationale: In general, denial of employment to cancer survivors who are qualified for the job solely because of their medical history violates most laws that prohibit discrimination against the handicapped. A handicap may be real or it may be perceived. But most federal laws apply only to employers who receive federal funding.

12. *Answer:* B

Rationale: As long as the employer has 20 or more employees, he must offer access to group medical coverage for those losing their jobs. During this grace period, the employee will assume the payment of insurance premiums and retain coverage for himself and his family. Social Security Disability Insurance is a monthly stipend that is available 6 months after a person qualifies as disabled. The FMLA offers workers 12 weeks of unpaid leave without losing their jobs. And the ADA offers limited job and insurance protection to persons perceived to be disabled, including those with cancer histories.

13. *Answer:* A

Rationale: Experiencing a life-threatening illness often heightens the desire to personally evaluate priorities and search for meaning throughout difficult times. Whereas some survivors become more religious, others may feel a deepened sense of spirituality or transformation. Yet this hardly describes everyone's experience with cancer. Because this is a very personal reaction to a difficult diagnosis, there can be as many negative effects as there are positive.

14. *Answer:* D

Rationale: Survivor's guilt is a normal reaction to surviving a life-threatening illness and is often triggered by a return to the clinic, hospital, or support group. Survivors can compare themselves to others with recurrent disease or to those who have died, and this can provoke mixed reactions and guilty feelings about doing well.

15. *Answer:* B

Rationale: Standardized guidelines for the follow-up care of adult cancer survivors are rare. Transfer back to primary care is decided on a case-by-case basis by either the referring oncologist or the insurance plan. Primary care physicians and other medical specialists see more long-term cancer survivors than oncologists, even though there are few guidelines to help with assessing long-term and late effects of cancer therapies.

16. *Answer:* A

Rationale: An exit interview will help develop a plan as to what life will look like after treatment is completed and, it is hoped, reduce some of the unknowns. The plan could include information about wellness promotion along with disease identification. This might include education on prevention and early detection, timelines for follow-up, identification of risk factors, and assessment of symptoms and recurrence. Honesty and education will prepare the survivor and family members for life after treatment.

17. *Answer:* D

Rationale: The Americans with Disabilities Act was enacted to expand coverage originally offered by the Federal Rehabilitation Act. Unfortunately, everyone is still not guaranteed protection by these combined acts.

18. *Answer:* A

Rationale: As greater numbers of survivors live longer after diagnoses of cancer, risks for problems related to their initial disease or therapy increase. Ideally, specialized clinics with professionals dedicated to assessing this ever-increasing population would be able to monitor long-term survivors, identify risks and early problems, and educate about prevention and control measures within an atmosphere of wellness.

19. *Answer:* C

Rationale: During the initial assessment, it is imperative that a medical history be as specific as possible to develop a follow-up surveillance and wellness plan. Also, insurance or method of paying for care is extremely important. After the initial health and financial assessment is concluded, you can then inquire as to her interest in doing community advocacy or volunteer work.

BIBLIOGRAPHY

Aziz, N.M. (2002). Cancer survivorship research: Challenge and opportunity. *American Society for Nutritional Sciences,* 3494S. (Presented as part of the International Research Conference on Food, Nutrition & Cancer for the American Society for Nutritional Sciences.)

Dow, K.H. (1990). The enduring seasons in survival. *Oncology Nursing Forum 17,* 511.

Ferrell, B.R., Dow, K.H., & Leigh S. (1995). Quality of life in long-term cancer survivors. *Oncology Nursing Forum 22,* 915.

Hoffman, B. (1999). *Working it out: Your employment rights as a cancer survivor (booklet).* Silver Spring, MD: National Coalition for Cancer Survivorship.

Koocher, G., & O'Malley J. (Eds.). (1981). The *Damocles syndrome: Psychosocial consequences of surviving childhood cancer.* New York: McGraw-Hill.

Leigh, S. (1992). Myths, monsters, and magic: Personal perspectives and professional challenges of survival. *Oncology Nursing Forum 19,* 1475.

Loescher, L.J., Welch-McCaffrey, D., Leigh, S.A., et al. (1989). Surviving adult cancer. Part 1: Physiologic effects. *Annals of Internal Medicine 3,* 411.

Maher, E.L. (1982). Anomic aspects of recovery from cancer. *Society of Scientific Medicine 16,* 907–911.

Mullan, F. (1985). Seasons of survival: Reflections of a physician with cancer. *New England Journal of Medicine 313,* 270.

Welch-McCaffrey, D., Loescher L.J., Leigh, S.A., et al. (1989). Surviving adult cancer. Part 2: Psychosocial implications. *Annals of Internal Medicine 3,* 517.

NOTES

6 Sexuality

EVELYN H. LARRISON

Select the best answer for each of the following questions:

1. Nurses should incorporate assessment of sexual functioning into cancer diagnosis and treatment because
    A. sexuality is a quality of life issue.
    B. clients won't ask about sex.
    C. cancer clients are getting younger.
    D. physicians should talk to clients about sexuality, not nurses.

2. Johnson's Behavioral Model (JBM) provides direction for appropriate nursing interventions by recognizing
    A. humans are biologic systems.
    B. once treatment is ended, effects dissipate.
    C. there are seven independent subsystems to consider.
    D. disturbance in one subsystem of sexual health affects other subsystems.

3. Mrs. S. is undergoing chemotherapy for breast cancer. When she asks about safe birth control, you tell her that
    A. an intrauterine device (IUD) is the safest method of birth control.
    B. contraceptive foam will increase vaginal lubrication.
    C. diaphragms are an effective form of birth control.
    D. a hormonal birth control pill is not appropriate for hormone-dependent tumors.

4. The PLISSIT (Permission, Limited Information, Specific Suggestions, Intensive Therapy) model for sexuality counseling
    A. can be used only by nurses with an advanced degree.
    B. does not require any knowledge about sexuality or how sexuality is affected by a diagnosis of cancer or the treatment for cancer.
    C. is a useful model for levels of nursing interventions based on the nurse's comfort and knowledge about the subject.
    D. is used primarily for clients with longstanding or severe problems with sexuality.

5. The first level of assessment "P" (Permission) in the PLISSIT model conveys the message that
    A. any sexual activity is appropriate behavior.
    B. discussing sexual issues is appropriate.
    C. they must remain sexually active.
    D. sexual discussions should be referred to other sources.

6. If cancer is diagnosed in a pregnant woman,

A. she should be counseled about the need for an immediate therapeutic termination of pregnancy.
B. her prognosis will be much worse, because pregnancy increases the rate of growth of malignancy.
C. diagnosis at an earlier stage of disease would be easier for a woman who was not pregnant.
D. she will need high-risk obstetric care and to have her diagnostic workup and treatment plan evaluated for risk to the fetus and herself.

7. Deciding on cancer treatment during pregnancy is influenced by
   A. risk to the fetus.
   B. anesthesia risks during surgery.
   C. inability to receive chemotherapy.
   D. the client's inability to have diagnostic procedures.

8. Molly is a 17-year-old client with newly diagnosed stage IIIB Hodgkin's lymphoma and will undergo chemotherapy. She openly admits that she has been sexually active. As her nurse, you would counsel her
   A. that she must stop all sexual activity.
   B. on the risks associated with becoming pregnant while receiving treatment.
   C. if she becomes pregnant, she can't be treated.
   D. that you will have to notify her parents of her sexual activity.

9. A physiologic sexual dysfunction caused by external pelvic irradiation in women is
   A. increased vaginal lubrication.
   B. radioactivity of the vagina.
   C. decreased elasticity of the vagina.
   D. decreased risk of vaginal infections.

10. A 45-year-old man is to undergo pelvic radiation for prostate cancer. Client education will include that
   A. his age reduces risk of sterility.
   B. more than 4 Gy results in temporary sterility.
   C. radiation below the diaphragm increases the risk of sterility.
   D. the use of condoms reduces radiation exposure to his partner.

11. A 30-year-old man has received Mechlorethamine, Oncovin (vincristine), procarbazine, and prednisone (MOPP) for lymphoma. After treatment he can expect that
   A. his fertility will not be affected by the treatment.
   B. he will be permanently sterile.
   C. his sperm count will recover within 1 year of treatment.
   D. he will need to monitor sperm counts for up to 4 years after treatment.

12. Sexual dysfunction resulting from chemotherapy
   A. results primarily from damage to the penis or vagina.
   B. is of little concern to "normal clients" but may be of importance to clients with a psychiatric history.
   C. indicates treatment should be discontinued.
   D. needs to be assessed, because sexuality issues can directly affect quality of life.

13. A 36-year-old woman is undergoing chemotherapy for ovarian cancer. She will be counseled that
   A. she may be affected sexually by premature menopausal changes.
   B. her libido will be increased.
   C. intercourse will be impossible because of pain.
   D. side effects of chemotherapy will not interfere with sexual activity.

14. Fertility after chemotherapy
   A. is not related to the age of the client when treated.
   B. is not influenced by the type of chemotherapy used.
   C. is more affected by combination versus single drug therapy.
   D. is permanent in men treated with Adriamycin (doxorubicin), bleomycin, vinblastine, dacarbazine (ABVD).

15. Which psychologic factor can affect sexual functioning?
   A. Anemia.
   B. Fatigue.
   C. Anxiety.
   D. Pain.

16. A sexual side effect of hormonal therapy in the male client is
    A. erectile dysfunction.
    B. increased libido.
    C. increased fertility.
    D. masculization.

17. Changes in sexual functioning occur as the result of
    A. prostatectomy.
    B. unilateral orchiectomy.
    C. head and neck surgery.
    D. oophoropexy.

18. Education and anticipatory guidance to prevent sexual dysfunction include
    A. assuming the client knows basic sexuality information.
    B. encouraging the couple to avoid discussing fears or concerns with each other.
    C. dispelling myths or misconceptions.
    D. using models or drawings to explain how sexuality can be affected.

19. A desired client outcome of nursing interventions to improve sexuality is
    A. client and partner recognize that sex is no longer a priority.
    B. client identifies potential or actual alteration in sexuality caused by disease or treatment.
    C. client identifies the need to sever relationships to protect partner from coping with terminal illness.
    D. client focuses on coping with treatment, not sexuality.

20. As a nurse caring for Mr. C. after an abdominoperineal resection, which of the following client's or significant other's concerns are most realistic to discuss with him?
    A. The variety of ways for sexual pleasure.
    B. Erectile dysfunction caused by the surgery.
    C. Ability to ejaculate with intercourse.
    D. Effect of surgery on his masculinity.

21. Mrs. J. is scheduled to have a mastectomy for breast cancer. Which of the following questions would be *most* appropriate for the nurse to ask when discussing the potential impact of surgery on sexuality?
    A. "Do you have any concerns about how the loss of your breast may affect how others see you?"
    B. "Some women have concerns about the effects the surgery will have on their sexual life. Do you have any concerns?"
    C. "Do you have any problems with your sexual life at this time?"
    D. "Some women don't see themselves as feminine after the surgery. Do you?"

22. Mrs. G. has been told to use a vaginal dilator after radiation therapy to the cervix. Which of the following statements is the most appropriate for the nurse to use in teaching Mrs. G.?
    A. Insert the dilator into your vagina as quickly as possible.
    B. Lubricate the dilator with an oil-based jelly.
    C. Leave the dilator inserted for 1 minute each time.
    D. Using a dilator prevents scarring and keeps the vagina open.

23. Mrs. T. is receiving radiation therapy to the pelvis. She states that she has not had intercourse for several weeks, although she desires sexual intimacy. Which of the following suggestions would be most appropriate for the nurse to make to Mrs. T.?
    A. "Let your partner know you are interested in having sex."
    B. "Limit the amount of time you and your partner initially spend on intercourse."
    C. "Ask your partner why he hasn't wanted to have sex."
    D. "Concentrate on pleasing your partner during intercourse."

24. Forty-five-year-old Oscar is recovering from radical head and neck surgery. His wife appears comfortable with giving him tracheostomy care and is ready for him to go home. As his nurse you counsel the couple that
    A. if she loves him, she shouldn't care how he looks.
    B. being able to talk isn't critical for sexual activity.
    C. they will need to learn interventions to cope with increased secretions.
    D. they will need to avoid sexual activity.

25. Nurses can contribute to client's sexual knowledge base by
    A. sharing their sexual (the nurse, the client, or both) experiences.
    B. providing them with erotic literature.
    C. researching resources on sexuality and cancer.
    D. providing Internet web sites.

26. Medical interventions for sexual dysfunction include
    A. psychotherapy.
    B. attendance at support groups.
    C. penile implants, vaginal reconstruction.
    D. incorporating cultural beliefs into intervention.

27. A nursing diagnosis specific to sexuality is
    A. impotence.
    B. disturbance in body image.
    C. vaginal stenosis.
    D. menopausal symptoms.

28. Mechanical devices to treat erectile dysfunction include
    A. penile injections.
    B. penile vacuum devices.
    C. Sildenafil (Viagra).
    D. Eros C.

29. Mr. J. is concerned about resuming sexual activity with his wife, who has received radiation and chemotherapy for uterine cancer. To counsel him, you need to know
    A. that he may "catch" cancer from her.
    B. that he may be exposed to radiation.
    C. the facts about how diagnosis and treatment can affect sexuality
    D. sexual intercourse will not be different than before treatment.

30. A sexual side effect of chemotherapy is
    A. alopecia.
    B. vaginal stomatitis.

    C. incontinence.
    D. retrograde ejaculation.

31. Miss S. has returned to your clinic for a follow-up visit after her colostomy for a bowel obstruction. She and her significant other are asking questions about resuming sexual activity. One suggestion you might give her is
    A. avoid anal intercourse.
    B. how to secure the ostomy bag for sexual activity.
    C. place a folded towel over the ostomy site.
    D. avoid face-to-face sexual positions.

32. A total abdominal hysterectomy, including ovaries, in a 40-year-old woman will cause
    A. fear of sexual intimacy.
    B. vaginal changes.
    C. total loss of sexual desire.
    D. destruction of self-concept as a woman.

33. Mrs. H. is undergoing chemotherapy for breast cancer. She confides in you that she has lost her desire for sex. You counsel her that
    A. the changes may be caused by medication.
    B. sex isn't important at this time.
    C. she feels this way because of her mastectomy.
    D. she shouldn't worry; it will come back.

34. Tom J. is receiving a continuous cisplatin infusion for treatment of testicular cancer. When you enter his room, you discover he and his partner engaged in sexual activity. Your best response would be:
    A. Report it to his physician.
    B. Instruct client and his partner to use condoms.
    C. Oral sex is a safe method of sexual satisfaction.
    D. Reprimand them for unacceptable behavior in a hospital.

ANSWERS

1. *Answer:* A
Rationale: The definition of quality of life includes sexual functioning. Cancer advocacy has resulted in more clients asking questions about sexual health. Sexuality is not an age issue.

2. *Answer:* D
Rationale: Disturbance in one subsystem affects other subsystems (fatigue may interfere with social life). Humans are seen as behavioral as well as biologic systems. Subsystems are not independent. The effects of cancer treatment can be extended over time; that is, childhood treatment of cancer could affect fertility in adulthood.

3. *Answer:* D
Rationale: Hormone-dependent tumors may grow in response to the hormone content of birth control pills. Use of an IUD or diaphragm carries a risk of infection in neutropenic clients. Foam may irritate vaginal mucosa, not increase lubrication.

4. *Answer:* C
Rationale: This model allows health care providers to obtain the information to plan interventions at the appropriate level based on their ability and identified client needs.

5. *Answer:* B
Rationale: Introducing the subject of sexuality to clients and their partners conveys acceptability that discussing sexuality is appropriate. It is not a blanket permission for all sexual behaviors. It should also include permission not to engage in sexual activity. All nurses are able to provide sexuality information at this level.

6. *Answer:* D
Rationale: The issue of termination would depend on the type of disease, doubling time of the malignancy, and the gestational age of the fetus. Diagnostic workups can be adjusted to reduce the amount of risk to the fetus. Different chemotherapy agents can be given during specific trimesters. Radiation therapy may be delayed until after delivery.

7. *Answer:* A
Rationale: Decisions regarding treatment during pregnancy are based on the potential risk to the fetus. Modern anesthetics can be used safely during pregnancy, certain chemotherapies do not cross the placenta, and some diagnostic tests carry a reduced risk to the fetus, for example, magnetic resonance imaging and ultrasonography.

8. *Answer:* B
Rationale: Some chemotherapy agents are teratogenic. Interventions include birth control information. Rebellion may lead an adolescent to get pregnant to "be normal." Modification of therapy may allow treatment during pregnancy. Confidentiality is maintained at all times.

9. *Answer:* C
Rationale: Pelvic irradiation causes decreased elasticity of the vagina and thinning of vaginal tissues. External radiation therapy does not cause a body part to be "radioactive." Vaginal lubrication is decreased, causing an increased risk of vaginal infection.

10. *Answer:* C
Rationale: Twenty-five percent of men receiving radiation below the diaphragm are at risk for sterility. The age of the male does not affect risk of sterility, but more than 4 Gy results in permanent sterility. A client receiving radiation is not radioactive after treatment.

11. *Answer:* D
Rationale: Fertility may reverse as late as 4 years after treatment. Eighty percent of men who receive MOPP have fertility affected but will not be permanently sterile.

12. *Answer:* D
Rationale: Sexual dysfunction resulting from chemotherapy is usually temporary and can be related to nausea, fatigue, decreased

vaginal lubrication, body image changes from alopecia, among others.

13. *Answer:* A

Rationale: Premature menopause caused by chemotherapy can affect libido, body image, and ability to engage in sexual intercourse. Libido will be decreased; intercourse is possible with use of vaginal lubricants, and side effects of chemotherapy such as fatigue and vaginal changes will affect sexual functioning.

14. *Answer:* C

Rationale: Combination therapies carry a greater risk of posttreatment infertility. Fertility is usually recovered after ABVD treatment, and age and type of chemotherapy influence future fertility.

15. *Answer:* C

Rationale: All other answers are physiologic responses.

16. *Answer:* A

Rationale: Hormonal therapy causes decreased libido and fertility and may cause feminization.

17. *Answer:* A

Rationale: Nerve damage during prostatectomy may cause erectile dysfunction. Unilateral orchiectomy preserves some hormone production, and oophoropexy removes the ovary from radiation exposure. Head and neck surgical changes in appearance may affect self-image but not sexual function per se.

18. *Answer:* C

Rationale: Myths or misconceptions can escalate anxiety and interfere with sexual functioning.

19. *Answer:* B

Rationale: Client and partner need to be educated about the potential sexual side effects of cancer and its treatment. Cancer is not always a terminal illness, and clients need reinforcement that sexuality remains an important part of life.

20. *Answer:* B

Rationale: Client and significant others should be informed of the possibility of erectile dysfunction after surgery. The degree of erectile dysfunction is related to the extent of the surgery and success of nerve-sparing procedures. After the degree of dysfunction is established, a variety of means of achieving sexual pleasure can be discussed. Retrograde ejaculation is a side effect of an abdominoperineal resection but is a moot point if he cannot achieve an erection. He will probably not internalize the effect of these changes on his self-concept of masculinity before leaving the hospital.

21. *Answer:* B

Rationale: The correct answer provides permission for sexual concerns. By using "some women..." an opportunity is provided for the client to express her individual concerns.

22. *Answer:* D

Rationale: Using a vaginal dilator after radiation treatments keeps the vagina open for sexual intercourse and future vaginal examinations. The dilator must be inserted slowly using a water-soluble lubricant and kept in place for 10 minutes.

23. *Answer:* A

Rationale: Often the partner is reluctant to initiate sexual activities for fear of hurting the client or because the partner assumes that the client does not want to have sex.

24. *Answer:* C

Rationale: Interventions to contain increased secretions will make the couple more comfortable. There is no physical reason to avoid sexual activity. Answer "A" places a judgmental burden on his wife, and speech is not necessarily important for intimacy.

25. *Answer:* C

Rationale: There are many appropriate nursing publications about sexuality. Sharing one's sexual experiences or providing erotic literature is inappropriate. Searching for sexual information via the Internet may result in receiving pornographic material.

26. *Answer:* C

Rationale: Penile implants and vaginal reconstruction are medical interventions. The other choices are psychologic interventions.

27. *Answer:* B
Rationale: All the rest are medical diagnoses.

28. *Answer:* B
Rationale: Penile injections and sildenafil (Viagra) are medical treatments. Eros C is used for female sexual dysfunction.

29. *Answer:* C
Rationale: Nurses need to know the facts about how diagnosis and treatment can affect sexuality. It is a myth that he can catch cancer from his wife. He will not be exposed to radiation after treatment, and she will have vaginal changes resulting from surgery and treatment.

30. *Answer:* B
Rationale: Vaginal and oral stomatitis are side effects of some chemotherapies. Alopecia may cause a change in self-image but not in sexual functioning per se. Retrograde ejaculation and incontinence are surgical side effects.

31. *Answer:* B
Rationale: Management of ostomy appliances by securing the bag or changing position will help prevent accidental spilling of contents. Discuss anal intercourse at a later time, unless they specifically introduce the subject. A folded towel placed above the ostomy acts as a bridge over the ostomy site. There are no restrictions to sexual positions.

32. *Answer:* B
Rationale: Loss of ovarian function results in vaginal changes of decrease elasticity and lubrication, which may make sexual intercourse painful. A hysterectomy does not cause a total loss of sexual desire, and although fear of sexual intimacy and changes in self-concept may occur, they are a psychological response and are not present in every woman having a hysterectomy.

33. *Answer:* A
Rationale: Many of the medications used to control side effects may cause changes in libido (e.g., antihistamines, antiemetics). A nurse should not negate a client's interest in sexual activity by dismissing her concern or saying it will come back. Although a mastectomy may cause a change in self-concept resulting in a loss of libido, the surgery itself does not affect libido.

34. *Answer:* B
Rationale: Most chemotherapy is excreted from the body in the first 72 hours. During this time they should use condoms. Oral sex should be avoided unless using condoms. His physician should know about the activity so that he can reinforce safety issues, and although the activity may be inappropriate in a hospital setting, it is not a primary focus if it is done in a private setting.

BIBLIOGRAPHY

Bruner, D., & Iwamoto, R. Altered sexual health in cancer. www.cancersource.com. Retrieved May 20, 2002.
Grossfeld, L., & Cullen, M. (2000). Sexuality and fertility issues. In Moore-Higgs, G. (Ed.). *Women and cancer: A gynecologic oncology nursing perspective.* Sudbury, MA: Jones and Bartlett Publishers, pp. 467-500.
Krebs, L.U. (2000). Sexual and reproductive dysfunction. In C.H. Yarbro, M.H. Frogge, M. Goodman, & S.L. Groenwald (Eds.). *Cancer nursing principles and practice* (5th ed.). Sudbury, MA: Jones and Bartlett Publishers, pp. 831-853.
Larrison, E. (2002). Causes and treatments of sexual dysfunction in the gynecologic oncology patient. *Women's Oncology Review 2,* 135-142.
Schover, L. (1996). *Sexuality and cancer: For the woman who has cancer and her partner.* Atlanta: American Cancer Society.
Schover, L. (1996). *Sexuality for the man who has cancer and his partner.* Atlanta: American Cancer Society.
Susman, E. (2001). Recognizing female sexual dysfunction as a complication of chemotherapy. *Oncology Times 23,* 46.
Winks C., & Semans, A. (1994). *The new vibrations guide to sex* (2nd ed.). San Francisco: Cleis Press.

7 Supportive Care: Dying and Death

MOLLY LONEY

Select the best answer for each of the following questions:

1. Mr. S. has been admitted for pain control because of bone metastases from advanced prostate cancer. He is still seeking aggressive treatment. Which of the following types of care is indicated?
   A. Acute care.
   B. Palliative care.
   C. Rehabilitative care.
   D. Hospice care.

2. In orienting Mr. S. and his family, which of the following best describes what they can expect?
   A. Holistic end-of-life care with an interdisciplinary team.
   B. Entry into a clinical trial to manage pain and extend life.
   C. Referral to physical therapy for muscle-strengthening exercises.
   D. Symptom control to enhance quality of life.

3. An important first step in caring for Mr. S. is
   A. assessing Mr. S.'s pain.
   B. assessing how Mr. S.'s family is coping.
   C. talking with Mr. S. and his family about hospice.

   D. Developing a therapeutic relationship with Mr. S. and his family.

4. In managing Mr. S.'s pain, which of the following immediate treatments would you anticipate?
   A. An opioid.
   B. A steroid.
   C. An antidepressant.
   D. A radiopharmaceutical.

5. In monitoring Mr. S.'s response to treatment, which of the following would be important to watch for?
   A. Seizures.
   B. Unrelieved pain.
   C. Diarrhea.
   D. Anuria.

6. Best practice interventions for managing Mr. S.'s pain include
   A. providing relaxation with music.
   B. encouraging ambulation three times a day.
   C. providing analgesia around the clock.
   D. medicating only when he complains of pain.

7. A key barrier to effective pain management in clients with cancer is
   A. difficulty in assessing pain.
   B. older clients not wanting to complain.

C. physicians' undertreatment of pain.

D. effects of cancer or its treatment.

8. Mr. S. may experience constipation from which of the following factors?

A. Anorexia.

B. Hypernatremia.

C. Enlarged prostate.

D. Spinal cord compression.

9. Common causes of urinary retention or incontinence in clients with cancer include

A. dehydration.

B. stress from diagnosis.

C. constipation.

D. diarrhea.

10. While receiving chemotherapy and radiation therapy for ovarian cancer, Mrs. J. has developed diarrhea. Priority care includes

A. using a perianal skin barrier.

B. starting on intravenous antibiotics.

C. monitoring for hypercalcemia.

D. teaching Mrs. J. about reducing fiber in her diet.

11. Understanding dyspnea means recognizing that it

A. is rarely associated with anxiety.

B. can arise from tumor, metastasis, or anemia.

C. always responds to inhalers or oxygen therapy.

D. can be measured with pulmonary function tests.

12. Pharmacologic management of dyspnea may include

A. a steroid.

B. a muscle relaxant.

C. an antibiotic.

D. nebulized morphine.

13. Which of the following interventions can help relieve dyspnea in a 45-year-old athletic man with lung cancer and pleural effusion?

A. Breathing through the nose.

B. Exercising the upper body while sitting erect.

C. Leaning over a pillow on an over-the-bed table.

D. Lying flat on the unaffected side with legs straight.

14. Nurses can make a difference in supporting coping in terminally ill clients with cancer and their families by

A. avoiding any discussion about death or dying.

B. helping clients and families get a second opinion.

C. encouraging clients to drink fluids every 2 hours.

D. offering information about how symptoms can be controlled.

15. Important distinctions between anorexia and cachexia include which of the following:

A. Anorexia is an irreversible loss of fat and muscle.

B. Cachexia is a reversible loss of protein metabolism.

C. Anorexia is a reversible decrease in appetite with weight loss.

D. Cachexia is always a consequence of vitamin and electrolyte deficits.

16. Supportive care for a client with end-stage cancer and anorexia focuses on

A. teaching the family how to give tube feedings.

B. suggesting small meals with liquid supplements.

C. letting the client choose what he/she eats and drinks.

D. teaching the family about the use of total parental nutrition.

17. Miss B. was admitted today with stage IV gastric cancer and severe nausea and vomiting. Which of the following initial treatments would you anticipate her physician to order?

A. Octreotide (Sandostatin).

B. An antianxiety medication.

C. Nasogastric tube to suction.

D. Surgery for possible bowel obstruction.

18. Dietary changes that can help minimize nausea and associated vomiting may include

A. mealtime distraction.

B. clear, nonacidic liquids.

C. warm or room temperature foods.

D. salty, sweet, or high-protein foods.

19. Miss B.'s severe nausea and vomiting continues. She may be experiencing which of the following complications?
    A. Diarrhea.
    B. Obstruction.
    C. Imminent death.
    D. Spinal cord compression.

20. It is important to teach family members of a terminally ill client with cancer that dehydration can indirectly increase the client's comfort by
    A. decreasing risk of confusion.
    B. increasing gastric secretions with less vomiting.
    C. decreasing bleeding from the nose, gums, or lungs.
    D. decreasing pulmonary edema and gurgling breathing.

21. Providing comfort to a client with end-stage cancer with dehydration includes
    A. vital signs every 2 hours.
    B. oral care every 2 hours while awake.
    C. ambulating down the hall every 8 hours.
    D. coughing and deep breathing every 2 hours while awake.

22. Factors contributing to anxiety in clients at the end of life include
    A. loss of familiar surroundings.
    B. chemotherapy and radiation therapy.
    C. loss of normal routine and family contact.
    D. concerns about diagnosis and risk of metastases.

23. Mary C., a 32-year-old with stage IV colon cancer, has been admitted with a very distended stomach and abdominal pain. She complains of chest tightness, dyspnea, heart palpitations, and irritability and is afraid of being left alone. Mary's complaints are most likely symptoms of
    A. anxiety.
    B. ascites.
    C. depression.
    D. liver failure.

24. On her second hospital day, Mary says "I'm just not worth anything to anyone...I'm just a burden to my family. I can't keep on living like this. If I had a gun..." Mary's comments are signs of
    A. fear.
    B. anxiety.
    C. depression.
    D. change in mental status.

25. What priority intervention is needed to address Mary's safety needs?
    A. Antianxiety medication.
    B. Antidepressant medication.
    C. Assess for any suicidal plans.
    D. Ask Mary's family to stay with her overnight.

26. Delirium in clients with cancer is characterized by
    A. short-term memory loss.
    B. clonic and myoclonic tremors.
    C. permanent disorientation and confusion.
    D. abrupt or fluctuating change in level of consciousness.

27. Possible causes of delirium may include which of the following:
    A. Antibiotics.
    B. Antiemetics.
    C. Bowel obstruction.
    D. Urinary tract infection.

28. A classic sign of delirium in clients facing imminent death is
    A. indigestion.
    B. agitation.
    C. heart palpitations.
    D. lack of coordination.

29. Nursing interventions to support a client with cancer and delirium may include
    A. keeping the environment calm.
    B. giving opioids prn for sedation.
    C. moving the client to a chair in the nursing station.
    D. keeping the lights off in the client's room during the night.

30. Signs of a client's impending death may include which of the following:
    A. Thirst.
    B. Erythema of the skin.
    C. Fitful sleeping at night.
    D. Talking about going on a trip.

31. Physical signs that become high priorities for care when death is imminent include
    A. pain, insomnia, and restlessness.
    B. dyspnea and decreased urine output.
    C. pain, restlessness, dyspnea, and agitation.
    D. dyspnea, insomnia, and dysphagia.

32. Best practice guidelines in using sedation for symptom control at the end of life include
    A. recognizing that sedation is never indicated.
    B. titrating the dose until symptoms are controlled.
    C. recognizing that sedation interferes with a peaceful death.
    D. administering a minimal dose for the first 24 hours.

33. Mr. W. has been hospitalized for the past 2 days for malignant pleural effusion. His breathing has progressively become more rapid, shallow, and moist. Important nursing interventions include which of the following?
    A. Changing his position every 2 hours.
    B. Educating his family about a living will.
    C. Helping him use an incentive spirometer.
    D. Contacting his doctor for an anticholinergic order.

34. The oncology nurse can help promote communication among Mr. W. and his family members by which of the following:
    A. Avoid repeating information.
    B. Encourage them to tell their own stories about the situation.
    C. Encourage them to avoid talking about their worries and fears.
    D. Suggest they talk with another end-of-life client and family.

35. Mr. W. has continued his labored, shallow breathing through the night with increasing restlessness. How can the nurse help the family support Mr. W.'s dying peacefully?
    A. Encourage his entire family to spend the night with him.
    B. Tell his family to request mechanical ventilation in the intensive care unit.

C. Encourage his family to say good-bye and tell him it's okay to let go.
    D. Tell his family that their presence may be making Mr. W. more restless.

36. Major family reorganization associated with Mr. W.'s terminal phase of cancer includes
    A. searching for meaning.
    B. searching for a new spouse.
    C. setting long-term family goals.
    D. selling the family's house and business.

37. At the end of life, families look to oncology nurses for which of the following?
    A. Skilled comfort care.
    B. Skilled high-tech care.
    C. Advice on how to grieve.
    D. Friendship and a listening ear.

38. In meeting their spiritual needs at the end of life, terminally ill clients with cancer search for
    A. life goals, hope, reassurance, and answers.
    B. life goals, religion, connections, and answers.
    C. meaning, hope, connections, and forgiveness.
    D. meaning, religion, reassurance, and forgiveness.

39. Which of the following statements are true about cultural and spiritual values?
    A. They are defined by an individual's religion.
    B. They are influenced by the hospital environment.
    C. They are defined by a family's socioeconomic status.
    D. They may influence preferences for end-of-life and postmortem care.

40. Oncology nurses can help meet their client's spiritual needs at end-of-life by
    A. praying over the dying client.
    B. referring all spiritual questions to the chaplain.
    C. offering advice from their own religious beliefs.
    D. finding time to allow the client to talk about spiritual concerns.

41. An important task of bereavement involves
   A. denying the loss.
   B. justifying the loss.
   C. experiencing the pain of grieving.
   D. replacing the lost person or object.

42. Bereavement support for Mr. W.'s family following his death includes
   A. assessing his family's religious practices.
   B. scheduling his family members for physical examinations.
   C. teaching his family what caused Mr. W.'s illness.
   D. teaching his family about the normal response to grief.

43. Common manifestations of grief over the loss of a loved one may include
   A. restlessness and dyspnea.
   B. exhaustion and insomnia.
   C. weight gain and diaphoresis.
   D. hyperactivity and palpitations.

44. Factors that place Mr. W.'s family at risk for developing complicated grief include
   A. short course of Mr. W.'s terminal illness.
   B. Mr. W.'s diagnosis of metastatic lung cancer.
   C. guilt over past relationship conflicts with Mr. W.
   D. enjoying life again—3 months after Mr. W.'s death.

NOTES

ANSWERS

1. *Answer:* B
Rationale: Palliative care is defined as care that provides symptom management, comfort, and support to clients living with a life-threatening illness. Hospice care is care that is initiated when the client has less than 6 months to live.

2. *Answer:* D
Rationale: Mr. S.'s palliative care focuses on controlling symptoms to enhance his quality of life in managing the effects of advanced disease.

3. *Answer:* A
Rationale: Symptoms that cause the greatest client distress should be addressed first by the interdisciplinary team. Once Mr. S.'s pain is assessed and intervention is initiated, the next priority is developing a therapeutic relationship with Mr. S. and his family.

4. *Answer:* A
Rationale: Opioids are the drugs of choice in treating severe pain. Other treatment for bone pain may include using a steroid and radiopharmaceutical.

5. *Answer:* B
Rationale: Ongoing evaluation includes determining whether the pain is not responding to the current intervention and monitoring for side effects of opioids such as constipation, nausea and vomiting, and sedation.

6. *Answer:* C
Rationale: Pain management focuses first on round-the-clock dosing with analgesics. Relaxation with music may also be helpful as a supplement to analgesia.

7. *Answer:* C
Rationale: A key barrier to effective pain management is physicians' undertreatment of pain. Other barriers include difficulty in measuring pain and older clients not wanting to complain.

8. *Answer:* D
Rationale: Constipation may be caused by spinal cord compression, opioid use, hypercalcemia, low-fiber diet, dehydration, reduced defecation, and depression.

9. *Answer:* A
Rationale: Urinary retention and incontinence in clients with cancer can be caused by dehydration and by spinal cord damage, increased weakness and confusion, urinary tract infections, and side effects of medications.

10. *Answer:* A
Rationale: Priority care in responding to Mrs. J.'s diarrhea includes using a skin barrier to prevent skin breakdown, teaching Mrs. J.'s about adding fiber to her diet to increase bulk, and assessing for a possible bowel obstruction as the diarrhea's underlying cause. Hypercalcemia, not hyperkalemia, can also cause diarrhea.

11. *Answer:* B
Rationale: Dyspnea is always associated with anxiety. Dyspnea may be caused by cancer, metastases, or anemia, and is always associated with anxiety. Dyspnea may respond to oxygen therapy, but not always. Dyspnea is a subjective symptom that cannot be detected by an outside observer or diagnostic tests.

12. *Answer:* A
Rationale: Pharmacologic management of dyspnea includes treating the underlying cause first and then providing symptom management with a steroid and bronchodilator. There is no evidence to support the use of nebulized morphine or a muscle relaxant (unless caused by muscle spasms in the chest).

13. *Answer:* C
Rationale: Relief of dyspnea for a 45-year-old athletic man with lung cancer and pleural effusion can include sitting up using a table to support the arms and body, elevating the head of the bed, limiting exercise, pacing activities, and pursed-lip breathing.

14. *Answer:* D
Rationale: Nurses can make a difference in supporting coping in terminally ill clients and their families by offering information about how symptoms can be controlled, active listening, and helping open up communication about concerns and preferences with death and dying.

15. *Answer:* C
Rationale: Anorexia is a decrease in appetite resulting in weight loss and may be reversible. Cachexia is a metabolic syndrome associated with cancer that results in loss of fat, muscle, and bone mineral content.

16. *Answer:* C
Rationale: Supportive nursing care for a client with end-stage cancer and anorexia focuses on letting the client eat what he/she wishes. Enteral and parenteral nutrition are avoided in palliative care. If the client is interested, small meals with liquid supplements may be suggested.

17. *Answer:* C
Rationale: Initial interventions to address Miss Barnes's severe nausea and vomiting should include intravenous antiemetics from different classes and a nasogastric tube. Octreotide and total parenteral nutrition are not considered initially. Given her advanced disease, total parenteral nutrition may not be considered.

18. *Answer:* B
Rationale: Dietary changes that can help minimize nausea and vomiting include clear liquids, nonacidic foods/fluids, cold foods or food at room temperature, and avoiding salty, sweet, or fatty foods.

19. *Answer:* B
Rationale: Unrelieved and severe nausea and vomiting can be caused by malignant bowel obstruction.

20. *Answer:* D
Rationale: It is important to teach family members of a terminally ill client with cancer that dehydration can actually increase the client's comfort by decreasing urine output, decreasing gastric secretions, decreasing pulmonary secretions and edema, and decreasing ascites and peripheral edema.

21. *Answer:* B
Rationale: Providing comfort for a client with end-stage cancer and dehydration should include providing mouth care at least every 2 hours. Frequent monitoring of vital signs, ambulation, coughing, and deep breathing are not considered part of comfort care.

22. *Answer:* C
Rationale: Factors most contributing to anxiety in clients at the end of life include loss of normal routine/control, separation from loved ones, burden on family, and an uncertain future. Loss of familiar surroundings can cause grieving but is not a major source of anxiety. Concerns about chemotherapy, radiation therapy, diagnosis, and risk of metastases are more common during the acute phase of cancer and its treatment.

23. *Answer:* A
Rationale: Mary's symptoms are classic manifestations of anxiety (i.e., dyspnea, chest tightness, palpitations, irritability, and fear).

24. *Answer:* C
Rationale: Mary's comments are now symptoms of depression (i.e., hopelessness, helplessness, worthlessness, guilt, and suicidal thoughts).

25. *Answer:* C
Rationale: Priority interventions to meet Mary's safety needs should start with assessing for suicidal thoughts/plan, before requesting an antidepressant from the doctor or asking family to stay with Mary. Mary's symptoms needing attention are now her depression and suicidal thoughts, not her anxiety.

26. *Answer:* D
Rationale: Delirium in clients with cancer is best defined as an alteration in the level of consciousness, which may occur abruptly or may fluctuate. Delirium may involve an intermittent loss of short-term memory. Permanent disorientation and confusion is seen in dementia, not delirium.

27. *Answer:* D
Rationale: Possible causes of delirium may include steroids, infection, opioids, organ failure, metabolic changes, and the effects of disease on the central nervous system.

28. *Answer:* B
Rationale: A classic sign of delirium is agitation, often with restlessness. Indigestion, heart palpitations, and lack of coordination are not seen with everyone experiencing delirium.

29. *Answer:* A
Rationale: Supporting clients with delirium should involve providing a calm environment, reviewing the client's history for contributing medications, and keeping the lights on at night. Opioids can cause delirium.

30. *Answer:* D
Rationale: Signs of a client's impending death may include mottling of the skin and talking about going away on a trip. Dying clients complain of a dry mouth, not thirst. Time sleeping actually increases.

31. *Answer:* C
Rationale: Physical symptoms that become high priorities for care when death is imminent include pain, dyspnea, restlessness, and agitation. Each of these symptoms causes distress for the client and family, affecting quality of life.

32. *Answer:* B
Rationale: Guidelines for using sedation when death is imminent should include obtaining consent from the client or family and titrating the sedating medication's dose until symptoms of terminal restlessness and agitation are controlled. Sedation can actually help promote quality of life and death.

33. *Answer:* D
Rationale: Key comfort measures for Mr. W. and his family include reviewing with his family what to expect as death approaches and asking the doctor for an anticholinergic order to dry his secretions and prevent suffering from gurgling. Discussion about a living will should have occurred before this point. Changing his position every 2 hours will not reduce his secretions as he approaches the end of life.

34. *Answer:* B
Rationale: Communication among Mr. W. and his family can best be promoted by encouraging them to tell their stories in sharing their experiences throughout his illness. Information often needs to be repeated, rather than avoided. Openly talking about their fears can support their communication and grief. Their priority needs to focus on communication within their own family at end of life.

35. *Answer:* C
Rationale: The nurse can help support the family in helping Mr. W. by encouraging them to say good-bye and give Mr. W. permission to let go. Rapid shallow breathing does not equate terminal restlessness, so sedation or restricting family visitors is not indicated.

36. *Answer:* A
Rationale: Major family reorganization during the terminal phase of a family member's illness involves redefining family roles, searching for meaning, and living day to day. Setting long-term goals, finding a new spouse, and selling the house and business are not priorities during the terminal phase.

37. *Answer:* A
Rationale: At the end of life, families look to the oncology nurse for skilled comfort care and open, honest communication. Families need a listening ear, but not a nurse as a friend. Because everyone grieves in his or her own way, no advice can be given on how best to grieve.

38. *Answer:* C
Rationale: Spiritual needs of terminally ill clients include meaning, hope, connections or relationships, and forgiveness.

39. *Answer:* D
Rationale: Cultural and spiritual values influence how individuals view and make sense of grief and may influence preferences for end-of-life care (including postmortem care). They are defined by an individual's or family's ethnic background, but not religion or

socioeconomic status. The hospital culture doesn't influence cultural and spiritual values.

40. *Answer:* D

Rationale: Nurses can best support dying clients in meeting their spiritual needs by finding ways to allow clients to talk about their spiritual fears and concerns. It is important for the nurse to remain nonjudgmental and objective. Once concerns are shared, referral to a chaplain is appropriate.

41. *Answer:* C

Rationale: Tasks of bereavement include accepting the reality of the loss, experiencing the pain of grief, and adjusting to the new environment without the loved one. Denial and justifying are manifestations, not tasks, of bereavement. Replacing the loss may occur but is also not a task of bereavement.

42. *Answer:* D

Rationale: Assessment should focus on manifestations of grief and social supports, not specific religious practices. Although family members need to talk through what happened, teaching them what caused Mr. W.'s illness should have occurred at time of diagnosis. Bereavement support for the family following Mr. W.'s death should also include teaching the family about the normal grief response. Bereavement support does not involve scheduling his family for routine physical examinations.

43. *Answer:* B

Rationale: Common manifestations of grief associated with the loss of a loved one may include exhaustion, insomnia, weight loss, palpitations, social withdrawal, restlessness, and anxiety. Dyspnea is not a common manifestation of grief.

44. *Answer:* C

Rationale: Risk factors for Mr. W.'s family developing unresolved or complicated grief may include guilt over past relationship conflicts with Mr. W. Other risk factors may include reawakening of an old loss, multiple losses, angry/ambivalent relationship with the deceased, social isolation, lack of financial support, and history of physical and/or mental illness.

BIBLIOGRAPHY

Berger, A., Porternoy, R., & Weissman, D. (Eds.). (2002). *Principles and practices of palliative care and supportive care.* Philadelphia: Lippincott Williams & Wilkins.

Ferrell, B., & Coyle, N. (Eds.). (2001). *Textbook of palliative nursing.* New York: Oxford University.

Hermann, C., & Looney, S. (2001). The effectiveness of symptom management in hospice patients during the last seven days of life. *Journal of Hospice and Palliative Nursing 3*(3), 86-96.

Klagsbrun, J. (2001). Listening and focusing: Holistic health care tools for nurses. *Nursing Clinics of North America 36*(1), 115-129.

Leahy, M. (Ed.). (2002). *Study guide for the generalist hospice and palliative nurse.* Dubuque, IA: Kendall Hunt.

Matzo, M., & Sherman, D. (Eds.). (2001). *Palliative care nursing: Quality care to the end of life.* New York: Springer.

McCaffery, M., & Pasero, C. (1999). *Pain: Clinical manual.* St. Louis: Mosby.

8 Supportive Care: Rehabilitation and Resources

SUE L. FRYMARK

Select the best answer for each of the following questions:

1. The goal of preventive rehabilitation is to
   A. prevent cancer.
   B. reduce pain and nausea.
   C. restore strength and endurance.
   D. focus on clients who have a potential disability.

2. A major barrier to rehabilitation is
   A. medication management.
   B. available therapy equipment.
   C. competition between providers.
   D. the attitude that cancer is not curable.

3. Composition of the rehabilitation team is dependent on
   A. health care costs.
   B. national standards.
   C. caregiver availability.
   D. client need and resource availability.

4. Continuity of care depends on
   A. coordination.
   B. community standards.
   C. clients' independence.
   D. availability of rehabilitation resources.

5. The field of cancer rehabilitation is increasingly affected by
   A. government regulations.
   B. the size of the family unit.
   C. availability of a rehabilitation hospital.
   D. consumer awareness of wellness and quality of life.

6. Interdisciplinary planning and care is facilitated by
   A. insurance coverage.
   B. availability of meeting space.
   C. a local durable medical equipment company.
   D. mutual goal setting by client, family, and health care professionals.

7. Assessment of rehabilitation issues
   A. is completed at discharge.
   B. continues as needs change.
   C. is dependent on services available.
   D. is provided by the medical oncologist.

8. Caregiver demands have increased with
   A. the Family Medical Leave Act (FMLA).
   B. the expectations of the community.
   C. the need for rehabilitation services.
   D. the shift from hospitalized to ambulatory care.

9. Of all cancer, 77% occurs in
   A. minorities.
   B. the disabled.
   C. those 55 years and older.
   D. women.

10. Mr. J. has been diagnosed with advanced prostate cancer involving lesions of the bone and lungs, which has impaired his mobility, comfort, and endurance. A palliative goal of physical rehabilitation could be
   A. workplace modification.
   B. safe and comfortable mobility.
   C. restoration to full independence.
   D. reduction of cancer-related disability.

11. Mrs. C., who is diagnosed with metastatic breast cancer, is hospitalized and immobilized with a risk for pathologic fractures. Her rehabilitation plan would include
   A. stair climbing.
   B. aerobic exercises.
   C. antibiotic therapy.
   D. gentle range of motion and when safe, progressive safe mobility with family training.

12. Cancer rehabilitation assessment before cancer treatment will
   A. increase the cost of health care.
   B. meet accreditation requirements.
   C. add further anxiety for the family.
   D. identify potential and actual problems.

13. The client with cancer of the head and neck who undergoes surgery and subsequent radiation treatment will require the services of
   A. a psychiatrist.
   B. speech therapy.
   C. referral to Y-Me.
   D. vocational rehabilitation.

14. Cancer survivors may require cancer rehabilitation services years after treatment because of
   A. infections.
   B. family stress.
   C. other issues related to aging.
   D. long-term effects from cancer treatments.

15. Rehabilitation issues can go unaddressed as a result of
   A. professional conflicts.
   B. short hospitalizations.
   C. acute medical needs.
   D. lack of individual assessments.

16. Developmental needs should be considered among
   A. breast cancer survivors.
   B. kidney cancer survivors.
   C. economically disadvantaged survivors.
   D. young and elderly cancer survivors.

17. A community resource that can enhance body image and self-esteem is
   A. parish nursing.
   B. respite care.
   C. transportation services.
   D. American Cancer Society's "Look Good, Feel Better" program.

18. Mr. K. was treated for a soft tissue sarcoma requiring surgical resection and chemotherapy. His rehabilitation issues include impaired mobility and risk of lymphedema. His rehabilitation goals would be
   A. preventive.
   B. supportive.
   C. palliative.
   D. restorative and preventive.

19. Which factor can impede rehabilitation efforts?
   A. Low body weight.
   B. Family training.
   C. Inadequate pain control.
   D. Extended hospitalization.

20. Mr. S. has completed physical rehabilitation after his bone marrow transplant. He continues to experience fatigue. What would be an appropriate referral?
   A. Speech therapy.
   B. Comfort care team.
   C. Inpatient rehabilitation unit.
   D. Modified group exercise program.

21. Which of the following disciplines includes energy conservation, fine motor skills, and activities of daily living within their scope of practice?
   A. Dietitian.
   B. Psychiatrist.
   C. Enterostomal therapist.
   D. Occupational therapist.

22. Rehabilitation client teaching should consider

A. hydration.
B. income level.
C. level of independence.
D. language and cultural barriers.

23. Complementary services can
A. cure cancer.
B. reduce the cost of health care.
C. prevent the need for rehabilitation services.
D. promote physical and emotional wellness.

24. Cancer-related community programs are resources for
A. child care.
B. food and housing service.
C. symptom management.
D. information, education, and support.

25. Mrs. G.'s husband has advanced lung cancer. He had been hospitalized with acute respiratory distress. He is now considered stable and ready for discharge; however, he has become increasingly dependent and has a life expectancy of weeks. What would be an appropriate intervention?
A. Tube feedings.
B. Family planning conference.
C. Referral for Mrs. G. to a grief group.
D. Transfer to an inpatient rehabilitation unit.

26. Which of the following is not a functional health pattern?
A. Fatigue.
B. Mobility.
C. Cognition.
D. Activities of daily living.

27. Which of the following rehabilitation approaches builds self-esteem and self-confidence?
A. Team conferences.
B. Assistive device training.
C. Cognitive retraining.
D. Recognition of positive self-care behaviors.

NOTES

ANSWERS

1. *Answer:* D
   Rationale: The focus is on preventing disability by identifying clients at risk so preventive actions can be recommended to prevent or minimize disability.

2. *Answer:* D
   Rationale: There remains a common misconception that cancer is not curable, with an ineffable progression of disease that is not reversible. Many individuals assume rehabilitation is only for those who will not die of their disease, and since they believe cancer is not curable, they see no role. However, cancer rehabilitation can help individuals with all stages of cancer to maximize their independence and function within the limitations posed by their illness.

3. *Answer:* D
   Rationale: Although the other responses can have an impact on the team, the services of the team needed are based on the individual's needs and whether that rehabilitation team member is locally available.

4. *Answer:* A
   Rationale: Clients receive care in a variety of settings by a variety of disciplines so a coordinator will ensure communication across settings.

5. *Answer:* D
   Rationale: Despite the barriers to providing rehabilitation services, concern for quality of life is creating a demand for services. Wellness programs not only provide preventive and supportive rehabilitation efforts but also offer individuals a way to resume control of their health.

6. *Answer:* D
   Rationale: Care goals need to reflect the complexity of the client's needs, medically, socially, and emotionally, which therefore requires input from the client, family members, and team.

7. *Answer:* B
   Rationale: Assessment of needs is ongoing so if medical, social, and emotional situations change, any impact on rehabilitation issues could be addressed promptly to prevent further disability or distress.

8. *Answer:* D
   Rationale: Clients leave hospitals with more acute medical issues and complex care needs that often require continued technical care. Families are already often stressed with additional caregiving and family roles and may not feel confident in providing such care.

9. *Answer:* C
   Rationale: Cancer is more common in the elderly population.

10. *Answer:* B
    Rationale: The focus of palliative rehabilitation is on maximizing quality of living during end of life. This involves safe mobility, making daily life easier, and increasing comfort by reducing pressure from weight-bearing activity.

11. *Answer:* D
    Rationale: Immobilization increases the risk of further disability. Gentle range of motion is important until progressive mobility is permitted. Family training by a health care professional aware of the unsafe movements and weight-bearing issues is needed.

12. *Answer:* D
    Rationale: An assessment before treatment will establish baseline functioning and areas of risk for disability, which will assist in care planning and follow-up care.

13. *Answer:* B
    Rationale: There are preventive and restorative rehabilitation needs related to chewing, swallowing, speech, and saliva flow after surgery and radiation therapy to the head and neck area. A speech language pathologist can address these issues with clients. Some clients may benefit from a psychiatrist and/or vocational counselor later in the care plan. Y-Me provides support for those with breast cancer.

14. *Answer:* D
Rationale: Long-term effects such as lymphedema, impaired memory, disturbed sensory perception, cardiac changes, and bone loss generate new rehabilitation issues affecting quality of life. Options A, B, and C can be more appropriately addressed by other service providers and may or may not be related to cancer treatment.

15. *Answer:* D
Rationale: Individual assessments need to occur across the care continuum in conjunction with other medical issues. Options A, B, and C should not impede assessment for rehabilitation needs.

16. *Answer:* D
Rationale: Physical, functional, social, and emotional changes are common among these age groups, which can be further compounded by the impact of cancer treatments increasing the risk for disability.

17. *Answer:* D
Rationale: The "Look Good, Feel Better" program provides tips from experts in hair and skin care issues, but more importantly is done in a fun and supportive manner with others experiencing similar concerns.

18. *Answer:* D
Rationale: The goal of physical therapy is to restore mobility to a maximum level within the limitations posed by the surgery. A preventive goal involves client education about lymphedema and precautions to reduce risk.

19. *Answer:* C.
Rationale: Uncontrolled pain may be exacerbated with physical activity. It also creates anticipatory anxiety related to activity. Individuals are hesitant to participate in rehabilitation therapies for fear of increasing their pain. Reduced activity fosters additional problems. To remove this barrier, pain control is needed to promote physical activity and facilitate rehabilitation efforts.

20. *Answer:* D
Rationale: Fatigue often discourages individuals from physical activity. Because fatigue can continue for some time after transplant, a gentle but structured exercise program can facilitate physical activity. A group format offers support and further motivation to attend. A medical release is beneficial to alert individuals to any precautions warranted by their particular recovery.

21. *Answer:* D
Rational: Other disciplines may address these areas to some degree, but they are part of the educational and clinical practice of occupational therapy.

22. *Answer:* D
Rationale: To ensure understanding, an interpreter may be needed. Teaching may need to be adapted to cultural values and beliefs.

23. *Answer:* D
Rationale: Complementary services of exercise, nutrition, and stress management can help clients maintain and enhance their well-being after more acute and restorative rehabilitation.

24. *Answer:* D
Rationale: The strengths of these organizations are their cancer-related educational materials and peer support networks for cancer survivors and their families.

25. *Answer:* B
Rationale: Rehabilitation efforts are now palliative. A family conference will provide support and discussion of options for care. It can include assessment by the team of the family's emotional and physical abilities to care for Mr. G. If they are able, home care planning and family training can follow.

26. *Answer:* A
Rationale: Fatigue is a symptom that affects functional patterns.

27. *Answer:* D
Rationale: Disability can challenge self-esteem, so emphasis on strengths while learning to adapt to changes or until restoration is possible is important. Also, when individuals are overwhelmed with what they cannot do, they often need reminding what they can do.

BIBLIOGRAPHY

American Cancer Society. (2004). *Cancer facts and figures.* Atlanta: American Cancer Society.

Cheville, A. (2001) Rehabilitation of patients with advanced cancer. *Cancer 92*(suppl 4), 1039-1048.

Frymark, S.L. (1992). Rehabilitation resources within the team and community. *Seminars in Oncology Nursing 8,* 212-218.

Frymark, S.L. (1999). Cancer rehabilitation: The road to survivorship. *Oncology Issues 14*(6), 16-19.

Fucile, J. (1992). Functional rehabilitation in cancer care. *Seminars in Oncology Nursing 8,* 186-189.

Groenwald, S.L., Frogge, J.H., Goodman, M., & Yarbro, C.H. (Eds.). (1995). *A clinical guide to cancer nursing: A companion to cancer nursing.* Sudbury, MA: Jones and Bartlett Publishers.

Lundgren, J. (1999). A rehabilitation hospital-services for the oncology patient. *Oncology Issues 14*(6), 20-2.

Mellette, S.F., & Blunk, K. (1994). Cancer rehabilitation. *Seminars in Oncology 21,* 779-782.

O'Connor, K., & Blesch, K.S. (1992). Life cycle issues affecting cancer rehabilitation. *Seminars in Oncology Nursing 8,* 174-186.

Varricchio, C., & Aziz, N. (1999). Rehabilitation and survivorship. In R. Lenhard (Ed.). *Textbook of clinical oncology* (3rd ed.). Atlanta: American Cancer Society.

NOTES

9 Supportive Care: Support Therapies and Procedures

MARJORIE WHITMAN

Select the best answer for each of the following questions:

1. The primary reason for increased blood component therapy (BCT) is attributed to
   A. client demand.
   B. excessive community donations.
   C. advancement of surgical oncology techniques.
   D. increasing cure rates resulting from BCT.

2. Blood received from an autologous donor is
   A. human leukocyte antigen (HLA)-matched.
   B. collected during organ harvesting.
   C. collected from the intended recipient.
   D. collected and transfused within the same facility.

3. In addition to febrile and hemolytic complications of BCT, the nurse monitors the recipient's response for which potential complication?
   A. Allergic reactions.
   B. Fluid volume deficit.
   C. Deep vein thrombosis (DVT).
   D. Bone marrow suppression.

4. The client asks the nurse why BCT is indicated. After reviewing the client's complete blood count (CBC) data, the nurse recognizes which value as indicative of a need for BCT?
   A. Hematocrit greater than 55%.
   B. Platelets less than $10,000/mm^3$.
   C. Neutrophils equal to $9000/mm^3$.
   D. Red blood cell distribution width (RDW) index variation less than 3.5%.

5. The nurse is explaining a BCT procedure to a client. She correctly identifies an appropriate cognitive outcome as:
   A. Client believes the therapy will be helpful.
   B. Client understands the process of component infusion.
   C. Client describes signs and symptoms of reactions to therapy.
   D. Client relates to need for blood component therapy.

6. To decrease the incidence and severity of side effects from blood component therapy, the nurse will expect to
   A. administer cephalosporin 2 hours before administration.
   B. infuse 1000 ml bolus of normal saline (NS) after infusion.
   C. premedicate client with antipyretics and antihistamines as ordered.
   D. administer the components in 50 ml increments alternating with NS.

7. The nurse is preparing a BCT infusion. She knows that which of the following guidelines maximizes client safety?
   A. Use a gravity flow infusion line.
   B. Add medications through the Y-port slowly.
   C. Use the smallest gauge intravenous (IV) catheter available.
   D. With a second RN, check BCT product with client ID.

8. Shortly after a BCT transfusion is initiated, the client complains of flank pain. The nurse should immediately
   A. stop the infusion and withdraw the IV catheter.
   B. maintain the IV catheter with new tubing and NS.
   C. discard the tubing and bag in the biohazard container.
   D. flush the blood product in the tubing with NS, then remove the IV catheter.

9. To involve the client receiving BCT and the family in the plan of care, the nurse will
   A. include the social worker in all discussions.
   B. teach them to contact the physician for information.
   C. review the procedure for administering the blood component.
   D. caution them about touching items used by the client during the infusion.

10. The client is concerned about metabolic changes created by malignancy. The nurse discusses the impact of malignancy on the metabolism of
   A. vitamins and minerals.
   B. pharmaceutical products.
   C. protein and carbohydrates.
   D. mono- and polyunsaturated fats.

11. Although clients and their families often believe that parenteral nutrition is superior to oral or enteral nutrition, the most important reason for using the gastrointestinal (GI) tract is
   A. it is cheaper.
   B. it makes nutrients available faster.
   C. it protects the integrity of the bowel wall.

   D. it promotes adequate vascular fluid volume.

12. The nurse recognizes the need for more teaching when the client anticipating surgery states:
   A. I will need adequate protein after surgery.
   B. Increasing carbohydrates promotes healing.
   C. A variety of foods is the best source of essential nutrients.
   D. A high-fiber, low-fat diet is not appropriate during treatment.

13. Which of the following may impair the digestion of nutritional intake?
   A. Gastroparesis.
   B. Inability to prepare food.
   C. Poorly fitting dental prostheses.
   D. Vitamin and mineral deficiencies.

14. When the nurse reviews the nutrition-related laboratory data for the client with cancer, he or she expects to review
   A. erythrocyte sedimentation rate (ESR).
   B. serum bicarbonate.
   C. prothrombin and activated partial thromboplastin time (APTT).
   D. serum albumin and transferrin.

15. The client with evidence of malnutrition is likely to experience which of the following results?
   A. Beneficial weight loss.
   B. Shortened hospital stays.
   C. Prolonged wound healing.
   D. Increased tumor response to treatment.

16. A client is receiving enteral feedings per nasointestinal tube. The nurse monitors for complications by assessing for
   A. euthyroidism.
   B. aspiration and diarrhea.
   C. dehydration and dyspnea.
   D. hypoglycemia and edema.

17. Vascular access devices for planned short-term use include
   A. implanted ports.
   B. midline catheters.
   C. tunneled catheters.
   D. peripheral catheters.

18. The nurse is teaching a client and the family about the option of a peripherally inserted central catheter (PICC). He knows the client needs more teaching when the client describes the catheter as
   A. a silicone connection to an artery.
   B. inserted in the antecubital fossa in a vein.
   C. having decreased risks for pneumothorax.
   D. decreasing the need for intravenous sticks.

19. A client will receive a vesicant medication as part of the chemotherapy protocol. The nurse's plan to maintain safety during the infusion includes
   A. using a computer-controlled infusion pump.
   B. bringing the medication to 38° C before infusing.
   C. extending the time over which the medication infuses.
   D. maintaining aseptic technique when establishing venous access.

20. A client returns from surgery, where a tunneled catheter was implanted. The nurse finds the intravenous solution infusing at 30 ml/hr. The infusion rate can be increased to the ordered 125 ml/hr when which of the following tests confirms placement?
   A. Computed tomography (CT) scan.
   B. Endoscopy.
   C. Blood return on aspiration.
   D. Radiographic confirmation.

21. The oncology nurse is evaluating the potential for a client to receive an implanted venous access device. Which of the following concerns expressed by the client alerts the nurse to the need for further evaluation?

A. The client demonstrates ability to care for the device.
B. The client describes procedures for using the device.
C. The client expresses concerns about implantation of the device.
D. The client questions the need for anything more than short-term devices.

22. When changing the dressing on a cannulated implated port, the nurse uses which of the following rationale for the procedure?
   A. The procedure requires strict asepsis.
   B. The insertion site must be covered with opaque dressing.
   C. The change is a clean procedure because risk for infection is low
   D. The client should hold his breath while the iodine solution is applied.

23. A client is discharged from the ambulatory infusion center with an infusion system for continuous chemotherapy infusion. The client and family are confident about use of the infusion system because they know how to
   A. flush the line with sterile water every 12 hours.
   B. monitor the infusion system for proper functioning.
   C. attach a second line to the infusion for pain control.
   D. change the dose of the drug whenever the client sleeps.

24. Damage to implanted venous access catheters may occur as a result of
   A. nonsteroidal antiinflammatory drug (NSAID) use.
   B. bathing with the device in place.
   C. excessive pressure with infusions.
   D. lack of use for greater than 48 hours.

ANSWERS

1. *Answer:* C

Rationale: Advancement of surgical oncology techniques means that there is an increased number of procedures and refinement of existing procedures. Option A, client demand, would not be an appropriate reason to increase the use of BCT because Option B, unfortunately, rarely occurs, and if there were excessive blood supplies, it would not be an appropriate reason for increasing BCT. Providing BCT is a supportive, not a curative, therapy for those with cancer; therefore Option D is incorrect.

2. *Answer:* C

Rationale: Autologous donors are those who have their own blood preserved for use by themselves. The risk for incompatibilities is very low or nonexistent with autologous transfusion. Option A is incorrect. Tissue, not blood, has to be HLA-matched. Blood is matched according to blood type. Option B is also incorrect, because although bone marrow can be harvested after death, there is at this time no practical reason to do so, because all cadaver transplants have failed and no institutions are performing this procedure. Blood is not a tissue that can be donated after death has occurred, probably because it clots when circulation stops. Option D, the location of the blood donation and transfusion, is not relevant to compatibility of the blood.

3. *Answer:* A

Rationale: Allergic reactions to proteins in homologous blood components are a potential complication. Allergic reactions range from benign rashes to anaphylactic shock. Option B, fluid volume deficit, is unlikely because BCT adds volume to the intravascular system, creating a more likely risk of fluid volume excess. However, if shock with systemic vasodilation follows a transfusion reaction, fluids will have to be added to compensate for the volume deficit accompanying shock. Deep vein thrombosis, Option C, is not related to BCT. Malignancies are associated with increased risk for DVT, but these are not known to be related to BCT. Option D is not correct. BCT

does not suppress blood cell production in the bone marrow.

4. *Answer:* B

Rationale: Platelets less than $15,000/mm^3$ create a potential for serious bleeding disorder such as spontaneous hemorrhage. Option A, hematocrit greater than 55%, is not within the normal range for males or females. These values cited are abnormally high. Option C is incorrect. Neutrophils equal to $9000/mm^3$ are within the normal range. Option D is also incorrect. RDW index indicates variation in red blood cell size; a RDW index less than 3.5% reveals a homogeneous specimen of red blood cells without evidence of anemia.

5. *Answer:* C

Rationale: To evaluate the effectiveness of teaching or any intervention, the outcome must be measurable and observable. Option C reflects these qualities by incorporating the verb "describes." Options A, B, and D, while desirable outcomes, are subjective and difficult to evaluate. Evaluating cognitive behaviors is dependent on a measurable and observable response that verifies that the client understands the intended message.

6. *Answer:* C

Rationale: Premedicating with antihistamines decreases the risk of allergic reactions to BCT by stabilizing the receptors for histamine. This prevents vasodilation, increased capillary permeability causing edema, bronchoconstriction, itching, pain, and secretion of mucus. The use of antipyretics blocks release of the inflammatory cytokine stimulated by a hypersensitive reaction. These medications potentially increase the comfort of the client. Option A is incorrect. Prophylactic use of antibiotics would not address the potential side effects of BCT. If an infection were detected after infusion, an antibiotic for the specific organism would be identified and selected. Option B is an inappropriate intervention. Adding a 1000 ml bolus of normal saline after BCT could contribute to serious fluid volume overload. Option C is also incorrect. BCT products need to be infused as rapidly as possible to minimize degradation. Alternating NS with the BCT product would prolong the infusion and not produce a desirable effect.

7. *Answer:* D

Rationale: Two licensed professional health care professionals must verify that the BCT product is correctly labeled and dated and that it matches information on the client's blood identification band, usually worn as a bracelet. The client's name must be spelled correctly and the blood group and type identified on both the product and client identifiers. Option A is incorrect because the method of infusion is not the priority intervention to maximize safety. Gravity infusions, although not the preferred method, may be used if controlled infusion pumps are not available. Option B is incorrect. Never add medications to BCT infusions! Doing so risks hemolytic reactions in the BCT product. Option C is an incorrect choice. Intravenous therapy guidelines recommend larger catheters for viscous infusions such as BCT products. BCT products must be infused within 4 hours' maximum time to prevent degradation of the components.

8. *Answer:* B

Rationale: Although most BCT is administered using a Y-port tubing with normal saline (NS) infusing through one of the ports and the BCT product through the other, this tubing should not be used. New tubing and NS should be attached to the IV catheter to keep the line open. The Y tubing should be discontinued immediately to prevent infusion of additional BCT product. Option A is not correct. The client will need fluid and medications to address the reaction, and intravenous access should not be terminated. Option C is incorrect because any BCT product associated with a serious client reaction must be returned to the blood bank for analysis to determine the cause of the reaction. Flushing the BCT product in the tubing into the cleint increases the client's exposure to potentially life-threatening reactions. Discontinue and send the tubing and the BCT product to the blood bank.

9. *Answer:* C

Rationale: By reviewing the procedure with the client and family, the nurse provides information and opportunity to prepare and reassure them about safety and efficacy of the treatment. Option A is incorrect if the client has consented to the transfusion. Social workers may become involved if complications develop about consenting to transfusion and a referral is considered helpful. Option B is incorrect. Although physicians are good sources of information, nurses do not defer to physicians for client education on routine procedures. Option D is also incorrect. Clients receiving BCT products are not contagious relative to the BCT product infusing. If the client has a previously diagnosed contagious disease, of course the family should be advised about sources of contagion and methods to prevent spread.

10. *Answer:* C

Rationale: Cancer cell division and growth are associated with increased protein metabolism and hyperglycemia, presumably to meet the energy demands of malignant tumors. Carbohydrate metabolism is altered in malignant states, leading to hyperglycemia. Option A is incorrect. Vitamin and mineral deficiencies are not associated with malignancies, although individual clients may develop deficiencies or require additional amounts. Option B is also incorrect. If liver function is adequate, medications are metabolized normally by liver enzymes. Fortunately, clients with malignancy benefit from antihypertensives, antibiotics, and other medications. Option D is not correct. Malignant metabolism is associated with increased protein metabolism, not increased fat metabolism.

11. *Answer:* C

Rationale: Using the GI tract maintains the integrity and functioning of the bowel wall. A healthy bowel provides the benefits of regulated absorption of nutrients and stimulation of the immune system, which protects the blood from contaminants in food, thus reducing the risk of infection. Option A is incorrect. Parenteral nutrition is far more costly than oral or enteral nutrition. Option B is incorrect. Parenterally infused nutrients are introduced directly into the circulation, making that route the quickest method for speedy delivery. A potential drawback to the constant level of nutrients infused may be an alteration in the normally intermittent hormone release and may provoke a higher metabolic rate. Option D is the correct answer because it is not unique to oral and enteral nutrition; parenteral nutrition affords the same benefit of supporting adequate vascular fluid volume.

12. *Answer:* B
Rationale: This statement suggests an erroneous understanding of the role of carbohydrates. Carbohydrates are energy sources; proteins supply the amino acids necessary for tissue repair and healing. Carbohydrates are not the best source of energy; the body's need for calories is most efficiently supplied by fats. Proteins, vitamins, and minerals are associated with healing, and Options A and C demonstrate that understanding. Option D is true but does not indicate a need for more teaching. High-fiber, low fat diets are associated with low protein intake, which is inappropriate for the high-energy healing necessary after surgery.

13. *Answer:* A
Rationale: Gastroparesis, slowing of gastric contractions caused by neuropathies, impairs the mechanical and chemical digestive process. Options B and C are associated with ingestion rather than digestion and therefore are incorrect. Option D, vitamin and mineral deficiencies, is associated with absorption and metabolism rather than digestion. Digestion is the process of preparing ingested food for absorption and metabolism.

14. *Answer:* D
Rationale: Serum albumin and transferrin reflect protein stores in the body. Option A is incorrect. ESR is a measure of sedimentation of red cells that accelerates with inflammation and infection. Option C is indirectly related to nutrition. The liver manufactures these components of the anticoagulation process. Without adequate amino acids, synthesis of these proteins may lag, especially in liver disease. Option B is incorrect. Bicarbonate is an indicator of serum pH, an important buffer of acidity.

15. *Answer:* C
Rationale: Malnutrition deprives the body of the components for wound healing. Option A

is incorrect. Malnutrition associated with malignancy deprives the client of necessary elements for the immune system and for healing and results in loss of lean muscle mass rather than reduction of fat stores. Option B is incorrect. Lengthened hospital stays are a complication of malnutrition. Option D is incorrect and implies that malnourishment is an appropriate therapy for malignancy. Clients need good nutrition to tolerate the side effects and adverse reactions associated with cancer treatment.

16. *Answer:* B
Rationale: The hyperosmolar enteral feedings are introduced slowly to promote tolerance and absorption of the formula, avoiding diarrhea. Aspiration caused by reflux of the liquid formula is a potential risk that is decreased by elevating the head of the bed 30 to 45 degrees or higher as tolerated. Option A is incorrect. Euthyroid means normal thyroid hormone levels. Enteral feeding formulas do not correct thyroid excesses or deficiencies. Option C is also incorrect. Dehydration is a condition corrected by enteral feedings, and unless there is congestive heart failure, the fluid provided in the enteral feeding remains in the vascular system, not causing dyspnea. Option D is not correct. If the client develops hypoglycemia, it is related to excessive insulin, either endogenous or exogenous. Edema is not a side effect of enteral feeding. Edema may accompany congestive heart failure or inadequate albumin to hold water in the vascular system. Enteral feedings are a good source of essential amino acids, promoting synthesis of albumin by the liver.

17. *Answer:* D
Rationale: Peripheral catheters are intended for short-term use, and the site must be rotated every 96 hours to avoid complications. Midline catheters, Option B, are intended for intermediate-term use and may be kept 2 to 6 weeks. Options A and C are catheters for long-term use. Inserted surgically, these catheters may remain in place and be used for months or years if no complications such as infection develop.

18. *Answer:* A
Rationale: The client errs in believing that PICC lines are inserted in arteries. Although

the misunderstanding is not critical, the client needs more teaching. Option B is correct placement of a PICC line. Option C is correct because the insertion is in the antecubital fossa and the catheter is threaded through the brachial vein. The introducing needle remains in the antecubital fossa as the catheter is threaded into the superior vena cava. Option D is also correct. One of the advantages of PICC lines is their long-term viability, which decreases intravenous sticks.

19. *Answer:* D
Rationale: Maintaining aseptic technique does not guarantee that extravasation of a vesicant will not occur, but it does decrease the risk of infection at the insertion site of the IV catheter, promoting safety for the client. Option A is incorrect. Using an infusion pump promotes the correct rate of infusion but does not prevent extravasation of the medication. Until tissue pressure becomes significant, the pump will continue to introduce vesicants into interstitial space unless the client alerts the nurse to stop the infusion. Option B is incorrect. Warming vesicant medications does not prevent extravasation from a vein. Option C is also not correct. Extending the time over which the vesicant is infused will not safeguard against extravasation and by continuing the infusion may increase the risk of harm to the vein and possible infiltration.

20. *Answer:* D
Rationale: When radiologic confirmation of placement of the tip of the catheter in the superior vena cava (not in the right atrium of the heart, where it might trigger ectopic beats) is received, the infusion can be increased. Option A is not correct. CT scans are expensive and not necessary to confirm catheter placement. Option B is not correct. Endoscopy is a fiberoptic examination of the GI tract, not the thoracic vasculature. Option C is also incorrect. Blood return does not guarantee correct placement of the catheter tip. Blood may backflow into the catheter at any point during insertion.

21. *Answer:* D
Rationale: The client who does not consider his or her condition as necessitating long-term treatment may not be ready to commit to taking long-term treatments or coping with

the disease. Because cancer is often a chronic condition, clients must be aware that treatment may be ongoing for months or years. This client's understanding of his or her disease and the recommended treatment needs further evaluation. Options A, B, and C reflect a well-informed client who is comfortable expressing his or her concerns as well as learning to care for the device.

22. *Answer:* A
Rationale: Entering the skin by inserting the noncoring needle carries the risk of infecting the vascular central line. Option B is not correct. The dressing should not obscure a clear view of the insertion site to assess for redness, discharge, or migration of the catheter. Option C is incorrect because the risk for infection needs to be kept low by using strict aseptic technique. Infecting vascular central lines causes sepsis, a highly morbid complication. Option D is not correct. It is not necessary for the client to hold his or her breath while the iodine solution is applied. It is a good idea for the client to turn his or her head away from the insertion site while the dressing is changed to prevent the introduction of respiratory microbes onto the site.

23. *Answer:* B
Rationale: The client should be able to assess the system to determine that the power is on and the infusion is occurring. Option A is incorrect. Normal saline solution would be used, and when the infusion is ongoing, there is no need to flush the line. Option C is incorrect. These systems should be used only for their intended purpose. The nurse needs to assess the system and determine whether it is compatible and appropriate to be administered through a second line. Clients should not make that judgment independently. Option D is incorrect. Doses are programmed on the ambulatory infusion pumps with a sequence intended to prevent accidental or uninformed alteration by lay individuals. Changes in dose need to be made by the nurse when an order is changed or the infusion is complete.

24. *Answer:* C
Rationale: Fortunately, these implanted access devices are sturdy. To prevent excessive pressure, infusions are made with large-

volume syringes and with slow, steady rates. Option A is incorrect. NSAIDs do not damage the catheter **IF** they are administered in liquid form or tablets are powdered and dissolved in solution. Option B is incorrect. Clients with implanted devices can and should bathe regularly. Because the lines are centrally implanted, care must be taken to prevent infection or displacement, but clients are able to participate in ordinary activities of daily living. Option D is not correct. These catheters may go unused for several months without deteriorating or being damaged. Care must be taken to prevent obstruction with blood clots, but they can be dormant for long periods.

BIBLIOGRAPHY

Camp-Sorrell, D. (Ed.). 2004. Access device guidelines: Recommendations for nursing practice and education. (2nd ed.). Pittsburgh: Oncology Nursing Society.

Demark-Wahnefried, W., & Rimer, B.K. (1997). Weight gain in women diagnosed with breast cancer. *Journal of the American Dietetic Association* 97(5), 519-530.

Lehne, R.A. (2004). *Pharmacology for nursing care* (5th ed.). St. Louis: Saunders.

LeMone, P. & Burke, K. (2004). *Medical-surgical nursing: Critical thinking in client care* (3rd ed.). Upper Saddle River, NJ: Pearson/Prentice Hall.

Smith, S.F., Duell, D.J., & Martin, B.C. (2004). *Clinical nursing skills: Basic to advanced skills* (6th ed.). Upper Saddle River, NJ: Pearson/Prentice Hall.

Taylor, C., Lillis, C., & LeMone, P. (2001). *Fundamentals of nursing: The art & science of nursing care* (4th ed.). Philadelphia: Lippincott.

NOTES

10 Supportive Care: Pharmacologic Interventions

ROBERT J. IGNOFFO, CAROL S. VIELE, AND ZOE NGO

Select the best answers for the following questions:

1. Mrs. J. has breast cancer and is being treated with chemotherapy. The white blood cell count 10 days after her last treatment is $800/mm^3$. Her physician prescribes prophylactic antibiotics to be given at home. Which is an appropriate statement for you to teach Mrs. J.?
   A. Discontinue daily temperature monitoring during antibiotic therapy.
   B. Take all daily antibiotic doses between 8 AM and 5 PM.
   C. Notify the physician of any rash or fever.
   D. Chills are an expected side effect of antibiotic therapy.

2. Amphotericin B and fluconazole are two common agents used for the treatment of
   A. *Staphylococcus*.
   B. *Candida albicans*.
   C. *Streptococcus*.
   D. *Escherichia coli*.

3. Aminoglycosides are used in conjunction with other antimicrobials to treat infections in clients with cancer. The major toxicity of aminoglycosides is
   A. hepatotoxicity.
   B. cardiac toxicity.
   C. nephrotoxicity.
   D. neurotoxicity.

4. Acyclovir is commonly used to treat
   A. pseudomonas pneumonia.
   B. herpes simplex infection.
   C. pulmonary aspergillosis.
   D. megalovirus retinitis.

5. Mrs. C. is receiving cefepime for an infection. The nurse teaching Mrs. C. and her family regarding signs and symptoms of hypersensitivity reactions would instruct them to observe for which of the following?
   A. Shortness of breath, hives, itchiness
   B. Increased thirst.
   C. Decreased urine output.
   D. Increased urine output.

6. The most frequent side effect of clients receiving voriconazole (Vfend) is
   A. constipation.
   B. vaginitis.
   C. visual changes.
   D. slow heart rate.

7. The side effects associated with caspofungin acetate (Cancidas) are
   A. slow heart rate.
   B. rash/hives.
   C. rapid heart rate.
   D. visual changes.

8. Nonsteroidal antiinflammatory drugs (NSAIDs) suppress the inflammatory response by

A. inhibiting cyclooxygenase and the production of prostaglandins.
B. blocking opiate neurotransmitters.
C. causing tumor cell lysis.
D. increasing macrophage migration to the site of injury.

9. Mr. P. has coronary artery disease and takes one aspirin daily. He has recently had a diagnosis of metastatic lung cancer, and the physician has prescribed naproxen and dexamethasone for bone pain. Which of the following complications does not occur with naproxen or dexamethasone?
   A. Gastrointestinal ulceration.
   B. Bleeding.
   C. Fluid retention and renal insufficiency.
   D. Constipation.

10. A 16-year-old female has osteosarcoma with bone pain. She will be receiving a corticosteroid indefinitely. Client teaching should include discussion of which of the following side effects?
   A. Acne, weight gain, and moon face.
   B. Altered mental alertness.
   C. Diarrhea.
   D. Loss of appetite.

11. Mrs. T. is a 74-year-old woman who has metastatic lung cancer and complains of bone pain. Her cancer is being treated with docetaxel and irinotecan chemotherapy. Her pain is being treated with oxycodone hydrochloride (OxyContin) 30 mg twice daily, ibuprofen 600 mg orally three times daily, and amitriptyline 25 mg orally at bedtime for the last 4 weeks. She also complains of weight gain of 5 pounds and worsening constipation. The most likely explanation for this client's complaints is
   A. amitriptyline weight gain and ibuprofen-induced constipation.
   B. ibuprofen weight gain and OxyContin-induced constipation.
   C. OxyContin weight gain and docetaxel-induced constipation.
   D. Amitriptyline weight gain and irinotecan-induced constipation.

12. Which of the following anticancer drugs has a high emetogenic potential?

A. Paclitaxel (Taxol).
B. Vinorelbine (Navelbine).
C. Bleomycin (Blenoxane).
D. Dacarbazine (DTIC-Dome).

13. One reason for administering dexamethasone 20 mg intravenously (IV) before a chemotherapy regimen containing paclitaxel and carboplatin is to
   A. prevent allergic reactions to cisplatin.
   B. stimulate appetite after chemotherapy.
   C. improve antiemetic efficacy.
   D. decrease the chance of chemotherapy-induced diarrhea.

14. Mr. D. is to receive doxorubicin (Adriamycin) 60 mg/m^2 and cisplatin 100 mg/m^2 IV on day 1. An effective antiemetic regimen for this combination regimen is
   A. a 5-HT$_3$ antagonist plus metoclopramide plus diphenhydramine.
   B. metoclopramide plus dexamethasone plus diphenhydramine.
   C. a 5-HT$_3$ antagonist plus dexamethasone.
   D. a phenothiazine (e.g., prochlorperazine) plus a 5-HT$_3$ antagonist.

15. Mr. D. has two episodes of vomiting on day 3 after his cisplatin. Which of the following antiemetics is appropriate for treating his emesis?
   A. Granisetron 1 mg IV.
   B. Prochlorperazine 10 mg PR/PO.
   C. Lorazepam 0.5 mg sublingually.
   D. Diphenhydramine 25 mg PO/IV.

16. Mr. D. returns to the clinic for the next cycle of high-dose cisplatin. On the previous cycle of cisplatin, he had received granisetron 1 mg IV before cisplatin. He had two emetic episodes on day 1 and two emetic episodes on day 3. Which of the following would be the most rational therapy for this client?
   A. Granisetron 1 mg IV + dexamethasone 20 IV, both 30 minutes before chemotherapy followed by granisetron 1 mg PO qd and dexamethasone 8 mg PO bid for 3 days.
   B. Add prochlorperazine 10 mg IV on days 2 and 3 to Option A.
   C. Add lorazepam 1 mg IV or PO on days 2 and 3 to Option A.

D. Switch to aprepitant (Emend), 125 mg PO day 1, and 80 mg PO on days 2 and 3.

17. Nursing actions when selective serotonin antagonists (5-HT$_3$ antagonists like ondansetron or granisetron) are prescribed include
    A. administering diphenhydramine to prevent extrapyramidal symptoms (EPSs).
    B. monitoring vital signs for hypertension.
    C. administering acetaminophen for headache.
    D. teaching clients to take only as needed for nausea and vomiting.

18. The advantage of selective serotonin antagonists over metoclopramide or a phenothiazine is
    A. lower cost.
    B. absence of extrapyramidal side effects.
    C. absence of sedation.
    D. absence of anticholinergic effects.

19. Which of the following drugs does **not** augment antiemetics?
    A. Diphenhydramine.
    B. Dexamethasone.
    C. Lorazepam.
    D. Cimetidine.

20. You are mentoring a new oncology nurse about client education on prevention of chemotherapy-induced nausea and vomiting from high-dose cisplatin. Which of the following is an **incorrect** teaching point?
    A. Administer antiemetics before chemotherapy.
    B. Take prophylactic antiemetics on a scheduled basis for 3 or 4 days starting on the second day after chemotherapy.
    C. Avoid taking "prn" antiemetics for breakthrough nausea or emesis.
    D. Report persistent severe nausea or vomiting to your doctor or nurse.

21. In the treatment of chronic cancer pain, which of the following is **not** an accepted principle in the use of analgesic drugs?
    A. Choose the lowest dose of analgesic to control a client's pain.
    B. Give the analgesic around the clock on a scheduled basis.

    C. Prevent constipation from narcotics with a stool softener plus a stimulant cathartic.
    D. Add an NSAID if a client has bone pain.

22. Which of the following opioid analgesics is more likely to cause respiratory depression?
    A. Meperidine.
    B. Acetaminophen.
    C. Methadone.
    D. Morphine.

23. When administering morphine sustained-release (SR) tablets to a client through a nasogastric feeding tube, the nurse should
    A. crush the tablets and administer concurrently with the tube feeding.
    B. clamp the tube for 30 minutes, crush the tablets, and then administer.
    C. find an alternative route of administration (e.g., intrarectally or vaginally).
    D. crush the tablets and add to tube feeding solution.

24. Mr. C. is taking aspirin for rheumatoid arthritis and is also receiving 5-FU, doxorubicin, and methotrexate for colon cancer. What risk may be increased significantly as a result of drug interaction?
    A. Increased risk of cardiac toxicity.
    B. Increased risk of methotrexate toxicity.
    C. Increased risk of diarrhea.
    D. Increased risk of aspirin toxicity.

25. Mr. C. is being discharged on SR morphine and acetaminophen. Which of the following instructions would you question?
    A. Take both morphine and acetaminophen around the clock.
    B. Increase fluid and fiber intake to prevent constipation.
    C. Use SR morphine for breakthrough pain.
    D. Avoid driving hazardous vehicles that require mental alertness.

26. Which of the following agents is effective for controlling opioid-induced constipation?
    A. Cimetidine.
    B. Lansoprazole.
    C. Senna plus a stool softener.
    D. Loperamide (Imodium).

27. A sedative hypnotic agent with minimal daytime hangover is:
   A. triazolam.
   B. phenobarbital.
   C. chlordiazepoxide.
   D. diazepam.

28. A major disadvantage of using a barbiturate as a sedative/hypnotic agent is
   A. rebound anxiety.
   B. loss of concentration and depression of affect.
   C. tolerance builds quickly.
   D. high incidence of Stevens-Johnson syndrome.

29. In a client with brain metastases, phenytoin (Dilantin) may be a necessary prophylactic medication if the client is receiving which of the following drugs?
   A. Granisetron and dexamethasone.
   B. Prochlorperazine and meperidine.
   C. Acetaminophen and codeine.
   D. Naproxen and dexamethasone.

30. The following is true about hematopoietic growth factors. They
   A. exert biologic effects such as enhancing differentiation or maturation of immunologic cell lines.
   B. promote tumor activity by stimulating bone marrow stem cells.
   C. are used for primary treatment of breast cancer.
   D. do not affect duration of neutropenia.

31. Which nursing action is recommended when administering a hematopoietic growth factor (HGF)?
   A. Add albumin in the carrier solution.
   B. Instruct the client to use NSAIDs for bone pain.
   C. Shake the vial vigorously during reconstitution.
   D. Administer the HGF before chemotherapy.

32. Granulocyte colony-stimulating factor (G-CSF) acts by

A. decreasing phagocytic activity.
B. stimulating precursors committed to neutrophil lineage.
C. interacting with specific receptors on erythroid burst-forming units.
D. regulating megakaryocytopoiesis.

33. A common side effect of filgrastim (G-CSF) is
   A. sedation.
   B. liver dysfunction.
   C. constipation.
   D. bone pain.

34. Mr. L. immigrated to the United States from Hong Kong 3 years ago and speaks limited English. He is 57 years old, has lung cancer, and is seen in a clinic in Chinatown for his chemotherapy. After seeking a traditional Chinese herbalist to treat his anxiety. Mr. L. turned to his Western physician, who prescribed diazepam for him. In Chinese clients receiving diazepam, which of the following may apply?
   A. Mr. L. probably needs a lower dose of diazepam.
   B. Chinese herbs interact with diazepam.
   C. Mr. L. should increase the dose of diazepam as needed.
   D. Mr. L. should take the diazepam with tea.

35. Which of the nursing considerations below is appropriate when caring for cultural clientele?
   A. Herbal preparations are commonly used, but some may cause side effects and interact with prescribed medications.
   B. Clients from different cultural and ethnic backgrounds routinely consult with traditional healers.
   C. Biologic variations among racial groups have little effect on drug metabolism rates, drug responses, and side effects to drugs.
   D. Cultural beliefs have little influence on the self-medicating behavior of clients.

ANSWERS

1. *Answer:* C
Rationale: Rash, fever, and nausea may indicate a reaction to the antibiotic or may indicate another infectious process. The physician would need to be aware of these symptoms to treat the client properly.

2. *Answer:* B
Rationale: These are antifungal agents, and *Candida* is a fungal organism.

3. *Answer:* C
Rationale: The major toxicity of aminoglycosides is nephrotoxicity. Careful monitoring of antibiotic levels (peak and trough), serum creatinine levels, and urine output is indicated to maximize treatment while minimizing toxicity.

4. *Answer:* B
Rationale: Acyclovir is an antiviral agent indicated in the treatment of herpes simplex virus and varicella zoster virus. Pseudomonas pneumonia is a bacterial infection. Pulmonary aspergillosis is a fungal infection. Acyclovir is not effective against cytomegalovirus retinitis.

5. *Answer:* A
Rationale: Cephalosporins cause allergic reactions, which are manifested by shortness of breath, hives, and itching. The other options are not associated with allergic reactions.

6. *Answer:* C
Rationale: Visual disturbances in the form of difficulty tolerating bright light or sunlight have been noted with voriconazole. Clients may also report double vision and visual hallucinations. Counsel clients to avoid night driving and to wear sunglasses when in sunlight. Additional side effects include nausea, vomiting, diarrhea, tachycardia, and hypersensitivity.

7. *Answer:* B
Rationale: The main side effects noted from caspofungin, an antifungal agent, have been reported as those related to histamine release, which may manifest as rash or hives.

8. *Answer:* A
Rationale: The mechanism of action of NSAIDs involves the inhibition of cyclooxygenase and thus the production of prostaglandins. This break in the cascade in turn suppresses the inflammatory response of white blood cell and macrophage migration to the site of injury and results in or contributes to symptom relief. Antiinflammatory agents do not work centrally by blocking opiate neurotransmitters and do not cause tumor cell lysis.

9. *Answer:* D
Rationale: The combined interaction and potential side effects of aspirin, naproxen, and dexamethasone put Mr. T. at higher risk of gastrointestinal ulceration, bleeding, and fluid retention and urinary insufficiency. Constipation is not a common side effect.

10. *Answer:* A
Rationale: Acne, weight gain, moon face, and an increase in appetite are common side effects of corticosteroids. For a teenage girl especially, these side effects will more than likely affect her body image. Diarrhea and CNS sedation are not common side effects of corticosteroids.

11. *Answer:* B
Rationale: NSAIDs are associated with fluid retention caused by an inhibition of the renin-aldosterone system. Thus weight gain can occur taking an NSAID. Most opioid analgesics inhibit peristalsis and therefore may lead to constipation.

12. *Answer:* D
Rationale: On the Hesketh scale of emetogenic potential, dacarbazine is a level 5 emetogen and is as severe as cisplatin in causing nausea and vomiting. The other three agents have mild to no emetogenic potential.

13. *Answer:* C
Rationale: Dexamethasone improves antiemetic efficacy by approximately 20% for both moderate and highly emetogenic

chemotherapy. It is also used before taxanes (docetaxel and paclitaxel) for preventing and treating hypersensitivity reactions. It has no effect on allergic reactions to cisplatin.

14. **Answer:** C
Rationale: The use of a 5-HT$_3$ antagonist such as ondansetron, granisetron, or dolasetron plus dexamethasone produces approximately 60% complete control (no emesis, no rescue) in clients treated with highly emetogenic chemotherapy.

15. **Answer:** B
Rationale: Prochlorperazine is an effective treatment for breakthrough emesis. 5-HT$_3$ antagonists and lorazepam or diphenhydramine do not have proven efficacy. Lorazepam is useful for anticipatory nausea or vomiting, and diphenhydramine is useful to prevent dystonic reactions from metoclopramide.

16. **Answer:** A
Rationale: The client is experiencing both acute and delayed vomiting. The addition of a dexamethasone to the 5-HT$_3$ antagonist might improve both acute and delayed episodes. Prochlorperazine is used for treatment of nausea, not prevention. Lorazepam is not a proven effective antiemetic. It is useful for preventing anticipatory emesis and anxiety. Aprepitant (Emend) is effective for acute and delayed emesis but should be added to a 5-HT$_3$ antagonist plus dexamethasone.

17. **Answer:** C
Rationale: 5-HT$_3$ antagonists can cause headache, which can be effectively treated with acetaminophen. EPS side effects do not occur with selective serotonin antagonists (5-HT$_3$). Principles of nursing management include the administration of antiemetics prophylactically to cover the onset, peak, and duration of action of each antineoplastic agent. Waiting to administer antiemetics only when a client vomits is not recommended.

18. **Answer:** B
Rationale: Selective serotonin antagonists, although more expensive than substituted benzamides and phenothiazines, do not have EPSs as a notable adverse side effect. Thus they have a major advantage over metoclopramide and phenothiazines, which also are sedating and have anticholinergic side effects.

19. **Answer:** D
Rationale: Diphenhydramine, dexamethasone, and lorazepam are all often used to augment antiemetics. Cimetidine is an H$_2$ blocker that is not indicated for augmentation of antiemetics.

20. **Answer:** B
Rationale: Prophylactic antiemetics should be administered before chemotherapy.

21. **Answer:** A
Rationale: The principle of dosing of opioid analgesics is that the dose necessary to control pain varies widely among clients. So, the effective dose is that which controls pain and may not be the lowest dose possible. Also, selection of the dose should be based on the previous effectiveness of analgesics used, not on a set fixed dose. Around-the-clock dosing, preventing gastrointestinal side effects, and using an NSAID for bone pain are reasonable approaches.

22. **Answer:** D
Rationale: Morphine is the most potent and CNS-depressing of the agents listed and thus has the potential of causing the most respiratory depression.

23. **Answer:** C
Rationale: Finding an alternative route is the best solution. Sustained-release tablets cannot be crushed. Other options involving tube feeding can compromise pain relief by increasing transit time and decreasing gastrointestinal absorption of the tablets.

24. **Answer:** B
Rationale: Aspirin competes with methotrexate for protein binding sites and kidney excretion, thus liberating more methotrexate into the circulation. This can result in increased blood levels of methotrexate and enhanced toxicity, especially to the bone marrow. Other drugs that compete with methotrexate include sulfonamides, penicillins, NSAIDs, and probenecid. These drugs should not be given concurrently with methotrexate.

25. *Answer:* C

Rationale: SR morphine has too slow an onset of action to be useful for breakthrough pain. Immediate-release opioids like morphine solution or hydromorphone are preferred. Around-the-clock dosing on analgesics is recommended in chronic pain. Increased fluid and fiber intake are useful adjuncts to prevent narcotic-induced constipation.

26. *Answer:* C

Rationale: Opioids cause constipation by slowing peristalsis. Agents that stimulate the gastrointestinal tract include senna derivatives and metoclopramide. Another approach is to use a peristaltic antagonist like low-dose naloxone. In addition, stool softeners aid in allowing for easier movement of bowel contents.

27. *Answer:* A

Rationale: Triazolam is a short-acting sedative-hypnotic agent with minimal daytime hangover effect. Chlordiazepoxide and diazepam are indicated more for anxiety, seizure control, and alcohol withdrawal. Phenobarbital is a long-acting sedative.

28. *Answer:* C

Rationale: Tolerance to the sedating properties of barbiturates occurs rapidly and allows for rapid titration of the drug. Stevens-Johnson syndrome does occur, but it is rare. Rebound anxiety and loss of concentration and depression of affect are not usual side effects of barbiturates.

29. *Answer:* B

Rationale: The use of a phenothiazine (prochlorperazine) or high-dose meperidine in a client with brain metastases might lower the seizure threshold. Thus phenytoin might be used as a prophylactic anticonvulsant in a client with brain metastases. Neither granisetron and dexamethasone nor naproxen and dexamethasone lower the seizure threshold. Although codeine may lower the seizure threshold, Option B is the best answer, because prochlorperazine lowers the seizure threshold and normeperidine (the metabolite of meperidine) may also lower the seizure threshold.

30. *Answer:* A

Rationale: Hematopoietic growth factors for the myeloid line enhance the production of granulocytic myeloid cells. It is thought that they do not promote tumor activity by stimulating bone marrow stem cells. They are not used as a primary treatment for breast cancer, and they can shorten the duration of neutropenia.

31. *Answer:* B

Rationale: An NSAID is effective for bone pain. Vials of proteins like filgrastim (G-CSF) should not be shaken vigorously because this will degrade the protein. Hematopoietic growth factors should be given 24 hours **after** chemotherapy.

32. *Answer:* B

Rationale: G-CSF increases phagocytic activity and stimulates production of neutrophils. It does not interact with the erythroid or platelet cell lines.

33. *Answer:* D

Rationale: Bone pain is the main side effect of filgrastim. This occurs as a result of expansion of granulocytic precursors in the client's bone marrow. Often, a client's peripheral white blood count will be correspondingly high.

34. *Answer:* A

Rationale: Because of biologic variations, the Chinese have been found to require a lower dose of benzodiazepines and are more sensitive to the sedative effects of this drug class.

35. *Answer:* A

Rationale: Several herbals are safe to use, but many may be deleterious and should be used with caution. St. John's wort is often used in depression but may increase the metabolism of other drugs that are used in the oncologic setting. Although traditional healers are frequently consulted, it cannot be assumed that clients will always consult these healers. Biologic variations are indeed a main reason that ethnic and cultural groups metabolize some drugs differently. Last, it is well reported that cultural beliefs have a substantial impact on the self-medicating behavior of clients, especially those with serious diseases.

BIBLIOGRAPHY

Beveridge, R.A. (Ed.). (2003). *Guide to selected cancer chemotherapy regimens and associated adverse events* (4th ed.). Thousand Oaks, CA: Amgen.

Bociek, R.G., & Armitage, J.A. (1996). Hematopoietic growth factors. *CA: Cancer Journal for Clinicians, 46*(3), 165-184.

Cleri, L.B. (1995). Serotonin antagonists: State of the art management of chemotherapy-induced emesis. *Oncology nursing: Patient treatment and support 2*(1), 1720.

Cleri, L.B., & Haywood, R. (2002). *Oncology pocket guide to chemotherapy* (5th ed.). St. Louis: Elsevier.

DiGregorio, G.J., Barbieri, E.J., Sterling, G.H., et al. (1994). *Handbook of pain management* (4th ed.). West Chester, PA: Medical Surveillance.

Dorr, R.T., & Van Horn, D. (1994). *Cancer chemotherapy handbook* (2nd ed.). Norwalk, CT: Appleton & Lange.

Malseed, R.T., Goldstein, P.J., & Balkon, N. (1995). *Pharmacology: Drug therapy and nursing considerations* (4th ed.). Philadelphia: JB Lippincott.

Pitler, L.R. (1996). Hematopoietic growth factors in clinical practice. *Seminars in Oncology Nursing 12*(2), 115-129.

Rhodes, V.A., Johnson, M.H., & McDaniel, R.W. (1995). Nausea, vomiting, and retching: The management of the symptom experience. *Seminars in Oncology Nursing 11*(4), 256-265.

Skidmore-Roth, L. (2005). *Mosby's nursing drug reference.* St. Louis: Elsevier.

Spratto, G.R., & Woods, A.L. (2004). *PDR Nurse's drug handbook.* Clifton Park, NY: Thomson, Delmar Learning.

NOTES

11 Supportive Care: Nonpharmacologic Interventions

DENISE MURRAY EDWARDS

Select the best answer for each of the following questions:

1. Which of the following reasons do oncology clients give as their motivation for seeking complementary and alternative (CAM) medicine?
    A. Decrease cost.
    B. Increase availability.
    C. Recommended by physician.
    D. Decrease discomforts of treatment.

2. A client in your clinic made an appointment with a practitioner of traditional Chinese medicine (TCM). In this system, the belief is that most health problems are caused by
    A. too much rich food.
    B. negative thoughts of others.
    C. deficiency or stagnation of Qi.
    D. an opposition of yin and yang.

3. The lack of which of the following is considered the cause of seasonal affective disorder (SAD)?
    A. Vitamin A.
    B. Sunlight.
    C. Exercise.
    D. Hormones.

4. Imagery is a mind-body intervention that a nurse might recommend to a client to be used for
    A. an alternative to conventional medicine.

    B. distracting the listener from stressful stimuli.
    C. changing the underlying reality of the situation.
    D. a decreased sense of control and responsibility.

5. It is estimated that 80% of the world's population use herbs for medicinal purposes. Clients seldom volunteer their use of herbs to health care providers. These facts are *most* essential to the nurse when
    A. developing client intake forms.
    B. restocking the outpatient clinic.
    C. planning for future inservice programs.
    D. talking to pharmaceutical representatives.

6. Ms. L. tells you she has been having problems with insomnia and has started taking valerian for sleep. You notice she has a history of allergies. While you are establishing your relationship and before you begin your client teaching, what is the most important piece of information you need?
    A. How long have you been taking it?
    B. Are you taking any other herbs?
    C. Have you used this herbal before?
    D. Have you tried pharmaceuticals for sleep?

7. A client has experienced an acute trauma to his ankle. There is no open wound. What nonpharmacologic intervention would you use first?
   A. Heat.
   B. Cold.
   C. Water.
   D. Stabilization.

8. An artificially induced alteration of consciousness, characterized by increased suggestibility and receptivity to suggestion, is
   A. hypnosis.
   B. focusing.
   C. meditation.
   D. mindfulness.

9. A hospital/clinic may have available a list of licensed/certified complementary clinicians that may be helpful in preventing/treating symptoms. Making this list available to clients is considered
   A. a referral.
   B. a consult.
   C. a liability concern.
   D. client collaboration.

10. There may be agencies or individuals in your community offering potentially dangerous "alternative" medicine practices. To protect clients from harm by these practitioners, it is best to
   A. warn clients about the growing numbers of fraudulent and dangerous "treatments" they are likely to hear about during your first meeting with them.
   B. establish an open and nonjudgmental atmosphere for discussing alternative treatments.
   C. tell clients not to take any herbs or supplements or visit any nontraditional healers.

   D. give clients handouts on possible interactions with chemotherapy and vitamins and herbs.

11. Knowing the country of origin of the material used in which of these CAM interventions could give the well-informed nurse important data about the probable quality of the treatment?
    A. Needle acupuncture.
    B. Aromatherapy.
    C. Herbs.
    D. Yoga.

12. One of the common goals of practitioners of healing touch, acupuncture, Reiki, therapeutic touch, and reflexology is
    A. employing the six senses.
    B. increasing mindfulness meditation.
    C. teaching clients to increase relaxation.
    D. restoring harmony and balance in energy.

13. After a massage, in addition to a feeling of relaxation, a client often experiences an increased sense of well-being. This is most likely due to
    A. decreased fatigue.
    B. release of endorphins.
    C. restoration of harmony.
    D. increased sense of balance.

14. Complementary and alternative medicine includes all practices and ideas that promote health and well-being as defined by the
    A. users of these practices.
    B. American Medical Association.
    C. American Holistic Nurses Association.
    D. Agency for Health Care Policy and Research.

ANSWERS

1. *Answer:* D
   Rationale: CAM has been shown to minimize some of the discomforts associated with standard therapy. CAM interventions are an added expense, eliminating Option A; are not easily available, eliminating Option B; and, because the physician seldom discusses CAM with the client, Option C is not appropriate.

2. *Answer:* C
   Rationale: Qi (pronounced chee) is the vital energy or life force that animates all living beings and the entire universe. Options A and B are not concepts in TCM, a system that looks at the whole person's energy and is not based on magical influences. Yin is associated with the feminine, passive, dark, and inner qualities, while yang represents the masculine, active, light, and outer qualities. These entities exist as polarities. Consequently, Option D represents the normal state.

3. *Answer:* B
   Rationale: Sunshine causes the body to produce melatonin, a precursor of serotonin, and a brain chemical responsible for mood. Vitamin A, exercise, and hormones do not have seasonal effects.

4. *Answer:* B
   Rationale: Imagery is used as a distraction. A nurse would never recommend a complementary intervention in place of conventional medicine, nor would imagery have the power to change reality. The goal is to increase the client's sense of control and responsibility.

5. *Answer:* A
   Rationale: This information is essential in developing assessment tools. The nurse typically would not be dispensing herbs/supplements. It could be helpful (but not most important) in planning for future inservice programs, and not important in talking to pharmaceutical representatives.

6. *Answer:* C
   Rationale: Because the nurse wants to establish this relationship and protect the client, she must first turn to the client's experience with the supplement. Options A, B, and D may be useful pieces of information but certainly not the most important in establishing the potential for allergy.

7. *Answer:* B
   Rationale: Cold reduces swelling. Heat brings fluid to the area, which is not the initially desired response. Water and stabilization are not considered nonpharmacologic interventions.

8. *Answer:* A
   Rationale: Hypnosis is considered artificially induced. Focusing, meditation, and mindfulness are all self-induced.

9. *Answer:* D
   Rationale: Having available a list of licensed/certified CAM clinicians for client referral is an excellent example of client collaboration. The definitions of either a referral or a consult do not work here. It would be within the knowledge of most nurses that handing a client a list of names is not a liability concern.

10. *Answer:* B
    Rationale: The goal of establishing communication with a client regarding CAM is to keep the information flowing, whereas the other three options may shut down that communication.

11. *Answer:* C
    Rationale: Country of origin, thus far, has been important only in the quality of herbs.

12. *Answer:* D
    Rationale: All of these are considered energy work with the goal as restoring harmony and balance in energy. There is no goal in common compatible with Options A, B, or C.

13. *Answer:* B
    Rationale: The research on massage consistently identifies an increase in endorphins connected to a sense of well-being. There is no information to support decreased fatigue,

restoration of harmony, or an increased sense of balance as the source of this increased sense of well-being.

14. *Answer:* A

Rationale: None of the three other groups have created their own definitions.

BIBLIOGRAPHY

Adler, P., Good, M., Roberts, B., & Snyder, S. (2000). The effects of tai chi on older adults with chronic arthritis pain. *Journal of Nursing Scholarship 32*(4), 377.

Benson, H. (1996). *Timeless healing: The power and biology of belief.* New York: Scribner.

Blanchard, C., Courneya, K., & Laing, D. (2001). Effects of acute exercise on state anxiety in breast cancer survivors. *Oncology Nursing Forum 28*(10), 1617-1621.

Blumenthal, M. (Ed.). (1998). *The complete German Commission E monographs: Therapeutic guide to herbal medicine.* Austin, TX: American Botanical Council.

Brennan, B. (1993). *Light emerging: The journey of personal healing.* New York: Bantam Books.

Caudill, M. (1995). *Managing pain before it manages you.* New York: The Guilford Press.

Cooke, B., & Ernst, E. (2000). Aromatherapy: A systematic review. *British Journal of General Practice 50,* 493- 496.

Courneya, K. S., Keats, M.R., & Turner, A.R. (2000). Physical exercise and quality of life in cancer patients following high dose chemotherapy and autologous bone marrow transplantation. *Psycho-Oncology 9,* 127-136.

Cousins, N. (1979). *Anatomy of an illness as perceived by the patient: Reflections on healing and regeneration.* New York: W.W. Norton & Company.

Decker, G. (Ed.). (1999). *An introduction to complementary and alternative therapies.* Pittsburgh: Oncology Nursing Society.

Dibble, S., Chapman, J., Mack, A., & Shih, A. (2000). Acupressure for nausea: Results of a pilot study. *Oncology Nursing Forum 27*(1), 41-47.

Eastman, C., Young, M., Fogg. L., et al. (1998). Bright light treatment of winter depression: A placebo-controlled trial. *Archives of General Psychiatry 55,* 883-889.

Ehman, J., Ott, B., Short, T., et al. (1999). Do patients want physicians to inquire about their spiritual beliefs or religious beliefs if they become gravely ill? *Archives of Internal Medicine 23,* 1803-1806.

Eisenberg, D., Davis, R., Ettner, S., et al. (1998). Trends in alternative medicine in the United States. (1990-1997). Results of a follow-up national survey. *Journal of the American Medical Association 280,* 1569-1575.

Ginandes, C., & Rosenthal, D. (1999). Using hypnosis to accelerate healing of bone fractures; a randomized controlled pilot study. *Alternative Therapies in Health and Medicine 5*(2), 67-75.

Grealish, L., Lomasney. A., & Whiteman, B. (2000). Foot massage: A nursing intervention to modify distressing symptoms of pain and nausea in patients hospitalized with cancer. *Cancer Nursing 23*(3), 237-243.

Gross, J., Ott, C., Lindsey, A., et al. (2002). Postmenopausal breast cancer survivors at risk for osteoporosis: Physical activity, vigor and vitality. *Oncology Nursing Forum 29*(9), 1295-1262.

Grunewald, J., Brendler, T., & Jaenicke, C. (Eds.). (1998). *PDR for herbal medicines.* Montvale, NJ: Medical Economics Co.

Halstead, M., & Roscoe, S. (2002). Restoring the spirit at the end of life: Music as an intervention for oncology nurses. *Clinical Journal of Oncology Nursing 6*(6), 332-336.

Highfield, M. (2000). Providing spiritual care to patients with cancer. *Clinical Journal of Oncology Nursing 4*(3),115-120.

Johnson, P. (2002). Use of humor and its influences on spirituality and coping in breast cancer survivors. *Oncology Nursing Forum 29,* 691-695.

Lengacher, C., Bennett, M., Kip, K., et al. (2002). Frequency and use of complementary and alternative medicine in women with breast cancer. *Oncology Nursing Forum 29*(10), 1445-1452.

Lewis, L. (1999). Acupuncture: Another therapeutic choice? *Patient Care.*

Linz, K., Penson, R., Chabner, B., & Lynch, T. (2002). A staff dialogue on caring for an intensely spiritual patient: Psychosocial issues faced by patients, their families, and caregivers. *The Oncologist 7*(2), 16-22.

Murray Edwards, D. (Ed.). (2002). *Voice massage: Scripts for guided imagery.* Pittsburgh: Oncology Nursing Society.

O'Mathuna, D. (2000). Evidence-based practice reviews of therapeutic touch. *Journal of Nursing Scholarship 32*(3), 279-285.

Pan, C., Morrison, R., Ness, J., et al. (2001). Complementary and alternative medicine in the management of pain, dyspnea, and nausea and vomiting near the end of life: A systematic review. *Journal of Pain & Symptom Management 20,* 374-387.

Rexillius, S., Mundt, C., Erickson, M., & Agrawal, S. (2002). Therapeutic effects of massage therapy and healing touch on caregivers of patients undergoing autologous hematopoietic stem cell transplant. *Oncology Nursing Forum 29*(3), 1-15.

Rusy, L., & Weisman, S. (2000). Complementary therapies for acute pediatric pain. *Pediatric Clinics of North America 47,* 589-599.

Smith, M., Casey, L., Johnson, D., et al. (2001) Music as a therapeutic intervention for anxiety in patients receiving radiation therapy. *Oncology Nursing Forum 28*(5), 855-862.

Smith, M., Kemp, J., Hemphill, L., & Vojir, C. (2002). Outcomes of therapeutic massage for hospitalized cancer patients. *Journal of Nursing Scholarship 34*(3), 257-262.

Sparber, A., Bauer, L., Curt, G., et al. (2000). Use of complementary medicine by adult patients participating in cancer clinical trials. *Oncology Nursing Forum 27*(4), 623-630.

Stephenson, N., Weinrich, S., & Tavakoli, A. (2000). The effects of foot reflexology on anxiety and pain in patients with breast and lung cancer. *Oncology Nursing Forum 27*(1), 67-72.

VanFleet, S. (2000). Relaxation and imagery for symptom management: Improving patient assessment and individualizing treatment. *Oncology Nursing Forum 27*, 501-507.

White, J. (2001). Music as an intervention: A notable endeavor to improve patient outcomes. *Nursing Clinics of North America 36*, 83-92.

White, P.F. (1997). Are nonpharmacologic techniques useful alternatives to antiemetic drugs for the prevention of nausea and vomiting? *Anesthesia Analgesia 84*, 712-714.

Winstead-Fry, P., & Kijek, J. (1999) An integrative review and meta-analysis of therapeutic touch research. *Alternative Therapies in Health and Medicine 5*(6), 58-67.

Wint, S., Eshelman, D., Steele, J., & Guzzetta, C. (2002). Effects of distraction using virtual reality glasses during lumbar punctures in adolescents with cancer. *Oncology Nursing Forum 29*(1), 1-12.

Wolfson, L. (1996). Balance and strength training in older adults: Intervention gains and tai chi maintenance. *Journal of American Geriatric Society 44*, 498-506.

NOTES

PART TWO

PROTECTIVE MECHANISMS

12 Alterations in Mobility, Skin Integrity, and Neurologic Status

JENNIFER DOUGLAS PEARCE

Select the best answer for each of the following questions:

1. Which laboratory result is most important in the client with impaired skin integrity?
    A. Hemoglobin (Hgb) 9.5 g/dl and hematocrit (Hct) 30%.
    B. Albumin (serum) 2.9 g/dl.
    C. Amylase (serum) 70 Somogyi unit/dl.
    D. Blood urea nitrogen (BUN) 20 mg/dl.

2. Which statement by the client receiving radiation therapy would indicate that further teaching is necessary?
    A. "I can wash around these markings while I am receiving therapy."
    B. "An oral sponge soaked in saline can be used after meals."
    C. "I use an alcohol-based skin lotion for my itchy skin."
    D. "A warm oatmeal bath can help relieve my itching."

3. The client with impaired skin integrity is receiving an antineoplastic medication that causes myelosuppression. For which of the following should the nurse assess the client?
    A. Diarrhea.
    B. Infection.
    C. Constipation.
    D. Dysrhythmias.

4. Which activity is most related to tertiary prevention in a client with impaired physical mobility?
    A. Educating.
    B. Promoting.
    C. Immunizing.
    D. Rehabilitating.

5. Which is the most appropriate nursing action in the client with cancer who is at risk for fungal infection?
    A. Apply povidone-iodine (Betadine) to moist areas.
    B. Dry the skin folds of the client.
    C. Bathe the client daily.
    D. Keep the client's room cool.

6. Mr. S. is cognitively impaired and has a loss of bowel and bladder control. What is the most appropriate nursing action to prevent skin breakdown?
    A. Inspect and wash the perineal area at frequent intervals.
    B. Remind the client to use the call light for assistance.
    C. Apply an adult diaper.
    D. Turn and position the client every 4 hours.

7. Which nursing action is used to support and communicate with the cognitively impaired client with cancer who is receiving chemotherapy?

A. Call the client by a term of endearment when addressing him or her.
B. Identify the client using the identification band.
C. Identify yourself and give a simple explanation to the client.
D. Avoid touching the client to decrease the risk of anxiety.

8. During a bed-to-chair transfer, the nurse sits the client with impaired physical mobility on the side of the bed. What is the rationale for this action?
A. Allow the client to breathe normally after the activity.
B. Provide time for the client's heart rate to return to normal.
C. Allow the nurse to breathe normally after the activity.
D. Prevent dizziness and the potential for falls.

9. What is the priority nursing diagnosis for the client with hip pinning 1 week after surgery?
A. Risk for altered skin integrity related to immobility.
B. Risk for infection related to hip pinning.
C. Activity intolerance related to bed rest.
D. Altered role performance related to surgery.

10. The client with cancer has surgery with hip pinning. The skin around the pin site is swollen, red, and crusty with dried drainage. What is the nurse's most appropriate action?
A. Decrease the traction weight.
B. Apply a new dressing.
C. Observe the site for 24 hours.
D. Notify the physician.

11. The client with osteogenic sarcoma has had a below-the-knee amputation. Which nursing intervention will be most appropriate to help the client adjust to the new body image?
A. Visit with the client often and sit during conversation.
B. Arrange to have the hospital chaplain visit.
C. Use empathetic touch during conversation with client.

D. Arrange for a survivor with similar health issues to visit with client.

12. The client with a history of breast cancer has a seizure during a clinic visit. Which nursing intervention should be implemented first?
A. Prevent injury.
B. Observe and record characteristics of seizure.
C. Insert an oral airway.
D. Reorient client to environment when awakened.

13. A client with a history of prostate cancer is admitted to the emergency room with numbness and tingling of the legs. Which is the most appropriate nursing action?
A. Immobilize the body and instruct the client not to flex his head.
B. Reassure the client that the change in sensation is temporary.
C. Turn client every 2 hours and check his skin.
D. Initiate a complete neurologic examination.

14. The client has a spinal cord compression as a result of metastatic disease. To maintain the integrity of the skin, the nurse should
A. give range-of-motion exercises to the extremities.
B. set up regular bowel and bladder programs.
C. log roll every 2 hours and check skin.
D. monitor for edema of extremities.

15. Which is an example of tertiary prevention for a client with spinal cord compression with lower leg paralysis?
A. Establish an individualized rehabilitation program.
B. Initiate bowel retraining.
C. Check for bladder distention.
D. Use aseptic technique for intermittent catheterization.

16. The client has had a brain tumor. Which intervention should the nurse use, if the client has a temperature of 99.8° F (38°C); pulse 130, and blood pressure 150/90?
A. Cluster activity for longer periods of rest.
B. Monitor vital signs every 4 hours.

C. Maintain the client's head of bed at 30°.

D. Keep suctioning equipment at the bedside.

17. Which of these medications should alert the nurse to a client's increased risk for osteoporosis?

A. Insulin.

B. Acetaminophen.

C. Aspirin.

D. Corticosteroid.

18. Which assessment finding would support the nursing diagnosis of impaired physical mobility?

A. Curvature of the spine.

B. Muscle atrophy in lower extremity.

C. Generalized decreased upper muscle mass.

D. Bilateral hypertrophy of paired muscle groups.

19. A client with metastatic bone disease is receiving chemotherapy. Her calcium level is 10.6 mg/dl. Which is the most appropriate action of the nurse?

A. Assess the client's muscle strength.

B. Institute seizure precautions.

C. Notify the physician.

D. Document the results.

20. The nurse anticipates and prepares which drug of choice to treat the client with increased intracranial pressure (ICP)?

A. Morphine.

B. Mannitol.

C. Vinblastine.

D. Prednisone.

21. Before the administration of doxorubicin (Adriamycin), which of the following is important for the nurse to assess?

A. Gastrointestinal (GI) system.

B. Neurologic status.

C. Intravenous (IV) system access.

D. Renal function.

22. What is appropriate documentation before administration of doxorubicin?

A. Central line patent, aspirated blood return without difficulty.

B. Client reports pain and burning at IV site.

C. Skin intact, warm and dry to touch, turgor elastic.

D. Redness and swelling noted at IV site, angiocath discontinued.

23. Which statement would indicate to the nurse that the client needs additional information about vincristine?

A. "I will call the nurse if I experience any muscle weakness."

B. "I should drink lots of water to decrease the risk of constipation."

C. "I will call my nurse at the first sign of numbness and tingling."

D. "I will see a hair stylist for a hair prosthesis before I lose my hair."

24. One goal for the client with posttherapy confusion is safety. Which of the following is the best nursing intervention to achieve this outcome?

A. Medicate with oral lorazepam.

B. Assign a sitter from the nursing pool.

C. Use physical restraints.

D. Invite a family member to sit with the client.

25. When communicating with a cancer client who is confused, the nurse should

A. speak in a soft, low, reassuring voice and identify self.

B. speak in a high, hurried tone of voice.

C. touch the client before speaking.

D. avoid direct eye contact when working with the client.

26. Planning care for the client with delirium should include:

A. Remove the calendars from the client's environment, because they increase confusion.

B. Allow family photos only if the client can identify the people in them.

C. Encourage the client to consistently use assistive devices such as eyeglasses and hearing aids.

D. Maximize the client's exposure to environmental sounds, such as alarms, to remind him that he is in the hospital and not at home.

27. The client has a nursing diagnosis of impaired physical mobility related to calcium loss resulting from bed rest. The nurse knows that calcium is necessary for strong bones and teeth. What is another necessary function of calcium?
    A. Keeping the stomach acidic.
    B. Muscle contraction.
    C. Preventing blood clotting.
    D. Production of insulin.

28. The client receiving radiation therapy is on a high-protein diet. The nurse evaluates the client's understanding of the diet plan when the client selects which meal?
    A. Peanut butter on graham crackers with milk.
    B. Red beans and rice.
    C. Bacon, lettuce, and tomato sandwich.
    D. Low-fat, sugar-free butter pecan yogurt with sprinkles.

29. The client has carcinoma of the liver. Which is the appropriate nursing care?
    A. Administration of vitamins A, D, E, and K.
    B. Administration of vitamins A, B, and C.
    C. High-carbohydrate, low-fat diet.
    D. High-fat, low-protein diet.

30. The client with liver cancer has some blood work drawn. The appropriate nursing action is
    A. place a thick bandage on the area.
    B. apply a pressure dressing on the area.
    C. apply pressure until the area stops bleeding and apply pressure dressing.
    D. have the client apply pressure to the area.

31. When is it appropriate for the nurse to begin client and family education regarding the neurotoxic effects of chemotherapeutic agents?
    A. Upon client's request.
    B. Before treatment.
    C. As symptoms appear.
    D. After the physician's request.

32. What is the rationale for assessing deep tendon reflexes of a client receiving vincristine?

A. To assess adherence and effectiveness to the rehabilitation plan.
B. To determine deep tendon reflex stability and improvement.
C. Neuropathies may indicate that the dosage or schedule of chemotherapy administration should be modified.
D. Strong deep tendon reflexes indicate that the chemotherapy is combating target cells effectively.

33. A client with brain metastasis is on seizure precautions. The nurse should verify that the client is on bed rest, side rails are raised, and anticonvulsant medication is ordered. What would be an additional precaution?
    A. An aide to sit at the bedside.
    B. Padded tongue blade available.
    C. An oral airway available.
    D. Padded side rails.

34. The client recently has been informed of his metastatic cancer. Which of the following is an appropriate nursing intervention?
    A. Discuss a regular exercise schedule with the client.
    B. Plan activities for diversional therapy.
    C. Provide opportunity for the client to share his feelings.
    D. Have client attend occupational therapy with other clients.

35. The client with breast cancer is in her fourth week of radiation therapy. The client reports scaling, dryness, and pruritus. The nurse responds:
    A. The skin reaction is totally unexpected and should be reported.
    B. The skin reaction is expected and reviews care with client.
    C. That radiation be discontinued until the condition has healed.
    D. Ulceration is the next step in the skin reaction.

36. Which characteristics of the skin make it sensitive to the effects of radiation and chemotherapies?
    A. The presence of mucus-producing glands.
    B. Rapidly dividing epithelial cells.
    C. Sensitivity to heat, cold, and pain.
    D. The porous nature of the skin.

37. The client is on bed rest. The nurse obtains a prescription for compression stockings to prevent which condition?

   A. Thrombophlebitis.
   B. Cellulitis.
   C. Foot drop.
   D. Stasis dermatitis.

38. Which discharge instruction is most important for a client receiving biologic response modifiers therapy?

   A. Increase your vitamin K.
   B. Eat no more than 2000 calories a day.
   C. Increase intake of high-fiber foods.
   D. Take frequent rest periods for fatigue.

NOTES

ANSWERS

1. *Answer:* B
   Rationale: Albumin is important for maintaining adequate protein, which is essential to tissue repair. A low albumin is indicative of malnutrition. Option A is incorrect because a low Hgb and Hct are indicative of acute blood loss, anemia, and kidney disease. Option C is incorrect because a high amylase is indicative of pancreatic problems. Option D is an elevated BUN, which may be indicative of dehydration or possible renal disorder.

2. *Answer:* C
   Rationale: Alcohol is drying to the skin and will increase the risk of itching. Options A, B, and D are all appropriate responses by a client receiving radiation therapy.

3. *Answer:* B
   Rationale: Most antineoplastic medications cause myelosuppression. With leukopenia there is increased risk for infection. A client with impaired skin integrity is at greater risk because of the break in the first line of defense, the skin. Option A is incorrect because diarrhea may occur as a side effect of antineoplastic medication. It is not related to myelosuppression. Option C is incorrect because most antineoplastic medications cause diarrhea, not constipation. Option D is incorrect because some antineoplastic medications can cause cardiotoxicity. It is not related to myelosuppression.

4. *Answer:* D
   Rationale: Rehabilitation activities that help maintain and restore function are tertiary prevention activities. Option A is incorrect because education is provided at all levels of prevention for informed decision making. Options B and C are related to primary prevention, which includes preventing and protecting persons from disease.

5. *Answer:* B
   Rationale: Attention to the skin folds that are dark, moist, and retain wetness will decrease the risk of fungal infection. Option A will cause drying to the skin, which may increase the risk of breaks in the skin. Option C is incorrect because bathing is necessary, but without careful drying of skin folds, fungal infections can occur. Option D is incorrect because a cool room will reduce perspiration; however, skin folds are moist and conducive to the growth of fungi.

6. *Answer:* A
   Rationale: Urine or stool on the skin can irritate the skin and increase the risk of skin breakdown. Option B is an unrealistic expectation for a cognitively impaired client. Option C is incorrect because an adult diaper may increase the risk of skin breakdown because the moisture is in constant contact with the skin and the perineal area may not be checked frequently. Option D is incorrect because turning and positioning should be implemented more frequently to decrease the risk of skin breakdown.

7. *Answer:* C
   Rationale: When working with the cognitively impaired client, it is important for the nurse to reorient the client to person, place, and time. Option C helps achieve this goal. Option A is inappropriate and is not best practice. Option B is standard procedure but does not contribute to reorienting or maintaining cognitive function in the client. Option D is essential to nursing care; neglecting to touch the client will increase his or her anxiety.

8. *Answer:* D
   Rationale: Orthostatic hypotension can result when moving from a lying to a sitting position. Sitting at the side of the bed allows the client to adjust to the change in position. Options A and B are not primary purposes of the nurse's action. Option C is inaccurate.

9. *Answer:* B
   Rationale: A break in skin integrity, because of surgery, places an immocompromised client at risk for infection. Option A is incorrect because there is an actual break in the skin integrity due to the surgical incision. Option C is incorrect because the client is not on bed rest; physical therapy is encouraged.

Option D may be a problem, but it is not the priority diagnosis at this time.

10. *Answer:* D
Rationale: A swollen, red, draining wound is indicative of inflammation and possible infection. Infected pin sites in an already compromised client can lead to osteomyelitis and should be treated immediately. Option A is not a nursing action, Option B may be done after the site is seen by the physician, and Option C, observing the site for 24 hours, is too long to wait in an immunocompromised client.

11. *Answer:* D
Rationale: Visits allow the client to derive strength and hope from a person with similar experiences, and provide an opportunity to ask questions. Options A, B, and C may be appropriate but not the most therapeutic toward adjustment to the amputation.

12. *Answer:* A
Rationale: The first priority is to protect the client and prevent injury. This can be done by cradling the client's head during the seizure and preventing further trauma. Option B is also important but not the first priority. Option C may cause damage to the client's mouth and teeth. Option D is appropriate after the client has been awakened.

13. *Answer:* D
Rationale: A neurologic examination will determine motor, sensory, and reflex loss caused by spinal cord compression resulting from prostate cancer metastasis to the spine. Options A and C may be necessary, if the neurologic examination indicates spinal cord injury. Option B may be false reassurance.

14. *Answer:* C
Rationale: Changing positions decreases the pressure in the area and decreases the risk of skin breakdown. The log-roll technique will prevent further injury. Options A and D decrease the risk for circulatory complications, and Option B controls factors to decrease the risk of autonomic dysreflexia.

15. *Answer:* A
Rationale: Tertiary prevention deals with restorative and rehabilitative care. Options B,

C, and D are all primary level preventions to prevent further complications such as constipation and urinary distention that can lead to bladder infection, and they decrease the risk of infection.

16. *Answer:* C
Rationale: Elevation of the head promotes venous drainage and prevents increased intracranial pressure. Options A, B, and D would not decrease or prevent increased intracranial pressure.

17. *Answer:* D
Rationale: Chronic use of corticosteroids increases resorption of minerals from the bone, decreasing bone density and increasing the risk for osteoporosis. Options A, B, and C have no effect on the musculoskeletal system.

18. *Answer:* B
Rationale: Muscle atrophy can occur when a client has a painful joint condition. Disuse atrophy occurs as the client avoids joint movement to prevent pain. Options A, C, and D are not related to physical mobility.

19. *Answer:* D
Rationale: This is an expected normal level. Options A, B, and C are not necessary because the level is a normal finding.

20. *Answer:* B
A client with ICP elevation requires an osmotic diuretic, which is a hyperosmolar agent. Option A is useful to decrease pain, which is a noxious stimulant that ultimately increases ICP. However, there are insufficient data presented to support that the client has pain. Option C is a chemotherapeutic agent and as such does not decrease ICP. Option D is a steroid, but not the drug of choice for increased ICP.

21. *Answer:* C
Rationale: Adriamycin is a vesicant. Infiltration may lead to extravasation and necrosis of the tissues. Option A is incorrect because GI upset can be treated and would not delay administration of the medication. Options B and D are not required before the administration of this drug.

22. *Answer:* A
Rationale: Vesicants are best administered through large veins with generous blood flow to decrease the risk of infiltration. Options B and D are indications of nonfunctioning IVs. Option C is appropriate documentation for intact skin.

23. *Answer:* D
Rationale: Alopecia is not a side effect of vincristine. Options A, B, and C are side effects of vincristine.

24. *Answer:* D
Rationale: Family provides a familiar face and may decrease the client's anxiety, fear, and restlessness. Options A, B, and C are also appropriate, but a family member is the best intervention.

25. *Answer:* A
Rationale: When the client does not fully comprehend what is happening, the nurse's facial expressions and tone of voice can create a comfortable, reassuring atmosphere. Options B and C: Confusion may be increased if the nurse communicates alarm by the tone of voice and actions. Option D: verbal and nonverbal acts of the caregivers should be congruent to decrease the client's agitation, which may further increase confusion.

26. *Answer:* C
Rationale: Assistive devices limit the distortion of sights and sounds and decrease the client's anxiety, which decreases the delirium. Options A, B, and D increase the risk of maintaining or increasing the client's delirium.

27. *Answer:* B
Rationale: Calcium acts as a catalyst in initiating and controlling muscular contractions and relaxation. Option A is incorrect because calcium does nothing for stomach acidity. Option C is incorrect because calcium aids in the formation of blood clots. Option D is incorrect because calcium does nothing for insulin production.

28. *Answer:* A
Rationale: Peanut butter is an excellent source of protein, and milk complements it.

Option B is incorrect because red beans are also a good source of protein; rice is a carbohydrate. Option C is incorrect because there is no protein in this selection; there is carbohydrate and fat. Option D has some protein found in the yogurt and pecans, but peanut butter and milk have more.

29. *Answer:* A
Rationale: The liver may be unable to produce the fat-soluble vitamins; supplements will aid with clotting and other essential functions. Option B is incorrect because production of water-soluble vitamins may be affected by the client's appetite, but not directly by the liver function. Option C is incorrect because this diet is deficient in protein, essential for healing. Option D is also deficient in protein and requires less fat.

30. *Answer:* C
Rationale: If the liver is severely damaged, there may be alterations in clotting, and additional pressure may be necessary to ensure that clotting occurs. Option A is not sufficient to stop bleeding. Option B is incorrect because application of a dressing without ensuring that the bleeding has stopped is unsafe practice. Option D is incorrect because the client may not be able to apply sufficient pressure to stop the bleeding.

31. *Answer:* B
Rationale: Early detection of these neurologic effects may mean the difference between the symptoms being treatable and reversible. Options A, C, and D are all incorrect and constitute unsafe care.

32. *Answer:* C
Rationale: Vincristine can cause neurotoxicity with possible footdrop from muscle weakness. Early detection of neuropathies allows for manipulation of dosages and may prevent irreversible neurologic damage.

33. *Answer:* D
Rationale: Padded side rails may cushion the client's movement and decrease the risk of injury. Option A is not necessary. Options B and C are discouraged; they may increase the risk of oral injury.

34. *Answer:* C

Rationale: The client needs time to talk and time to explore and share his feelings. Option A is not advisable at this time until the interdisciplinary plan of care has been discussed. Options B and D may be needed eventually, but handling feelings is the more immediate concern.

35. *Answer:* B

Rationale: This is a normal skin reaction that occurs between the fourth and fifth weeks of therapy related to dose, type of machine, location of treatment, and concomitant chemotherapy. Option A is inaccurate. Option C is also inaccurate. Option D is a chronic reaction and may be seen 10 to 20 years after treatment.

36. *Answer:* B

Rationale: Both chemotherapy and radiation act best on rapidly dividing cells, of which skin is one. Options A, C, and D are not affected by chemotherapy.

37. *Answer:* A

Rationale: Stasis of blood and muscle inactivity with decreased pumping action leads to stasis of blood, which may lead to thrombus formation. Compression or antiembolism stockings may support venous return through compression of superficial veins and redirection of blood flow to deeper veins. Option B is caused by infection in the skin and subcutaneous tissue. Option C may be caused by chemotherapeutic agents or damage to the common peroneal nerve. Option D is treated with bed rest, antibiotics, and steroid therapy.

38. *Answer:* D

Rationale: Clients receiving biologic response modifiers may experience fatigue, flulike symptoms, and anorexia. Options A, B, and C are not side effects of these drugs.

BIBLIOGRAPHY

Bush, N.J., & Hartkopf-Smith, L. (2002). Clinical highlights: Normeperidine neurotoxicity. *Oncology Nursing Forum 29*(4), 634.

Flounders, J., & Ott, B.B. (2003). Oncologic emergency modules: Spinal cord compression. *Oncology Nursing Forum 30*(1), E17-E23; www.ons.org.

Haisfield-Wolfe, M., & Rund, C. (2000). A nursing protocol for the management of perineal-rectal skin alterations. *Clinical Journal of Oncology Nursing 4*(1), 15-21.

Ignatavicius, D. (2002). Rehabilitation concepts for acute and chronic problems. In D.D., Ignatavicius, & L. Workman, (Eds.). *Medical-Surgical nursing: Critical thinking for collaborative care* (4th ed.). Philadelphia: W.B. Saunders, pp. 119-136.

Landier, W. (2001). Continuing education: Childhood acute lymphoblastic leukemia: Current perspectives. *Oncology Nursing Forum 28*(5): 823-833.

Lovejoy, C.N., Tabor, D., & Deloney, P. (2000). Cancer-related depression. Part II: Neurological alterations and evolving approaches to psychopharmacology. *Oncology Nursing Forum 27*(5), 795-810.

Lovejoy, C.N., Tabor, D., Matteis, M, & Lillis, P. (2000). Cancer-related depression. Part I: Neurologic alterations and cognitive-behavioral therapy. *Oncology Nursing Forum 27*, 667-680.

Olsen, L.D., Raub, W., Bradley, C., et al. (2001). The effects of aloe vera gel/mild soap versus mild soap alone in preventing skin reactions in patients undergoing radiation therapy. *Oncology Nursing Forum 28*(3), 543-547.

Stafford–Fox, V., & Guindon, K. (2000). Cutaneous reactions associated with alpha interferon therapy. *Clinical Journal of Oncology Nursing 4*(4): 164-168.

Sweeney, C. (2002). Understanding peripheral neuropathy in patients with cancer: Background and patient assessment. *Clinical Journal of Oncology Nursing 6*(3), 163-166.

13 Myelosuppression

DAWN CAMP-SORRELL

Select the best answer for each of the following questions:

1. The immune system of a client with cancer may be depressed because of the following:
    A. Nutritional status.
    B. Continuous narcotic drip.
    C. Administration of growth factors.
    D. Taking iron supplements.

2. During the nadir period from chemotherapy, the client should be instructed to avoid all drugs that inhibit platelet function. Such drugs include
    A. aspirin and ibuprofen.
    B. iron supplements.
    C. vitamins.
    D. morphine.

3. When implementing a teaching plan for the client with low absolute neutrophil count (ANC), the nurse should plan to emphasize the following:
    A. Have fresh flowers in the room.
    B. Infection precautions.
    C. Avoid hand washing.
    D. Strenuous exercise.

4. Clients who are at high risk for becoming neutropenic include
    A. clients who have normal bone marrow function.
    B. clients with tumor invasion of the bone marrow.
    C. clients with a high positive nitrogen balance.
    D. clients who received radiation to the lower left calf for sarcoma.

5. Growth factors for neutrophils are usually initiated when
    A. chemotherapy dose is reduced.
    B. anemia persists.
    C. a client experienced a previous febrile neutropenic episode with chemotherapy administration.
    D. a client is undergoing radiation.

6. Clients at high risk for development of thrombocytopenia include those with
    A. high doses of interferon.
    B. normal bone marrow function.
    C. hypercoagulation disorders such as paraneoplastic syndromes.
    D. growth factor administration.

7. The most common method for transmitting infectious organisms to clients is
    A. direct contact.
    B. indirect contact.
    C. airborne transmission.
    D. blood transfusion.

8. Risk factors for infection include
    A. altered mucosal barriers.

B. trimming fingernails and toenails.
C. daily bathing.
D. strict hand washing.

9. Hemorrhage can result from
   A. chemotherapy administration.
   B. platelet count of 120,000/mm^3.
   C. hematocrit of 30%.
   D. disseminated intravascular coagulation (DIC).

10. Fever can result from
    A. strict hand washing.
    B. biotherapy agents.
    C. all chemotherapy agents.
    D. good personal hygiene.

11. Clients who experience the following are at a high risk for fever:
    A. An ANC of 2000/mm^3.
    B. Platelet count of 100,000/mm^3.
    C. Are 2 weeks postoperative.
    D. Have central nervous system and hepatic metastasis.

12. Ms. C. calls the clinic and reports a fever of 101° F (38.3° C) for the past 24 hours. This fever would not be uncommon if the client received any of the following:
    A. Bleomycin (Blenoxane) administration.
    B. Indomethacin for bone metastasis.
    C. Acetaminophen for headache.
    D. Chemotherapy peripherally.

13. Comfort measures that should be instituted when the client is experiencing a fever include
    A. have the client wear extra clothing.
    B. avoid use of acetaminophen.
    C. provide tepid sponge baths.
    D. avoid changing damp clothing.

14. Which of the following disorders is associated with anemia?
    A. Decrease in red blood cells (RBCs).
    B. Decrease in white blood cells (WBCs).
    C. Decrease in platelets.
    D. Decrease in myocytes.

15. Neutrophils arise from the following stem cell line:
    A. Lymphoid stem cells.
    B. Megakaryocyte stem cells.
    C. Myeloid stem cells.
    D. Epithelial stem cells.

16. Ms. D. presents to the clinic 20 days after treatment for a follow-up complete blood count. Her ANC remains below 500/mm^3. The nurse is concerned that Ms. D's prolonged neutropenia could lead to
    A. thrombocytopenia.
    B. disseminated intravascular coagulation.
    C. tumor lysis syndrome.
    D. sepsis.

17. The normal life span of platelets is
    A. 1 to 3 days.
    B. 4 to 5 days.
    C. 6 to 7 days.
    D. 8 to 10 days.

18. When 1 unit of platelets is administered in the presence of bleeding or when the platelet count is less than 10,000/mm^3, the nurse should monitor the platelet count for an overall increase of platelets by
    A. 10,000/mm^3.
    B. 20,000/mm^3.
    C. 30,000/mm^3.
    D. 40,000/mm^3.

19. Leukocyte-depleted filters are used in administering blood products to eliminate
    A. RBCs.
    B. platelets.
    C. WBCs.
    D. blood clots.

20. The following bleeding precaution orders have been written for a client with a platelet count of 10,000/mm^3. Which of the following orders should the nurse question?
    A. Avoid using a blood pressure cuff or tourniquet.
    B. Administer rectal acetaminophen for fever of 101° F (38.3° C).
    C. Apply firm pressure to venipuncture sites for 5 minutes.
    D. Administer stool softener twice a day.

21. The most important physical barrier against invasion of organisms is
    A. venous access device.
    B. skin.

C. oral cavity.

D. immune system.

22. The following neutropenic precautions have been written for a client with an ANC of $200/mm^3$. Which of the following orders should the nurse question?

A. Strict hand washing.

B. Daily personal hygiene.

C. Maintain fluid intake at 500 ml/8 hr.

D. Avoid enemas.

23. The potential sequelae of prolonged hemorrhage is

A. neutropenia.

B. infection.

C. shock.

D. blood clots.

24. A client is experiencing chills after receiving interleukin-2 (IL-2). The multidisciplinary team discusses how best to manage his chills and recommends that which of the following be administered?

A. Meperidine.

B. Indomethacin.

C. Acetaminophen.

D. Ibuprofen.

25. Normally, the body temperature is controlled by the thermoregulatory center located in the

A. kidney.

B. hypothalamus.

C. cerebellum.

D. parathyroid.

26. Granulocytes collectively include

A. neutrophils, basophils, and eosinophils.

B. neutrophils, lymphocytes, and basophils.

C. monocytes, lymphocytes, and eosinophils.

D. lymphocytes, neutrophils, and basophils.

27. Ms. B. presents to the clinic for her fourth course of chemotherapy for breast cancer. The ANC is $1000/mm^3$. What would be the next step?

A. Proceed with planned chemotherapy.

B. Admit Ms. B. to the hospital for hydration.

C. Begin antibiotics immediately.

D. Teach Ms. B. infection precautions and what symptoms should prompt her to call the physician or nurse.

28. Which measure would be important to follow for a client with an ANC less than $500/mm^3$?

A. Take a rectal temperature regularly.

B. Administer broad-spectrum antibiotics.

C. Send fresh flowers to the room.

D. Avoid bathing for 2 days.

29. Clients are at a severe risk of infection when the

A. hemoglobin value is less than 10 g/dl.

B. platelet count is less than $20,000/mm^3$.

C. ANC is less than $1500/mm^3$.

D. ANC is less than $500/mm^3$.

30. Clients are at a severe risk of bleeding when

A. neutrophils are 50%.

B. lymphocytes are 30%.

C. platelets are less than $20,000 mm^3$.

D. basophils are 0%.

31. Mr. H. returns to the clinic to receive his sixth course of etoposide (VP-16) and cisplatin (Platinol) for small cell lung cancer. After obtaining his blood counts, the platelet level is reported to be $30,000 mm^3$. What would be your next step?

A. Administer platelets immediately.

B. Teach Mr. H. about bleeding precautions and what symptoms should prompt him to seek medical attention.

C. Proceed with chemotherapy.

D. Call hospice for placement.

32. Nadir is a term used to describe

A. the highest point the WBCs reach after cancer treatment.

B. WBC lysis related to chemotherapy administration.

C. DNA content of the WBC.

D. the lowest point blood cells reach after a cancer treatment.

33. What is a major concern when administering amphotericin B?

A. Diarrhea.
B. Myelosuppression.
C. Fever and chills.
D. Hypersensitivity rash.

34. Ms. Z. arrives at the hospital emergency room with fever, chills, and malaise. Her signs and symptoms are indicative of
   A. anemia.
   B. thrombocytopenia.
   C. superior vena cava syndrome.
   D. infection caused by neutropenia.

35. The client should be instructed to contact the physician immediately if which of the following side effects occurs?
   A. Nosebleed that will not stop after applying pressure.
   B. Temperature of 99° F (37° C).
   C. One episode of nausea without vomiting after chemotherapy.
   D. Body hair begins to fall out after chemotherapy.

36. Which of the following drugs can produce a fever?
   A. Interferon, methotrexate, Adriamycin.
   B. Interferon, interleukin, vancomycin.
   C. Interleukin-2, penicillin, amphotericin B.
   D. Tumor necrosis factor, gentamycin, vancomycin.

37. Mr. S. presents to the clinic with a temperature of 102° F (38.3° C). What initial question would you ask in taking his history to determine risk for infection?
   A. Have you recently been treated for your cancer with chemotherapy, radiation, or biotherapy?
   B. Have you recently been outside the United States?
   C. Are you still taking your coumadin every day?
   D. Have you been experiencing dizziness, fatigue, or shortness of breath?

38. Ms. W. returns for her next chemotherapy treatment; however, her ANC is 1300/mm^3. Which cells of the WBC differential will predict the recovery of neutrophils?
   A. Eosinophils.
   B. Monocytes.

C. Basophils.
D. Neutrophils.

39. Myelosuppression is defined as the reduction in bone marrow function that results in a reduced release of which cells into the peripheral circulation?
   A. RBCs, megakaryocytes, and tumor necrosis factor.
   B. RBCs, WBCs, and platelets.
   C. WBCs, erythroblasts, and colony-stimulating factors.
   D. Platelets, RBCs, and interleukin.

40. Neutropenia describes a decrease in the number of circulating
   A. basophils.
   B. WBCs.
   C. neutrophils.
   D. RBCs.

41. Neutrophils are the first line of the body's defense against
   A. destroying viruses that invade the body.
   B. destroying bacterial infection.
   C. destroying fungal infection.
   D. destroying parasites.

42. Radiation to which of the following areas can result in myelosuppression?
   A. Ilia, vertebrae, ribs, skull, sternum, and long bones.
   B. Tibia, ribs, skull, and sternum.
   C. Ulna, sternum, and vertebrae.
   D. Skull, ribs, patella, and metacarpals.

43. The nurse should recognize that steroids will mask the occurrence of an infection by
   A. competing at the complement site with tumor necrosis factor.
   B. decreasing the production of B cells.
   C. preventing the migration of neutrophils to the bacteria.
   D. preventing the antigen and antibody reaction.

44. Antiviral mediations are usually administered to the febrile neutropenic client when
   A. the ANC is less than 500/mm^3.
   B. the fever continues for 3 days, after antibiotics are initiated.

C. the client has undergone high-dose chemotherapy.

D. mucosal lesions or viral disease is suspected.

45. Hematopoietic growth factors are administered to
   A. prevent neutropenia.
   B. prevent anemia.
   C. promote proliferation and differentiation of progenitor cells along multiple cell pathways.
   D. promote the proliferation and differentiation of interleukin.

46. When the client's nadir persists for more than 7 to 10 days, the risk increases for
   A. severe infection.
   B. compromised myelosuppression.
   C. resistant organisms to treatment.
   D. severe blood clots.

47. As the neutrophils decrease, the only sign of infection may be
   A. purulent drainage from a vascular access device.
   B. petechiae on the lower extremities.
   C. fever.
   D. dry, hacking cough.

48. The best measure to institute to prevent infection in the client with low ANC is
   A. encourage visitors.
   B. encourage the client to bathe every 2 days.
   C. strict hand washing.
   D. use of a laminar flow room.

49. Thrombocytopenia describes
   A. a decrease in the circulating platelets below $100,000/mm^3$.
   B. a decrease in the circulating WBCs below $1500/mm^3$.
   C. a decrease in the circulating neutrophils below $1000/mm^3$.
   D. a decrease in the circulating RBCs below $1000/mm^3$.

50. After chemotherapy administration, the platelet count usually decreases

A. before the WBCs decrease.
B. in 7 to 14 days after the administration of chemotherapy.
C. after the RBCs decrease.
D. in 28 days after chemotherapy administration.

51. Some medications that can alter platelet function are
   A. aspirin, indomethacin, and digoxin.
   B. milk of magnesia, heparin, and quinidine.
   C. senna, furosemide, and phenytoin.
   D. acetaminophen, sulfonamides, and penicillin.

52. If the client is at high risk for infection, measures that can be initiated to minimize the occurrence are
   A. inserting a urinary catheter to monitor the urine output.
   B. leaving all wounds to open air.
   C. encouraging daily personal hygiene, oral hygiene, and perineal care.
   D. flushing all lumens of a long-term catheter every 8 hours.

53. Hemorrhage describes the occurrence of
   A. platelet count less than $100,000/mm^3$.
   B. RBC count less than $100,000/mm^3$.
   C. abnormal internal or external bleeding.
   D. fibrinogen level less than 30 ml.

54. Consequence of prolonged hemorrhage includes
   A. shock.
   B. increase in fluid volume.
   C. decrease in circulating cancer cells.
   D. increase in cardiac output.

55. Prolonged fever and chills experienced by the client can lead to
   A. increase in fatigue.
   B. decrease in circulating cancer cells.
   C. increase in activity.
   D. decrease in the occurrence of infection.

ANSWERS

1. *Answer:* A
Rationale: Poor nutritional status contributes to a depressed immune system because the body lacks the necessary nutrients and protein to regenerate normal cells. Options B, C, and D do not interfere with the immune system.

2. *Answer:* A
Rationale: Aspirin and ibuprofen have the tendency to inhibit platelet function. Options B, C, and D do not interfere with platelet function.

3. *Answer:* B
Rationale: Infection precautions are important to emphasize in the teaching plan with a client with a low ANC. Options B, C, and D are incorrect points to include in teaching a client about low ANC, because fresh flowers and poor hygiene contribute to infection while exercise has no relationship to infection.

4. *Answer:* B
Rationale: Clients with tumor invasion of the bone marrow are at a higher risk for neutropenia because of a smaller reserve of normal cells. Clients with a high negative nitrogen balance are at a high risk for neutropenia because of poor nutritional status. Clients who receive radiation to a major bone marrow production site such as the sternum, skull, pelvic, or long bones will be at a risk for becoming neutropenic.

5. *Answer:* C
Rationale: If the chemotherapy dose is reduced and will not compromise the goal of cancer treatment, growth factor is not recommended. However, if the dose cannot be reduced, growth factor would be prescribed. Growth factors for neutrophils are not prescribed for anemia or clients undergoing radiation.

6. *Answer:* C
Rationale: Clients who have a hypercoagulation state from a paraneoplastic syndrome are at risk for thrombocytopenia. Although bio-therapy agents modulate the immune system, the potential for alteration of the blood cells remains unknown. The occurrence of thrombocytopenia after high doses of interferon has not been evident in clinical studies. Normal bone marrow function and growth factors do not place clients at risk for thrombocytopenia.

7. *Answer:* A
Rationale: Each method can transmit organisms to the client. The most common method to transmit infectious organisms is direct contact.

8. *Answer:* A
Rationale: Altered mucosal barriers such as mucositis increase the client's risk for infection. Options B, C, and D assist in preventing infections.

9. *Answer:* D
Rationale: A manifestation of DIC is hemorrhage. Hemorrhage does not occur from chemotherapy administration, platelet count greater than $100,000/mm^3$, or hematocrit above 30%.

10. *Answer:* B
Rationale: Biotherapy agents can cause fever. Only a few chemotherapy agents can cause a fever. Strict hand washing and good personal hygiene assists in preventing infections with subsequent fever.

11. *Answer:* D
Rationale: Clients with central nervous system and hepatic metastasis are at risk for tumor-induced fever. Clients with an ANC of $2000/mm^3$ are not at a high risk for a fever. Platelet counts do not contribute to a fever. Clients who are 2 weeks from an operative procedure are unlikely to experience a fever.

12. *Answer:* A
Rationale: A side effect of bleomycin is fever. Indomethacin and acetaminophen are often given to reduce tumor-induced fever. Giving chemotherapy peripherally does not produce a fever.

13. *Answer:* C
    Rationale: Reducing the amount of clothing worn by the client and administering acetaminophen can provide comfort during a fever episode. Changing damp clothing and providing tepid sponge baths can also provide comfort during a fever.

14. *Answer:* A
    Rationale: Anemia is a decrease in RBCs. A decrease in WBCs is associated with neutropenia. A decrease in platelets is associated with thrombocytopenia. A decrease in myocytes (cardiac cells) is associated with cardiotoxicity.

15. *Answer:* C
    Rationale: Neutrophils arise from the myeloid stem cells. Lymphoid stem cells give rise to lymphocytes. Megakaryocyte is an immature platelet. Epithelial stem cells give rise to skin cells.

16. *Answer:* D
    Rationale: Prolonged neutropenia can result in sepsis and septic shock. Options A, B, and C do not occur from prolonged neutropenia.

17. *Answer:* D
    Rationale: The normal life span of platelets is 8 to 10 days.

18. *Answer:* A
    Rationale: One unit of platelets should increase the peripheral blood level approximately 10,000 to 12,000 cells/mm^3.

19. *Answer:* C
    Rationale: Leukocyte-depleted filters are used to eliminate WBCs from the blood product to prevent alloimmunization.

20. *Answer:* B
    Rationale: Invasive procedures such as rectal medications should be avoided in clients with thrombocytopenia. Options A, C, and D are bleeding precautions.

21. *Answer:* B
    Rationale: The most important physical barrier against invasion of organisms is the skin. Breakdown of the skin is a portal entry for organisms.

22. *Answer:* C
    Rationale: Adequate hydration and a high-calorie, high-protein diet must be maintained. Options A, B, and D are neutropenic precautions.

23. *Answer:* C
    Rationale: The potential sequela of prolonged hemorrhage is shock. Neutropenia, infection, and blood clots are not associated with hemorrhage.

24. *Answer:* A
    Rationale: Meperidine is administered to relieve chills. Options B, C, and D are administered as a comfort measure for fever.

25. *Answer:* B
    Rationale: The thermoregulatory center is located in the hypothalamus.

26. *Answer:* A
    Rationale: Option A lists the cells referred to as granulocytes.

27. *Answer:* D
    Rationale: Option D is the correct response to teach Ms. B. what measures to take to prevent infection and when to call for medical assistance. A WBC count could reflect Ms. B.'s immune system's ability to fight infection, but an ANC is more reflective because the neutrophils can be low when the WBC count is normal. Option A is incorrect because most physicians do not administer chemotherapy if the ANC is less than 1500/ mm^3 or the WBC count is less than 1000/mm^3. Options B and C are incorrect because the client does not have a fever or signs of dehydration.

28. *Answer:* B
    Rationale: Options A, C, and D are not appropriate infection precautions. Broad-spectrum antibiotics should be administered to prevent further untoward effects of the infections such as sepsis.

29. *Answer:* D
    Rationale: Option D is correct. The risk for infection is higher when the ANC is below 1000/mm^3. Option A refers to anemia; Option B refers to thrombocytopenia; Option C, the ANC is not low.

30. *Answer:* C
Rationale: Options A, B, and D refer to the WBCs. Option C is correct because levels of platelets below 20,000/mm^3 increase the client's risk for severe bleeding.

31. *Answer:* B
Rationale: Option B is correct because the client is at risk for spontaneous bleeding and should follow bleeding precautions. Option A is incorrect. Unless the client is actively bleeding, platelets are usually administered for levels of 20,000/mm^3 or lower. Option C is incorrect. Chemotherapy is usually held if the platelet count is less than 100,000/mm^3. Option D is incorrect because there is no indication the patient is terminally ill.

32. *Answer:* D
Rationale: Options A, B, and C do not give the correct definition of nadir. Nadir refers to the lowest point.

33. *Answer:* C
Rationale: Amphotericin B can cause fever and chills during administration.

34. *Answer:* D
Rationale: These are signs of infection.

35. *Answer:* A
Rationale: A nosebleed that is difficult to control should alert the nurse that the client may have a low platelet count.

36. *Answer:* B
Rationale: All of these drugs can induce fever.

37. *Answer:* A
Rationale: This information would provide the nurse with the approximate time to expect the client's nadir and to suspect an infection with the presentation of fever.

38. *Answer:* B
Rationale: The monocyte count is usually elevated before the neutrophils recover.

39. *Answer:* B
Rationale: RBCs, WBCs, and platelets are mature cells that are released into the peripheral circulation from the bone marrow.

40. *Answer:* C
Rationale: A decrease in neutrophils in the blood is referred to as neutropenia.

41. *Answer:* B
Rationale: Neutrophils provide the first line of the body's defense against bacterial infection by localizing and neutralizing bacteria.

42. *Answer:* A
Rationale: Radiation of 20 Gy or more to the major bone marrow production sites will result in myelosuppression.

43. *Answer:* C
Rationale: Steroids prevent migration of neutrophils to the bacteria and the process of phagocytosis.

44. *Answer:* D
Rationale: Antiviral drugs are usually not initiated unless the client is undergoing a bone marrow transplant or the client exhibits signs of a virus such as an oral lesion.

45. *Answer:* C
Rationale: Hematopoietic growth factors promote the proliferation and differentiation of hematopoietic progenitor cells along multiple pathways. Growth factors do not prevent neutropenia or anemia but promote the production of the cells in anemic or neutropenic clients.

46. *Answer:* A
Rationale: When the client experiences a prolonged nadir, the risk for severe infection increases.

47. *Answer:* C
Rationale: Fever may be the only response to an infection because of the inhibition of phagocytic cells; therefore, erythema, inflammation, and drainage may be minimal or absent.

48. *Answer:* C
Rationale: Strict hand washing will prevent up to 90% of exogenous organisms that come into direct contact with the client.

49. *Answer:* A
Rationale: When platelet levels drop below 100,000/mm^3, the client has thrombocytopenia.

50. **Answer:** B
    Rationale: Platelet counts usually decrease in 7 to 14 days after administration of chemotherapy after the decrease in WBCs.

51. **Answer:** A
    Rationale: All of these drugs, aspirin, indomethacin, and digoxin, can alter platelet function.

52. **Answer:** C
    Rationale: Promoting meticulous hygiene can minimize the occurrence of organisms colonizing.

53. **Answer:** C
    Rationale: Hemorrhage is the result of abnormal internal or external bleeding.

54. **Answer:** A
    Rationale: Shock will occur with a decrease in fluid volume, which will result in decreased cardiac output and decreased tissue perfusion.

55. **Answer:** A
    Rationale: Prolonged fever and chills result in metabolic activity and oxygen consumption, which lead to an increase of fatigue.

BIBLIOGRAPHY

Adams, V.R. (2000). Adverse events associated with chemotherapy for common cancers. *Pharmacotherapy 20,* 96-103.

Barber, F.D. (2001). Management of fever in neutropenic patients with cancer. *Nursing Clinics of North America 36,* 631-644.

Begley, C.G., & Basser, R.L. (2000). Biologic and structural differences of thrombopoietic growth factors. *Seminars in Hematology 37*(Suppl 4), 19-27.

Boxer, L., & Dale, D.C. (2002). Neutropenia: Causes and consequences. *Seminars in Hematology 39,* 75-81.

Buchsel, P.C., Forgey, A., Grape, F.B., & Hamann, S.S. (2002). Granulocyte macrophage colony-stimulating factor: Current practice and novel approaches. *Clinical Journal of Oncology Nursing 6,* 198-205.

Dale, D.C. (2002). Colony-stimulating factors for the management of neutropenia in cancer patients. *Drugs 62*(Suppl 1), 1-15.

Demetiri, G.D. (2000). Pharmacologic treatment options in patients with thrombocytopenia. *Seminars in Hematology 37*(Suppl 4), 11-18.

Ellerhorst-Ryan, J.M. (2000). Infection. In C.H. Yarbro, M.H. Frogge, M. Goodman, & S. Groenwald (Eds.). *Cancer nursing: Principles and practice* (5th ed.). Sudbury, MA: Jones and Barlett Publishers, pp. 691-708.

Ezzone, S.A. (2000). Fever. In D. Camp-Sorrell & R. Hawkins (Eds.). *Clinical manual for the oncology advanced practice nurse.* Pittsburgh: Oncology Nursing Society, pp. 813-824.

Glauser, M.P. (2000). Neutropenia: Clinical implications and modulation. *Intensive Care Medicine 26,* S103-S110.

Gobel, B.H. (2000). Bleeding. In C.H. Yarbro, M.H. Frogge, M. Goodman, & S. Groenwald (Eds.). *Cancer nursing: Principles and practice* (5th ed.). Sudbury, MA: Jones and Barlett Publishers, pp. 709-736.

Koh, A., & Pizzo, P.A. (2002). Empirical oral antibiotic therapy for low risk febrile cancer patients with neutropenia. *Cancer Investigation 20,* 420-433.

Lynch, M.P. (2000a). Neutropenia. In D. Camp-Sorrell & R. Hawkins (Eds.). *Clinical manual for the oncology advanced practice nurse.* Pittsburgh: Oncology Nursing Society, pp. 693-698.

Lynch, M.P. (2000b). Thrombocytopenia. In D. Camp-Sorrell & R. Hawkins (Eds.). *Clinical manual for the oncology advanced practice nurse.* Pittsburgh: Oncology Nursing Society, pp. 703-707.

McCullough, J. (2000). Current issues with platelet transfusion in patients with cancer. *Seminars in Hematology 37*(Suppl 4), 3-10.

The Medical Letter. (2002). Pegfilgrastim (Neulasta) for prevention of febrile neutropenia. *The Medical Letter 44,* 44-45.

Ozer, H., Armitage, J. O., Bennett, C. L., et al. (2000). 2000 update of recommendations for the use of hematopoietic colony-stimulating factors: Evidence-based, clinical practice guidelines. *Journal of Clinical Oncology 18,* 3558-3585.

Rust, D. M., Simpson, J. K., & Lister, J. (2000). Nutritional issues in patients with severe neutropenia. *Seminars in Oncology Nursing 16,* 152-162.

PART THREE

GASTROINTESTINAL AND URINARY FUNCTION

14 Alterations in Nutrition

VALERIE KOGUT

Select the best answer for each of the following questions:

1. Which of the following is a key assessment factor of a client with xerostomia?
   - A. Overall status of teeth and gums.
   - B. Pattern of elimination.
   - C. Increased fatigue.
   - D. Pain.

2. Which of the following is a causative factor of anorexia?
   - A. Narcotics.
   - B. Candidiasis.
   - C. Diabetes.
   - D. Steroids.

3. Which of the following is a complication of xerostomia that would require medical intervention?
   - A. Aspiration pneumonia.
   - B. Infection in the oral cavity.
   - C. Constipation.
   - D. Weight gain of 10 pounds.

4. Which of the following is an important factor to consider in the assessment of taste alterations in persons with cancer?
   - A. Taste alterations can lead to anorexia.
   - B. Taste alterations can lead to positive nitrogen balance.
   - C. Taste alterations can lead to dysphagia.
   - D. Taste alterations can indicate disease progression.

5. Which of the following is appropriate for managing taste alterations?
   - A. Use commercial mouthwashes such as Scope or Listerine to eliminate the bacteria that cause bad taste.
   - B. Suggest that the client try meat served hot.
   - C. Have the client suck on sugar-free lemon drops or other smooth, flat, tart candies to stimulate saliva.
   - D. Suggest doing oral care once a week.

6. Which of the following interventions helps to relieve nausea?
   - A. Eating fatty or fried foods.
   - B. Drinking caffeinated beverages.
   - C. Medicating with an antiemetic each time vomiting is experienced.
   - D. Medicating with an antiemetic on a round-the-clock basis until nausea subsides.

7. Which of the following statements about the use of corticosteroids in the management of vomiting are true?
   - A. Beware of classic steroid side effects, even when used for a short time.
   - B. Corticosteroids work well in combination with other antiemetics from highly emetogenic chemotherapy drugs.
   - C. The use of corticosteroids can cause a decrease in appetite.
   - D. The use of corticosteroids can lead to dysphagia.

8. Which of the following is a sequela of pro-longed anorexia?
   A. Constipation.
   B. Increase of lean body mass.
   C. Visceral mass depletion.
   D. Increased immune function.

9. Which of the following is a sign or symptom of dehydration?
   A. Esophagitis.
   B. Poor skin turgor.
   C. Increased urinary output.
   D. Improved wound healing.

10. Which of the following would be a measure used to provide moisture to the oral cavity?
    A. Encourage the client to decrease the amount of liquids he or she drinks.
    B. Encourage the client to eat Popsicles.
    C. Encourage the client to eat hot and spicy foods.
    D. Encourage the client to eat foods that he or she enjoys.

11. Which of the following is a type of mucositis?
    A. Gingivitis.
    B. Enteritis.
    C. Dysphagia.
    D. Xerostomia.

12. Which of the following would be an appropriate nursing diagnosis for potential complications of dysphagia?
    A. Alterations in protective mechanisms.
    B. Alterations in safety related to potential for aspiration.
    C. Alterations in elimination.
    D. Alterations in skin integrity.

13. A sign and symptom related to the syndrome of inappropriate antidiuretic hormone (SIADH) is
    A. constipation.
    B. fluid retention.
    C. serum hypernatremia.
    D. low-grade fevers.

14. What is a hallmark sign of cachexia?
    A. Tissue wasting.
    B. Weight loss less than 10% of ideal body weight.

C. Nausea and vomiting.
D. Constipation.

15. Mr. M. will be having surgery in a week for prostate cancer. To help him get ready for the surgery, you tell him that
    A. surgery can increase his energy requirements 1.5 times what he normally needs.
    B. surgery, because of the bed rest required, will decrease his energy requirements.
    C. he should not be too concerned; surgery on his prostate should not have any direct involvement on his nutritional needs.
    D. nutritional problems resulting from his surgery will probably be long term.

16. Mr. S. has completed 2 weeks of radiation therapy and concomitant chemotherapy for carcinoma of the trachea. He complains of dysphagia, odynophagia, and occasional epigastric pain. He is most likely experiencing which of the following?
    A. Reflux.
    B. Tracheitis.
    C. Esophagitis.
    D. Bronchitis.

17. Which of the following chemotherapy agents is likely to potentiate the problem of esophagitis in clients also receiving radiation therapy to the esophagus?
    A. Cyclophosphamide (Cytoxan).
    B. 5-fluorouracil (5-Fu).
    C. Paclitaxel (Taxol).
    D. Busulfan (Myleran).

18. Mark has started radiation therapy to his right leg for a sarcoma. He experienced anorexia and slight nausea after his radiation treatment. You tell him that
    A. the waste products of tissue destruction are likely to cause his symptoms.
    B. because the radiation port does not include his stomach, it is not likely that his symptoms are related to the radiation.
    C. the likelihood is that the tumor is secreting substances that cause him to feel ill.
    D. the Cori cycle is breaking down the products of normal cell destruction and producing excess urea.

19. Betty has been given the diagnosis of unresectable lung cancer. She has not had an appetite for many weeks and is losing weight. What is the probable cause of her weight loss?
   A. Anorexia and cachexia are common manifestations of lung cancer.
   B. She is probably depressed over her situation.
   C. The chemotherapy and radiation cause weight loss.
   D. She most likely has liver disease, causing her loss of appetite.

20. Which of the following can be used to dissolve and break up thick saliva?
   A. Papain (found in papaya) and amylase (found in pineapple).
   B. Use of commercial mouthwashes.
   C. Drink caffeine-containing products such as coffee, tea, colas, and chocolate.
   D. Sialagogues.

21. Dan complains of a dry mouth after treatment and within several weeks develops thick, ropy saliva. Dan is experiencing the side effect of
   A. xerostomia.
   B. dysphagia.
   C. mucositis.
   D. trismus.

22. Miss M. is having radiation therapy as primary treatment for a pyriform sinus lesion. In describing xerostomia to Miss M., you are likely to discuss which of the following?
   A. The fact that the xerostomia is likely to be permanent.
   B. She can expect excessive saliva formation for at least 4 months after radiation.
   C. She will receive medication to minimize the severity of the xerostomia.
   D. Receiving chemotherapy will worsen the severity of the xerostomia.

23. Which of the following chemotherapy agents is associated with moderate to high incidence of emesis?
   A. Topotecan (Hycamtin).
   B. Busulfan.
   C. Idarubicin (Idamycin).
   D. Paclitaxel.

24. Your client is 30 years old and receiving doxorubicin and cyclophosphamide for her breast cancer. She feels jittery and nervous after her chemotherapy. She is taking ondansetron (Zofran) 24 mg, dexamethasone 10 mg, and prochlorperazine (Compazine) 15 mg according to her schedule. Which of the following actions would be most appropriate?
   A. Eliminate the dexamethasone from her protocol because it is making her jittery.
   B. Discontinue the prochlorperazine because she is allergic to it.
   C. Administer diphenhydramine (Benadryl) 25 mg with the prochlorperazine because she is young and likely to be sensitive to it.
   D. Discontinue both the dexamethasone and the prochlorperazine because either one can cause jitteriness and a hypersensitivity reaction.

25. Tom complains that food does not taste the same and that everything tastes like cardboard, especially red meat. This is best explained by the fact that persons with cancer may experience
   A. an increased threshold for sweet, sour, and salt and a decreased threshold for bitter foods.
   B. a decreased threshold for sweet, sour, and salt and increased threshold for bitter foods.
   C. difficulty digesting their foods.
   D. intolerance to bland foods.

26. Mr. J. is undergoing chemotherapy for high-grade testes cancer. He feels jittery, and his lab tests indicate low magnesium, albumin, and calcium. He is most likely experiencing which of the following complications of chemotherapy?
   A. Anorexia and weakness caused by chemotherapy.
   B. Low magnesium caused by cisplatin therapy.
   C. Low calcium caused by uremia syndrome.
   D. A paraneoplastic syndrome.

27. Which of the following metabolic disorders is common in clients receiving cisplatin therapy?
   A. Hyperkalemia.
   B. Hypomagnesemia.

C. Hypophosphatemia.
D. Hypercalcemia.

28. In trying to determine how much weight Paul has lost over what span of time, you learn that he is 5 feet 10 inches tall and weighed 170 pounds 1 year ago. Four months ago, he weighed 160 pounds, and now he weighs 132 pounds. What is the percentage of Paul's weight change in the past 4 months?
    A. 10%.
    B. 17%.
    C. 22%.
    D. 25%.

29. You want to choose an instrument that will give a complete diet history of a patient. The client has already told you that she doesn't pay much attention to what she eats and has a hard time remembering what she had for lunch yesterday. She is very upset about her recent diagnosis, which has changed her eating habits considerably. But she is willing to cooperate with you, and she understands the importance of being honest with you. The client is in the hospital now, but she will not be there for most of her treatment. You choose
    A. a calorie count.
    B. 24-hour dietary recall.
    C. a food frequency record.
    D. a diet diary.

30. Many women will gain weight and even become obese after adjuvant chemotherapy for breast cancer. What percentage of women on adjuvant chemotherapy for breast cancer gain weight?
    A. 10% to 20%.
    B. 30% to 35%.
    C. 40% to 70%.
    D. 80% to 90%.

31. Scott requests an appetite stimulant, and considering his condition, you are quite happy to find something appropriate for him. Scott is on an extensive chemotherapy regimen, is diabetic, and has not had problems with nausea or vomiting. Which of the following is the best possible medication for him?
    A. Cannabinoids.
    B. Corticosteroids.
    C. Metoclopramide (Reglan).
    D. Megestrol acetate (Megace).

32. Cancer-associated nutritional problems, rather than treatment-related nutritional problems, are best reversed by
    A. extensive nutrition counseling.
    B. self-care actions.
    C. medications.
    D. successful treatment of the tumor.

33. At what stage does nutritional intervention have the best chance to alter client outcome?
    A. Early, before treatment begins.
    B. Later, when the malignancy is aggressive.
    C. During treatment.
    D. After treatment has ended.

34. Mr. G. complains of pain in his throat and difficulty swallowing. The nurse practitioner suggests sucralfate (Carafate) suspension. The sucralfate is intended to accomplish which of the following?
    A. Pain control only.
    B. Promote healing by reducing infection.
    C. Promote comfort by numbing exposed nerve endings.
    D. Promote comfort and possibly healing by binding to exposed mucosa.

35. An elderly man presents with a thyroid mass and symptoms of dyspnea and dysphagia. Assessment indicates anaplastic carcinoma of the thyroid with metastases to the lung. His symptoms of dyspnea and dysphagia are most likely the result of
    A. infection caused by irritation of the oral mucosa.
    B. compressive effects of the tumor on the esophagus and larynx.
    C. a high concentration of iodine in the follicular cells of the thyroid.
    D. involvement of the parathyroid gland and associated hypocalcemia.

36. Dysphagia is the most common complaint of persons with which of the following?
    A. Tracheal cancer.
    B. Esophageal cancer.
    C. Skin cancer.
    D. Laryngeal cancer.

37. Your client has aspiration pneumonia from a tracheoesophageal fistula. The physician

has ordered scopolamine three to four times a day as needed. You explain to the client and family that the purpose of the scopolamine is which of the following?

    A. To decrease anxiety.

    B. To manage his nausea.

    C. To help manage dyspnea.

    D. To decrease the amount of secretions.

38. Betty has metastatic cancer. She complains she is having trouble eating and is steadily losing weight. Her doctor prescribes megestrol acetate 400 mg/day. Your teaching plans include which of the following?

    A. The purpose of the megestrol acetate is to increase her appetite.

    B. The purpose of the megestrol acetate is to treat her cancer.

    C. The side effects of megestrol acetate are edema and hyperglycemia.

    D. If she has congestive heart failure, she should not take megestrol acetate.

39. Miss P. has anorexia and says nothing tastes good. Which of the following medications would be most beneficial in helping her to combat her anorexia and gain weight?

    A. Steroids.

    B. Hydrazine.

    C. Dronabinol.

    D. Megestrol acetate.

40. Which of the following best explains the etiology of anorexia-cachexia syndrome?

    A. Uncontrolled nausea and vomiting.

    B. Loss of appetite resulting from food aversions.

    C. Reduced food intake resulting from tumor by-products.

    D. Multiple physiologic and metabolic abnormalities.

41. Xerostomia, a decrease in saliva secretion, is a side effect of

    A. oral surgery.

    B. busulfan administration.

    C. head and neck irradiation.

    D. bone marrow transplantation (BMT).

42. One of the primary problems with xerostomia is

    A. enamel decalcification.

    B. lack of pH balance in the mouth.

    C. diminished protection from fungal infections.

    D. increased esophageal and tracheal irritation.

43. An example of a chemotherapeutic agent that may cause a metallic taste during administration, leading to taste changes, is

    A. paclitaxel.

    B. etoposide.

    C. bleomycin

    D. cyclophosphamide.

44. Which of the following tests is used to determine protein status?

    A. Body mass index (BMI).

    B. Orthostatic vital signs.

    C. Daily weight.

    D. Midarm muscle circumference.

45. Mr. B. had an allogenic BMT 3 weeks ago and suffers from chronic diarrhea. A cause for his diarrhea is most likely which of the following?

    A. Graft-versus-host disease (GVHD).

    B. A high-fiber diet.

    C. Viral infection.

    D. Herpes simplex.

46. Which of the following antineoplastic agents can cause anorexia?

    A. Bleomycin (Blenoxane).

    B. Carboplatin (Paraplatin).

    C. Chlorambucil (Leukeran).

    D. Dacarbazine (DTIC-Dome).

47. Which of the following medications can cause mucositis and esophagitis?

    A. 5-fluorouracil.

    B. Busulfan.

    C. Docetaxel (Taxotere).

    D. Irinotecan (Camptosar).

48. Base of tongue resection can lead to which of the following postsurgical complications?

    A. Dry mouth.

    B. Nausea and vomiting.

    C. Compromised swallowing and aspiration potential.

    D. Diarrhea.

49. Which of the following interventions can be helpful in the management of a chyle fistula?

A. High-fat diet or formula.
B. Medium chain triglyceride formula or supplementation.
C. Use of a thickening agent.
D. Zinc sulfate lozenges.

50. Hypertriglyceridemia can be a postsurgical complication of which type of cancer?
    A. Esophagogastric.
    B. Pancreas.
    C. Gallbladder.
    D. Hepatocellular.

51. Which of the following foods are high in pectin?
    A. Chicken.
    B. Tuna.
    C. Salmon.
    D. Apples.

52. Which of the following herbal products has been helpful for clients with nausea and vomiting?
    A. Ginger.
    B. Echinacea.
    C. Milk thistle.
    D. Essiac.

53. Which of the following is a cause of anorexia?
    A. Hypocalcemia.
    B. Hyperkalemia.
    C. Hypernatremia.
    D. Tumor lysis syndrome.

54. Radiation therapy of 10 to 20 Gy results in what percent decrease in saliva?
    A. 10%.
    B. 25%.
    C. 50%.
    D. 75%.

55. Grade 1 mucositis is described as
    A. erythema of oral mucosa.
    B. isolated small white patches and ulcerations.
    C. confluent ulcerations covering less than 25% of oral mucosa.
    D. hemorrhagic ulceration.

56. Hypermagnesemia can be caused by
    A. adrenal insufficiency.
    B. antibiotics.
    C. liver failure.
    D. diuretics.

57. Nutritional education for a client with anorexia would include to:
    A. add nonfat dry milk powder to foods.
    B. consume three meals a day.
    C. drink liquids immediately before meals.
    D. increase the use of fresh fruits and vegetables.

58. A family member is caring for a bedbound hospice client. In teaching the caregiver about the client's food intake, it is important to
    A. encourage intake but not force the client to eat.
    B. offer dietary supplements every 4 hours.
    C. monitor the client's weight daily.
    D. eat six small meals every day.

59. A client with dysphagia is experiencing a high fever, coughing, and midchest discomfort. These symptoms suggest
    A. reflux.
    B. esophagitis.
    C. aspiration pneumonia.
    D. congestive heart failure.

60. Mucositis is more likely to occur in which of the following malignant conditions?
    A. Melanoma.
    B. Bladder cancer.
    C. Breast cancer.
    D. Leukemia.

61. Surgery can increase energy requirements by
    A. 1.2 times normal dietary requirements.
    B. 1.5 times normal dietary requirements.
    C. 1.75 times normal dietary requirements.
    D. 2 times normal dietary requirements.

62. Why must fluid status be monitored in clients with cancer, especially in those undergoing surgery, chemotherapy, or radiation?
    A. They usually don't drink extra fluid during the day.
    B. They always drink extra fluid at night.
    C. Their weights are not usually recorded daily.

D. Treatment methods may contribute to alterations in fluid status.

63. Which of the following diets would be indicated for clients with increased requirements due to illness or injury?

A. Regular diet.
B. Vegetarian diet.
C. Soft diet.
D. High-protein/high-calorie diet.

NOTES

ANSWERS

1. *Answer:* A
   Rationale: Xerostomia relates to conditions of the oral cavity.

2. *Answer:* A
   Rationale: Side effects of medications such as narcotics, antibiotics, and iron can cause anorexia. Uncontrolled diabetes and steroid use can cause hyperphagia. Hyperphagia is a period of overeating.

3. *Answer:* B
   Rationale: Xerostomia is dryness of the mouth and can lead to the infection of the oral cavity. Aspiration pneumonia is a complication of dysphagia, not xerostomia. Weight gain and constipation are not complications of xerostomia.

4. *Answer:* A
   Rationale: Taste alterations can lead to a decrease in intake, which can lead to negative, not positive, nitrogen balance from decreased protein intake.

5. *Answer:* C
   Rationale: Sialagogues (sugar-free lemon drops or smooth, flat, tart candies) stimulate production of saliva, which can improve taste. Commercial mouthwashes contain alcohol, which dries the mucosa and may lead to further taste changes and mucosal damage. Meat served hot would not affect the taste changes, and cold foods are usually better tolerated. Dysphagia and disease progression are not related to taste alterations.

6. *Answer:* D
   Rationale: Antiemetics, like pain medication, should be given around the clock to prevent nausea. Medicating after vomiting does little to relieve nausea that preceded the emesis. Fatty or fried food intake may contribute to nausea, and caffeine does not affect nausea.

7. *Answer:* B
   Rationale: Corticosteroids are frequently combined with antiemetics such as granisetron (Kytril). Classic steroid side effects are not seen when steroids are used short-term to manage nausea and vomiting. They increase appetite and do not cause dysphagia.

8. *Answer:* C
   Rationale: Lean body mass depletion, visceral mass depletion, and decreased functioning of the immune system can all be results of prolonged anorexia. Bowel movements may be less frequent because of the lack of food intake; constipation is not a side effect of anorexia.

9. *Answer:* B
   Rationale: Poor skin turgor is a classic sign of dehydration. Esophagitis is a side effect of chemotherapy or radiation, not dehydration. Decreased urinary output and depressed wound healing occur with bouts of dehydration.

10. *Answer:* B
    Rationale: Some of the foods a client may like may be moist; other may be dry, spicy, or hot and would irritate the oral mucosa. Popsicles will wet the mouth and numb the mucosa. Decreasing intake of liquids will cause less moisture to be present.

11. *Answer:* B
    Rationale: Enteritis is mucositis of the intestines. Gingivitis is inflammation of the gum tissues, usually of dental origin. Dysphagia is difficulty swallowing, and xerostomia is a dry mouth.

12. *Answer:* B
    Rationale: One of the potential complications of dysphagia is aspiration. Elimination and skin integrity are not involved in swallowing.

13. *Answer:* B
    Rationale: Primary symptoms of SIADH are manifestations of water intoxication. Serum sodium would be low, not high, and fever is not associated.

14. *Answer:* A
    Rationale: Tissue wasting is the hallmark sign of cachexia. Weight loss of greater than

10% of body weight is significant for protein-calorie malnutrition. The other answers may occur but are not signs.

15. *Answer:* A
Rationale: Surgery can increase his energy requirements 1.5 times what his normal nutritional requirements are.

16. *Answer:* C
Rationale: The early symptoms of esophagitis include difficulty and pain on swallowing and epigastric pain. Esophageal pain that worsens indicates progressing esophagitis. The other answers involve different parts of the body.

17. *Answer:* B
Rationale: 5-fluorouracil produces an additive toxic effect with irradiation.

18. *Answer:* A
Rationale: Anorexia is probably related to the presence in the client's system of the waste products of tissue destruction. This side effect is systemic and not specific to the site of irradiation. The tumor does not secrete substances that would make the client anorectic. Radiation-induced cell changes are not "normal cell destruction."

19. *Answer:* A
Rationale: Anorexia and cancer cachexia are common manifestations of lung cancer; other factors are contributory.

20. *Answer:* A
Rationale: Papain and amylase are enzymatic agents that will break down the saliva. The other agents act as stimulants or increase the saliva or may be too drying.

21. *Answer:* A
Rationale: Xerostomia is a drying of the oral mucosa that results from loss of saliva due to damage that occurs to the salivary glands subsequent to radiation therapy. Dysphagia, mucositis, and trismus do not result in dry mouth. Trismus is contraction of the muscles of mastication. Dysphagia is inability to swallow or difficulty in swallowing.

22. *Answer:* A
Rationale: Some salivary function can return after the cessation of treatment, but the client should understand that xerostomia may be permanent. Medication is not always indicated. Chemotherapy does not usually affect xerostomia.

23. *Answer:* C
Rationale: Idarubicin has moderate to high emetogenic potential. The other agents have minimal to mild emetogenic potential.

24. *Answer:* C
Rationale: Younger clients are more sensitive to the effects of the prochlorperazine. The combination of prochlorperazine and diphenhydramine can help decrease these effects.

25. *Answer:* A
Rationale: The recognized tastes (sweet, sour, and bitter) are common. These threshold changes can lead to meat and other food aversions. Digestion is not involved, and bland foods would be tolerated.

26. *Answer:* B
Rationale: Cisplatin frequently causes hypomagnesemia, which manifests as shaking. Daily magnesium supplementation is indicated during cisplatin therapy, and electrolyte levels should be monitored frequently.

27. *Answer:* B
Rationale: Mineral changes related to platinum chemotherapy include hypomagnesemia, hypokalemia, hyperphosphatemia, and hypocalcemia.

28. *Answer:* B
Rationale: The percentage of Paul's weight change can be determined by subtracting his actual weight from his usual weight and dividing the result by the usual weight. This number is multiplied by 100 to get the actual percentage.

29. *Answer:* D
Rationale: Because your client's eating habits have changed considerably and because she is not going to be staying in the hospital for most of her treatment, both the calorie count method and 24-hour recall method are inappropriate. A food frequency would not be ideal because the client has a hard time remembering what she ate. A diet diary would provide you with an extended record of your client's

eating habits that would rely on her cooperation and honesty.

30. *Answer:* C
    Rationale: From 40% to 70% of women with breast cancer receiving adjuvant chemotherapy gain weight, and some become obese.

31. *Answer:* D
    Rationale: Corticosteroids are not indicated in Scott's case because he is a diabetic, and both metoclopramide and cannabinoids are indicated in cases of clients experiencing chemotherapy-induced nausea, which Scott is not experiencing. Diabetics using megestrol acetate must monitor themselves closely; the drug is indicated in this case because it increases appetite, causes weight gain, and improves quality of life.

32. *Answer:* D
    Rationale: Treatment-induced nutritional problems are often handled successfully by medication and self-care actions. Cancer-associated nutritional problems are best resolved by successful treatment of the malignancy. Extended nutritional counseling may or may not be beneficial based on individual compliance.

33. *Answer:* A
    Rationale: Early nutritional intervention, while the tumor is still small, has the best chance to alter client outcomes.

34. *Answer:* D
    Rationale: The sucralfate suspension is used to treat radiation- and chemotherapy-induced esophagitis. Answer D is the most comprehensive of the choices.

35. *Answer:* B
    Rationale: Because anaplastic carcinoma of the thyroid can rapidly invade surrounding structures, symptoms may occur that are related to compressive effects of the enlarging mass on adjacent structures. Infection, increased iron, and decreased calcium levels are associated with dyspnea or dysphagia.

36. *Answer:* B
    Rationale: Dysphagia is one of the classic symptoms of esophageal carcinoma.

37. *Answer:* D
    Rationale: Scopolamine is used to manage excessive salivation and respiratory tract secretions and does not decrease anxiety, manage nausea, or help with dyspnea.

38. *Answer:* A
    Rationale: Megestrol acetate has been found to improve appetite, cause weight gain, control nausea, and improve quality of life among individuals with cancer.

39. *Answer:* D
    Rationale: Megestrol acetate increases appetite and lean body mass and decreases the breakdown of fat reserves. The other medications may affect appetite but rarely result in weight gain.

40. *Answer:* D
    Rationale: Multiple physiologic and metabolic abnormalities interact in the development of anorexia-cachexia syndrome, which cannot be correlated by increased food intake alone.

41. *Answer:* C
    Rationale: Radiotherapy to the head and neck region destroys taste buds and cells responsible for saliva secretion, resulting in xerostomia. Oral surgery does not destroy cells responsible for saliva secretion. Busulfan is a chemotherapeutic agent with no effects on saliva production, and BMT shows no salivary secretion effects.

42. *Answer:* A
    Rationale: Saliva inhibits decalcification of tooth enamel. The pH in the mouth is not normally "balanced." Diminished protection from fungal infections does occur but is not a primary problem. The esophagus and trachea are too far down in the gastrointestinal tract to be primarily affected from a decrease in saliva.

43. *Answer:* D
    Rationale: A common complaint during intravenous administration of drugs such as nitrogen mustard, cisplatin, and cyclophosphamide is that they cause a metallic taste.

44. *Answer:* D
    Rationale: Midarm muscle circumference is believed to be an accurate indicator of pro-

status that correlates with serum albumin levels. BMI and daily weight only show general nutritional status and do not distinguish between fat and protein stores. Vital signs are independent of protein status.

45. *Answer:* A
Rationale: After allogeneic BMT, diarrhea is a prominent manifestation of gastrointestinal GVHD. A high-fiber diet and herpes infection would not cause diarrhea in any client, and viral infections may cause diarrhea but only in an acute manner.

46. *Answer:* A
Rationale: Anorexia is one of the nutritional implications related to Dacarbazine (DTIC-dome).

47. *Answer:* A
Rationale: Mucositis and esophagitis are nutritional implications related to 5-fluorouracil.

48. *Answer:* C
Rationale: Compromised swallowing and aspiration potential are common postsurgical complications of base of tongue resection. Dry mouth, nausea and vomiting, and diarrhea are postsurgical complications that are not specifically related to base of tongue resection.

49. *Answer:* B
Rationale: Chyle fistula is defined as a leakage of lymphatic fluid from the lymphatic vessels, typically accumulating in the thoracic or abdominal cavities, but occasionally manifesting as an external fistula. Low-fat diet or formula and medium chain triglyceride formula can be helpful in the management of chyle fistula. There is no need to thicken food. The fistula will close on its own, and additional zinc is not needed.

50. *Answer:* D
Rationale: Hypertriglyceridemia is one of the common postsurgical complications for surgery for hepatocellular cancer. Surgery to the esophagus, stomach, pancreas, and gallbladder does not affect triglyceride levels.

51. *Answer:* D
Rationale: Plant foods are high in pectin (apples, bananas, oatmeal, rice, potatoes) and can be helpful in reducing the transit time in clients with dumping syndrome.

52. *Answer:* A
Rationale: Ginger has been found to be useful in treating motion sickness. Antiemetic properties are due to the local action on the stomach, not on the central nervous system.

53. *Answer:* D
Rationale: Metabolic causes of anorexia include hypercalcemia, hypokalemia, uremia, and hyponatremia (tumor lysis syndrome).

54. *Answer:* C
Rationale: As dose and percentage of tissue irradiated increases, damage to tissues increases. Ten to 20 Gy results in a 50% decrease in saliva.

55. *Answer:* A
Rationale: Grades of oral mucositis: Grade 1 – erythema of the oral mucosa, Grade 2 – isolated small white patches and ulcerations, Grade 3 – confluent ulcerations covering less than 25% of oral mucosa, Grade 4 – hemorrhagic ulceration.

56. *Answer:* A
Rationale: Hypermagnesemia can be caused by adrenal insufficiency and renal failure.

57. *Answer:* A
Rationale: The calories and protein content of food can be increased by adding nonfat dry milk to various foods. Several small meals a day would increase intake. Liquids before meals would decrease intake. Fresh fruits and vegetables are generally low-calorie, low-protein, and have a high satiety value, which would not help to reach the goal of increased food intake.

58. *Answer:* A
Rationale: Forcing a client to eat can be counterproductive. The other choices are too aggressive for someone in hospice care.

59. *Answer:* C
Rationale: Aspiration and aspiration pneumonia are common consequences of dysphagia. Aspiration pneumonia is characterized by coughing, gagging, fever, and chest pain.

60. *Answer:* D
Rationale: Mucositis is two to three times more likely to occur in hematologic

malignancies than in solid tumors like melanoma, bladder, and breast cancer.

61. *Answer:* B

Rationale: Surgery can increase energy requirements by 28 kcal/kg/day or 1.5 times normal dietary requirements.

62. *Answer:* D

Rationale: Fluid status must be monitored routinely in the client with cancer, especially in those undergoing surgery, chemotherapy, or radiation, because treatment methods may contribute to alterations in fluid status. Weight, intake and output, and laboratory data are appropriate measures to use in daily assessing hydration status.

63. *Answer:* D

Rationale: High-protein/high-calorie diets are used to provide protein and calorie-rich foods for individuals with increased requirements. A regular diet would not have enough calories or protein to meet increased needs. Vegetarian diets contain many foods that are not calorie- and high-quality protein-dense and may not be palatable for clients who do not normally follow them. A soft diet is limited and may not meet nutritional needs in the long term.

BIBLIOGRAPHY

Bloch, A.S. (1990). *Nutrition management of the cancer patient.* Rockville, MD: Aspen Publishers, Inc.

Bloch, A.S. (1997). Oncology. In L. K. Lysen (Ed.). *Quick reference to clinical dietetics.* Gaithersburg, MD: Aspen Publishers, Inc, pp. 96-106.

Bloch, A. S. (2000). *Oncology diet & nutrition patient education resource manual.* Gaithersburg, MD: Aspen Publishers, Inc.

Gosselin, T., & Pitz, S. (2000). Anorexia. In B.M. Nevidjon & K.W. Sowers (Eds.). *A nurse's guide to cancer care.* Philadelphia: Lippincott, pp. 319-333.

McCallum, P.D., & Polisena, C.G. (2000). *The clinical guide to oncology nutrition.* Chicago: American Dietetic Association Publications.

Rust, D.M., & Kogut, V.J. (2001). Anorexia & cachexia. In J.M. Yasko (Ed.). *Nursing management of symptoms associated with chemotherapy* (5th ed.). West Conshohocken, PA: Meniscus, Health Care Communications, pp. 41-62.

Walker M., & Masino K. (1998). *Oncology nutrition: Patient education materials.* Chicago: American Dietetic Association Publications.

15 Alterations in Elimination

ELISA RICCIARDI

Select the best answer for each of the following questions:

1. Mr. V. is a 68-year-old with prostate cancer. He has had a radical prostatectomy for stage II disease. He comes to the surgical oncology clinic for his 1-month follow-up and reports to the nurse that he has experienced urinary incontinence several times a day for the past week. Which statement made by Mr. V. indicates his understanding of his urinary symptoms?
   A. "Urinary incontinence commonly occurs after removal of the prostate, so I will probably always be incontinent."
   B. "The incontinence should have stopped by now, so I need to have an indwelling catheter, just like I did after my surgery."
   C. "Urinary incontinence may continue for several months but should improve with a scheduled voiding program and pelvic muscle exercises."
   D. "I need to take antibiotics, because my incontinence is probably caused by a bladder infection."

2. Mr. M., a 50-year-old with transitional cell carcinoma of the bladder, has received intravesical therapy with mitomycin. He is experiencing irritative bladder symptoms, including dysuria, daytime frequency, nocturia, and urgency. Which of the following is an appropriate outcome of symptom management for Mr. M.'s bladder disturbance?
   A. Voiding no more often than every hour during the day.
   B. Subjective report of relief from dysuria and bladder pain.
   C. Voiding no more than three times per night.
   D. Subjective report of urgent sensations less than three times per day.

3. Mrs. C. is a 61-year-old client with endometrial cancer. She recently underwent a total abdominal hysterectomy. She arrives at the emergency department with a temperature of 101° F (37.7° C) and complains of frequent severe dysuria, occasional urge incontinence, and low back pain. A urinalysis reveals the presence of white blood cells (WBCs) and red blood cells (RBCs). Mrs. C. is prescribed trimethoprim-sulfamethoxazole (Bactrim DS) and phenazopyridine (Pyridium). Which of the following should be included in the nurse's interactions with and teaching of the client?
   A. Verify that the client is not allergic to sulfa or other components of these medications.
   B. Inform her that her urine will have a bluish discoloration.
   C. Limit oral fluids to 1500 ml or less.
   D. Discontinue therapy when symptoms disappear.

4. Which of the following chemotherapy agents can cause neurotoxic side effects that may lead to difficulty or inability to reach the toilet before urination (functional incontinence)?
   A. Vincristine (Oncovin) and vinblastine (Velban).
   B. 5-Fluorouracil (5-FU) and bleomycin (Blenoxane).
   C. Methotrexate and doxorubicin (Adriamycin).
   D. Gemcitabine (Gemzar) and mitoxantrone (Novantrone).

5. Which of the following is a correct statement about the use of internal and external catheters to manage urinary incontinence?
   A. An internal or external catheter should be used at night to allow the client to get plenty to rest.
   B. Internal and external catheters should be used to prevent skin breakdown caused by incontinence.
   C. Catheters should never be used to manage incontinence.
   D. Catheters should be used as a last resort to manage incontinence.

6. Which of the following measures would be appropriate to avoid perianal skin breakdown in the client with fecal incontinence?
   A. Always use a fecal incontinence pouch.
   B. Clean the perianal area after every voiding or bowel movement with a soft washcloth and perianal cleaner; rinse thoroughly and pat dry.
   C. Use warm sitz baths four times a day to prevent breakdown.
   D. Keep the client on a clear liquid diet to decrease frequency of stools.

7. Ninety percent of all bowel obstructions occur in the
   A. sigmoid colon.
   B. transverse colon.
   C. small intestines.
   D. ascending colon.

8. Mr. D. is a 72-year-old with stage Dukes C colorectal cancer. He had a colon resection and has been receiving 5-fluorouracil (5-FU) for several weeks. He calls the cancer center and reports to the nurse that he has experienced constipation for the past few weeks. His last bowel movement was 4 days ago. He complains of abdominal distention, nausea, and onset of rectal bleeding this morning. Mr. D. is instructed to come to the clinic. What is the most likely cause of Mr. D.'s symptoms?
   A. Impaction from the constipating effects of 5-FU.
   B. Bowel obstruction, possibly from recurrent colorectal cancer.
   C. Change in dietary fiber intake and exercise.
   D. Chronic use of laxatives and enemas, which are no longer effective.

9. Mrs. H. is a 59-year-old client with advanced metastatic breast cancer. She is at home with hospice providing her care. She has severe bone pain and is taking opioids. Her daughter, who is her primary caregiver, states that Mrs. H. has begun to experience some constipation. Which statement indicates need for Mrs. H's daughter to have further instruction about a bowel program to prevent constipation?
   A. Mom needs to drink at least 8 glasses of fluid every day.
   B. Mom needs more fiber in her diet like whole-grain cereals and breads, legumes, nuts, and fresh fruits and vegetables.
   C. Some light exercise such as walking may help to keep Mom regular.
   D. Magnesium citrate used daily will help to prevent constipation.

10. Ms. O. is a 43-year-old client who has acute lymphocytic leukemia (ALL). She has completed induction therapy and is to begin consolidation with vincristine and prednisone. She has taken prednisone as part of earlier treatment. Information given to her about her new chemotherapy drug should include which of the following?
   A. May experience hot flashes.
   B. Bowel function should be monitored: stool softeners may be needed.
   C. Urine may become red.
   D. Stool should be monitored for presence of blood because of gastrointestinal ulceration.

11. Mr. J. has small cell lung cancer and is receiving combination chemotherapy. His

blood counts today are WBC 800/mm^3 platelets 32,000/mm^3, hemoglobin 12.7 g/dl , and hematocrit 38.1%. He reports that he has not had a bowel movement for 3 days. Which of the following is an appropriate intervention for this client?

A. Perform a rectal examination to check for impaction.

B. Give bisacodyl (Dulcolax) two to three tablets orally, now and repeat this evening. If no relief is obtained within 24 hours, call the doctor.

C. Administer soap-suds enemas until bowel is cleansed; then start stool softeners.

D. Give glycerin suppositories to relieve constipation and continue daily to prevent recurrence of constipation.

12. Mrs. I. is a 39-year-old client with ovarian cancer. She has completed chemotherapy and has undergone a second-look operation, which revealed no evidence of malignancy. She presents to the clinic for the first postoperative visit with a complaint of constipation. Which of the following statements indicates that she needs further teaching?

A. "Surgery can cause constipation because of the handling of the intestines."

B. "My pain pills may cause me to be constipated. I should increase my fluid intake and take stool softeners."

C. "My cancer must have returned and caused my bowels to close off."

D. "I've not been very active since my surgery. Walking may help my bowels to move."

13. Mr. G. is a 63-year-old client with metastatic carcinoma of the colon. His disease is refractory to 5-FU. He received his first dose of irinotecan (Camptosar) 2 days ago. He began having diarrhea 36 hours after his therapy. Which of the following is an appropriate intervention for management of diarrhea in this client?

A. Administer atropine or Lomotil to manage his diarrhea.

B. Administer loperamide (Imodium-AD) and monitor closely for dehydration and fluid-electrolyte imbalance.

C. Premedicate with dexamethasone before the next dose of irinotecan to prevent diarrhea.

D. Diarrhea is an expected side effect and requires no management.

14. What is the most common side effect of opioid analgesics when used to manage cancer pain?

A. Sedation.

B. Slowed respiratory rate.

C. Nausea and vomiting.

D. Constipation.

15. Which of these clients is at greatest risk for acute infectious diarrhea?

A. Mr. K., a 36-year-old client who has human immunodeficiency virus (HIV), just completed a 6-week course of antibiotics.

B. Mrs. N., a 66-year-old client with acute myelogenous leukemia (AML), currently in remission, who is traveling in the northeastern United States.

C. Miss B., an 8-year-old child, previously treated for rhabdomyosarcoma, in whom there has been no evidence of disease for the past 3 years.

D. Mr. R., a 70-year-old client with prostate cancer, receiving intramuscular leuprolide (Lupron) monthly.

16. Mr. L., a 52-year-old client with rectal cancer, has completed the first 2 weeks of radiation therapy to the rectum. He began experiencing loose, watery stools 3 days ago. Which statement indicates that Mr. L. needs further instruction about managing his diarrhea?

A. I should avoid food high in fiber, fatty foods, and rich desserts.

B. I will call the doctor if I have bloody or hard stools, can't keep down liquids, or have a temperature of 100.5° F (37.7° C) or greater.

C. I should drink less to make my bowel movements less watery.

D. I can use Imodium-AD to control my diarrhea.

17. The tumors that most commonly obstruct the bowel are

A. hepatic and colorectal.

B. ovarian and colorectal.

C. ovarian and endometrial.

D. pancreatic and ovarian.

18. Mrs. F. is a 43-year-old with advanced ovarian cancer. She presents to the clinic with complaints of abdominal distention, persistent cramping pain in the lower abdomen after eating, nausea, and no bowel movement for 3 days. On assessment, you note that the client has hypoactive bowel sounds. Which of the following does Mrs. F. most likely have?
    A. Partial bowel obstruction.
    B. Gastric outlet obstruction.
    C. Cholelithiasis.
    D. Bowel perforation with peritonitis.

19. Which factor is the most important in determining the consistency and volume of colostomy output?
    A. Amount and type of food eaten.
    B. Amount of fluid intake.
    C. Type of colostomy.
    D. How much mucus is produced.

20. Which client undergoing surgery most likely would require a urinary diversion and a fecal diversion?
    A. 50-year-old man with abdominoperineal resection for colorectal cancer.
    B. 46-year-old woman with pelvic exenteration for extensive gynecologic cancer.
    C. 42-year-old man with low anterior colon resection for rectal cancer.
    D. 63-year-old woman with total abdominal hysterectomy with bilateral salpingo-oophorectomy.

21. Which type of cancer produces Bence Jones proteins and damaging casts that result in renal dysfunction, often requiring hemodialysis?
    A. Testicular cancer.
    B. Cervical cancer.
    C. Small cell lung cancer.
    D. Multiple myeloma.

22. Which of the following chemotherapy agents requires aggressive hydration before, during, and after therapy to prevent renal toxicity?
    A. Daunorubicin (Cerubidine).
    B. 5-FU.
    C. Cisplatin (Platinol).
    D. Flutamide (Eulexin).

23. A potential complication of bowel obstruction is

    A. hyperkalemia.
    B. dyspepsia.
    C. fluid overload.
    D. bowel perforation.

24. Mrs. U. has breast cancer with bone metastases. Which condition commonly occurs with her disease and can cause the kidneys to lose the ability to concentrate urine?
    A. Hyperkalemia.
    B. Hypocalcemia.
    C. Hyponatremia.
    D. Hypercalcemia.

25. A critical change in the condition of a client with constipation that should be reported to the physician is
    A. inadequate fluid intake.
    B. absence of bowel sounds.
    C. cramping with enemas.
    D. failure to evacuate daily.

26. Which would be correct nutritional advice for a client prone to constipation?
    A. Include foods low in fiber and roughage in the daily diet.
    B. Take all narcotics with milk to reduce the incidence of gastrointestinal upset.
    C. Maintain fluid intake of 1000 ml/day to prevent dehydration.
    D. Include foods high in fiber and roughage in daily diet.

27. Which medication could cause constipation?
    A. Chloral hydrate.
    B. Digoxin.
    C. Morphine.
    D. Daunorubicin.

28. Ms. C. complains of abdominal bloating and cramping with no bowel movement for 5 days. She usually has a bowel movement every day. Bowel sounds are present. She received 80 mg of doxorubicin (Adriamycin) 10 days before this appointment. Recommendations include
    A. a soap-suds enema to relieve constipation immediately.
    B. a Fleet enema to stimulate peristalsis.
    C. an oral cathartic until bowel movement; then evaluate the need for daily stool softeners.

D. beginning daily stool softeners for constipation and mild narcotic for abdominal pain.

29. Mr. F. is receiving a combination therapy of 5-FU and radiation for colorectal cancer. He is most at risk for which of the following side effects?
    A. Peripheral neuropathy.
    B. Alopecia.
    C. Thrombocytopenia.
    D. Diarrhea.

30. Diarrhea can lead to fluid and electrolyte imbalance. Which of the following imbalances is of particular concern?
    A. Hypokalemia.
    B. Hypercalcemia.
    C. Hypophosphatemia
    D. Hyperkalemia.

31. Mrs. S. is receiving radiation therapy to her abdomen and asks for dietary instructions to decrease her diarrhea. You instruct her as follows.
    A. Eat a high-fiber diet that is high in protein.
    B. Eat what you want because diet has little or no effect on radiation-induced diarrhea.
    C. Begin a low-residue diet that is high in protein.
    D. Avoid solid foods and begin supplemental liquid feedings until diarrhea resolves.

32. Which of the following classes of chemotherapy drugs carries a high-risk potential for diarrhea?
    A. Vinca alkaloids.
    B. Antimetabolites.
    C. Hormonal agents.
    D. Nitrosoureas.

33. Ms. L. is at the nadir of her chemotherapy regimen. She is occasionally incontinent of urine, and her family requests that an indwelling urinary catheter be inserted. You explain this would not be wise at this time because
    A. Ms. L. is at increased risk for infection.
    B. it would be difficult for Ms. L. to regain her bladder function.

C. Ms. L. needs to become more independent with her daily activities.
D. the insertion of an indwelling urinary catheter would delay Ms. L.'s discharge.

34. Mrs. S. is an elderly, alert woman with metastatic breast cancer. She was admitted to your unit for management of treatment-induced congestive heart failure. On admission she is given 40 mg of furosemide (Lasix). Since she is elderly, frail, and in a strange environment, you are concerned about urinary incontinence. Your nursing plan would include
    A. providing adult diapers for the client so she will not have to worry about incontinence.
    B. inserting an indwelling urinary catheter to avoid incontinence.
    C. placing a commode at the bedside and instructing the client in its use.
    D. no special measures.

35. Mrs. P. is going home after a stay on the rehabilitation unit. She will be performing intermittent self-catheterization. Her discharge instructions include which of the following?
    A. Use a new catheter with each catheterization.
    B. Perform catheterization only when you feel the urge to void.
    C. Expect scant amount of blood in the urine as normal and no cause for alarm.
    D. Use catheters repeatedly as long as they are cleaned after each use.

36. When choosing an ostomy appliance for your client, which of the following should be considered?
    A. Size of appliance
    B. Location of stoma.
    C. Color of stoma.
    D. Preference of the ostomy nurse.

37. Mrs. J. has just undergone a cystectomy for bladder cancer and has an ileal conduit. As part of client teaching, the nurse should stress
    A. changing the ostomy appliance just before bedtime.
    B. attaching straight drainage tubing to the appliance every night for drainage.

C. removing the appliance for bathing.

D. using a permanent appliance that never needs changing.

38. Which of the following is a risk factor that can lead to renal dysfunction?

A. Radiation therapy has minimal effect on renal structures.

B. Fluid and electrolyte imbalances from some chemotherapy agents.

C. Hypocalcemia of malignancy causes loss of kidneys' ability to concentrate urine.

D. Renal hyperperfusion can promote renal damage.

39. In secretory diarrhea, the intestinal mucosa secretes excessive amounts of fluid and electrolytes. Which of the following can cause secretory diarrhea?

A. Enteral tube feedings.

B. Graft-versus-host disease.

C. Inflammatory bowel disease.

D. Bacteria such as *Escherichia coli* and *Clostridium difficile.*

40. According to the National Cancer Institute grading criteria, a client experiencing more than seven stools per day or has a need for parenteral support for dehydration is classified as

A. Grade 1.

B. Grade 2.

C. Grade 3.

D. Grade 4.

41. Mrs. W. has an abdominal perineal resection with sigmoid colostomy. She expresses a strong desire to irrigate her colostomy so she does not have to wear a pouch. In which of these situations would Mrs. W. be a candidate to learn colostomy irrigation?

A. She is to receive abdominal radiation.

B. She has a temporary colostomy.

C. She has a peristomal hernia.

D. She has a sigmoid colostomy that produces formed stool.

42. Which of these laxatives chemically stimulates smooth muscles of the bowel and increases contractions?

A. Senna.

B. Methylcellulose.

C. Docusate.

D. Sodium phosphate.

43. Which medication is frequently prescribed to alkalinize urine and decrease the incidence of renal dysfunction in clients receiving high-dose methotrexate?

A. Leucovorin.

B. Sodium bicarbonate.

C. Mesna (Mesnex).

D. Sodium thiosulfate.

44. Mrs. G. has a permanent sigmoid colostomy. She has been receiving chemotherapy, and her platelet count is $35,000/mm^3$. She has come to the clinic because she has noticed some bleeding of her stoma. Which of the following would be an appropriate intervention?

A. Instruct her to wear a tight binder over the stoma to apply pressure.

B. Instruct her to rub the stoma and peristomal skin vigorously to clean all the blood off.

C. Observe the client's pouch removal technique and application.

D. Reassure the client that bleeding from the stoma is normal.

45. Small bowel obstructions typically occur as a result of

A. nonsurgical adhesions.

B. volvulus.

C. diverticulitis.

D. gastrointestinal bleeding.

46. Which of these types of medications are prescribed to treat fecal incontinence?

A. Antispasmodics.

B. Anticholinergics.

C. Calcium antagonists.

D. Bulking agents.

ANSWERS

1. *Answer:* C
Rationale: Pelvic exercises and a scheduled voiding program are interventions frequently used for initial treatment of urinary incontinence. Option A is incorrect: Urinary incontinence is common after a radical prostatectomy and can last for several months. Option B is incorrect: An indwelling catheter is usually left in place for a few weeks, and then bladder retraining is started. Some incontinence may persist for several months. Interventions may include establishing a schedule for voiding, gradually increasing the intervals between voiding, and pelvic muscle exercises. Option D is incorrect: Incontinence is primarily caused by incompetence of the rhabdosphincter.

2. *Answer:* B
Rationale: The nurse determines the cause of the client's symptoms by asking him. Irritable bladder symptoms are related to the intravesical therapy with mitomycin. Option A is incorrect: Voiding should be no more often than every 2 hours during the day. Option C is incorrect: Voiding should be done no more than once per night for clients younger than 65 years of age. Option D is incorrect: There should be no reports of dysuria, bladder pain, or urgent sensations.

3. *Answer:* A
Rationale: Bactrim DS contains sulfa. Option B is incorrect. Pyridium will turn the urine red and can stain clothing. Option C is incorrect: Oral fluids should be increased to at least 2500 ml/day, rather than restricted, unless contraindicated (i.e., cardiac disease). A full course of therapy is needed to eradicate the infection.

4. *Answer:* A
Rationale: Vincristine and vinblastine can cause neurotoxic side effects that can lead to difficulty in reaching the toilet in time to urinate, also called functional incontinence. None of the other agents listed are associated with neurotoxicity.

5. *Answer:* D
Rationale: Internal and external catheters are appropriate to manage incontinence in some circumstances but should be reserved as the last resort. Option A is incorrect: Catheters are not typically used during the night to allow the client to rest. Bladder training techniques are recommended. Option B is incorrect: Skin protectants or barriers are used to prevent skin breakdown. Option C is incorrect: Catheters generally are reserved as a last resort for treatment of incontinence.

6. *Answer:* B
Rationale: Good skin care after each voiding or stool will optimize the perianal skin integrity. Option A is incorrect: Fecal pouches are generally used for constant liquid stooling and when skin integrity cannot be maintained using skin barriers. Option C is incorrect: Sitz baths are used to provide comfort and not prevent skin breakdown. Option D is incorrect: Clear liquids help prevent dehydration.

7. *Answer:* C
Rationale: Most obstructions occur in the small intestines, especially mechanical obstructions such as adhesions, hernias, tumors, intussusception, inflammatory bowel disease, and strictures. Large bowel obstructions occur less frequently than small bowel obstructions and commonly occur in the sigmoid colon. Causes of large bowel obstructions are cancer, volvulus, and diverticulitis.

8. *Answer:* B
Rationale: Symptoms are consistent with bowel obstruction, most likely recurrent colorectal cancer. Option A is incorrect: Constipation is not a side effect of 5-FU therapy. Diarrhea is the more likely effect of 5-FU. Option C is incorrect: Change in dietary fiber intake and exercise generally do not cause rectal bleeding. Option D is incorrect: Onset of rectal bleeding is not associated with chronic use of laxatives and enemas.

9. *Answer:* D
Rationale: Magnesium citrate is of little to no use in prevention of constipation. Its primary use is in the acute evacuation of the bowel. A total of 3000 ml/day of fluids is

recommended every day to decrease the incidence of constipation. High-fiber and high-residue diet are recommended. Exercise can help stimulate peristalsis.

10. **Answer:** B
Rationale: Vincristine side effects include neurotoxicity (peripheral neuropathies, cranial nerve neuropathy, central nervous system toxicity, constipation, paralytic ileus, and urinary retention). Option A is incorrect: Hot flashes are a frequent reported side effect of tamoxifen. Option C is incorrect: Adriamycin causes urine to appear red in color. Option D is incorrect: Oral and gastrointestinal ulceration are potential side effects of methotrexate.

11. **Answer:** B
Rationale: An oral cathartic is indicated to give the client timely relief. Option A is incorrect: Rectal examinations are contraindicated in clients who are neutropenic or thrombocytopenic. Options C and D are incorrect: Soap-suds enemas and suppositories are contraindicated in clients who are neutropenic or thrombocytopenic.

12. **Answer:** C
Rationale: Obstruction of bowel by tumor can cause constipation, but it is not likely, because her surgery showed no evidence of further disease. Option A is incorrect: Bowel manipulation during abdominal surgery can decrease peristalsis and motility, resulting in constipation. Option B is incorrect: Narcotics decrease bowel motility. Option D is incorrect: Immobility decreases bowel motility.

13. **Answer:** B
Rationale: Appropriate management of irinotecan-induced "late diarrhea" (occurring more than 24 hours after treatment) is loperamide. Clients should be monitored closely for dehydration and fluid-electrolyte imbalances. Option A is incorrect: Atropine, or Lomotil that contains atropine sulfate, is used to treat "early diarrhea" (occurring during the first 24 hours after treatment). Option C is incorrect: Dexamethasone as a premedication is used to prevent nausea and vomiting, not diarrhea. Option D is incorrect: Management of diarrhea consists of keeping skin clean, dry, and protected with a skin barrier.

14. **Answer:** D
Rationale: Constipation occurs in 40% of clients referred to a palliative care service and is the most common side effect from opioid therapy. Option A is incorrect: Sedation occurs in 20% of clients receiving an opioid therapy. Option B is incorrect. Slowed respiratory rate occurs in 25% of clients receiving an opioid therapy. Option C is incorrect: Nausea and vomiting occur in 15% of clients receiving an opioid therapy.

15. **Answer:** A
Rationale: The client with HIV is at greatest risk because his immune system is incompetent. He also recently took antibiotics, which places him at risk for overgrowth of *Clostridium difficile* or other organisms. Option B is incorrect: The AML is in remission, and therefore the client is not at increased risk for infectious diarrhea. It is less likely to occur for those who are traveling in the United States versus outside. Option C is incorrect: The rhabdomyosarcoma survivor is in remission and not at increased risk for infectious diarrhea. Option D: Infectious diarrhea is not a toxicity associated with leuprolide.

16. **Answer:** C
Rationale: The client should increase oral fluids, rather than restricting them to avoid dehydration. Option A is incorrect: A low-residue diet and Imodium-AD are used to manage radiation-induced acute diarrhea. Option B is incorrect: Bloody or hard stools, inability to keep liquids down, or a temperature of 100.5° F (38°C) or greater are symptoms that need to be reported to his physician. Option D is incorrect: Imodium-AD is frequently prescribed to control diarrhea.

17. **Answer:** B
Rationale: Ovarian and colorectal cancers most commonly cause bowel obstruction. Options A, C, and D are incorrect. Hepatic, endometrial, and pancreatic cancers do not commonly cause bowel obstruction.

18. **Answer:** A
Rationale: Her symptoms indicate a partial bowel obstruction. Option B is incorrect: Gastric outlet obstruction causes pain higher

in the abdomen and sour emesis that is not bile-colored. Option C is incorrect: Frequent symptoms associated with cholelithiasis are nausea and epigastric pain. Option D is incorrect: The characteristics of the client's pain are not consistent with bowel perforation and peritonitis, which cause a boardlike abdomen and increased pain on moving.

19. *Answer:* C
Rationale: The type of colostomy is the main determining factor. A cecostomy or ascending colostomy produces semifluid or mushy stool. A transverse colostomy drains mushy stool. A descending or sigmoid colostomy produces soft to formed stool and can be regulated by irrigation. Option A is incorrect: The amount and type of food eaten is not the most important factor in determining the consistency and volume of colostomy output. Option B is incorrect: The amount of fluid intake is not the most important factor in determining the consistency and volume of colostomy output. Option D is incorrect: Depending on the type of colostomy, typically minimal mucus is produced.

20. *Answer:* B
Rationale: Pelvic exenteration involves removal of all reproductive organs and adjacent tissues and frequently requires both a colostomy and urostomy because of advanced disease involvement of the colon, bladder, ureters, and other organs. Option A is incorrect: An abdominoperineal resection results in a descending or sigmoid colostomy. Option C is incorrect: The client does not typically have an ostomy when having a low anterior colon resection unless clear margins cannot be obtained or continence cannot be maintained. Option D is incorrect: No ostomy is created with a total abdominal hysterectomy with bilateral salpingo-oophorectomy.

21. *Answer:* D
Rationale: Bence Jones proteins are found almost exclusively in the urine of clients with multiple myeloma. Renal insufficiency and renal failure are common with end-stage disease.

22. *Answer:* C
Rationale: Cisplatin requires aggressive hydration before, during, and after therapy.

Option A is incorrect: Daunorubicin does not require aggressive hydration. The client experiences red urine. Option B is incorrect: 5-FU does not require aggressive hydration and is not associated with renal toxicity. Diarrhea and stomatitis are more common side effects. Option D is incorrect: *Flutamide* is more commonly associated with side effects of hepatoxicity and gynecomastia.

23. *Answer:* D
Rationale: Bowel perforation is a potential complication of bowel obstruction. Option A is incorrect: Hypokalemia can occur if there is a large loss of gastric secretions either through vomiting or nasogastric intubation. Option B is incorrect: Dyspepsia is not a symptom of bowel obstruction. Option C is incorrect: Fluid overload is not a possible complication to bowel obstruction.

24. *Answer:* D
Rationale: Hypercalcemia commonly occurs with metastatic breast cancer, multiple myeloma, squamous cell cancer of the lung and head and neck, renal cell cancer, lymphomas, and leukemia. Hypercalcemia interferes with the kidneys' ability to concentrate urine. Options A, B, and C are incorrect: Hyperkalemia, hypocalcemia, and hyponatremia do not commonly occur with breast cancer with bone metastases and cannot cause the kidneys to lose the ability to concentrate urine.

25. *Answer:* B
Rationale: Absence of bowel sounds may be a sign of obstruction, which is a potentially life-threatening complication. Option A is incorrect: Inadequate fluid intake is not a life-threatening complication. Option C is incorrect: Cramping with enemas is a normal response. Option D is incorrect: Failure to evacuate daily is not a life-threatening complication. Sometimes clients can have bowel movements every other day.

26. *Answer:* D
Rationale: High-fiber and roughage diets should be included in the diet daily to stimulate peristalsis and prevent constipation, thus, Option A is incorrect. Option B is incorrect: Milk can be constipating. Option C

is incorrect: Fluid intake should be 3000 ml/day.

27. *Answer:* C
   Rationale: Narcotics can cause constipation. Option A is incorrect: Common side effects of chloral hydrate are nausea and vomiting and drowsiness. Option B is incorrect: Side effects with digoxin are infrequent and typically occur if the client receives too much digoxin. Frequently reported side effects include nausea, vomiting, diarrhea, stomach pain, slow pulse, and changes in vision. Option D is incorrect: Side effects of daunorubicin are myelosuppression, nausea and vomiting, red urine, and stomatitis.

28. *Answer:* C
   Rationale: Constipation of 3 days or more is unusual in this client and demands immediate relief. Options A and B are incorrect. At 10 days after doxorubicin treatment, clients are susceptible to infection and should avoid rectal medications of treatments. Option D is incorrect. Narcotics can increase the risk of constipation. Stool softeners can take longer to provide relief than an oral cathartic.

29. *Answer:* D
   Rationale: Combined 5-FU and abdominal radiation therapy have a synergistic effect to cause diarrhea. Option A is incorrect: Peripheral neuropathy typically occurs with vincristine or vinblastine. Option B is incorrect: Alopecia can occur in the area that is being treated with radiation. Option C is incorrect: Thrombocytopenia may occur with radiation.

30. *Answer:* A
   Rationale: Diarrhea results in potassium loss. Option B is incorrect. Hypercalcemia is often seen in clients with breast cancer or multiple myeloma with bone metastases. Option C is incorrect: Hypophosphatemia is typically seen in clients being treated for diabetic ketoacidosis. Option D is incorrect: Hyperkalemia occurs when the kidney is unable to excrete potassium. This is often seen in acute or chronic kidney failure.

31. *Answer:* C
   Rationale: A low-residue diet will decrease irritation of the gastrointestinal tract.

Option A is incorrect: A high-fiber diet will increase irritation of the gastrointestinal tract. Option B is incorrect: Diet can affect radiation-induced diarrhea. Option D is incorrect: Client should consume solid foods that contain low residue and high protein.

32. *Answer:* B
   Rationale: Gastrointestinal alterations are a common toxicity of antimetabolites. Options A, C, and D are incorrect. Gastrointestinal alterations are not a common toxicity of vinca alkaloids, hormonal agents, and nitrosoureas.

33. *Answer:* A
   Rationale: Indwelling catheters are a source of infection. Option B is incorrect: Bladder training is recommended as a first-line treatment. Option C is incorrect: Bladder training will allow the client to become more independent. Option D is incorrect: Insertion of an indwelling catheter would not delay discharge because the client could be taught to manage the catheter at home. Indwelling catheters are a source of infection.

34. *Answer:* C
   Rationale: The client should be near a commode for easy access and for measurement of urine output. Option A is incorrect: Diapers would create difficulty in providing accurate measurement of urine output. Option B is incorrect: The preference is to do toilet training. Option D is incorrect: If no special measures are taken, the client could be at risk for falling, and accurate measurement of urine output would be difficult.

35. *Answer:* D
   Rationale: Self-intermittent catheterization is a clean, not sterile, technique. Option A is incorrect: Using a new catheter with each catheterization is not necessary because it is a clean, not sterile, technique. Option B is incorrect: Self-catheterization is performed on a schedule to maintain bladder tone. Option C is incorrect: Urine will typically be clean and yellow.

36. *Answer:* B
   Rationale: The location of the stoma is the most important factor to consider in determining the best type of ostomy appliance for the

client. Options A, C, and D are incorrect. Pouch selection is based on the consistency of effluent, stoma size, abdominal contour, and the degree of stomal protrusion.

37. *Answer:* B
Rationale: For the bladder to drain continuously, the conduit must be drained at night. Attaching tubing to the appliance promotes drainage and prevents leakage. Option A is incorrect: The ostomy appliance is not changed before bedtime. Tubing is attached to the appliance during the nighttime. Option C is incorrect: The appliance is not routinely removed for bathing. Option D is incorrect: The appliance barrier melts with wear from the urine. Permanent appliance is not typically used.

38. *Answer:* B
Rationale: Fluid and electrolyte imbalances from some chemotherapy agents can have an indirect effect on kidney function and can lead to renal failure. Option A is incorrect: Radiation therapy may cause permanent fibrosis and atrophy. Option C is incorrect: Hypercalcemia of malignancy causes loss of concentration by the kidneys. Option D is incorrect: Renal hypoperfusion promotes renal damage.

39. *Answer:* D
Rationale: Bacteria such as *Escherichia coli* and *Clostridium difficile* are causes of secretory diarrhea. Option A is incorrect: Enteral tube feedings are nonabsorbable substances in the intestine, which draws water into the intestinal lumen by osmosis. Option B is incorrect: Diarrhea caused by graft-versus-host disease is a result of hypermobility (limited absorption caused by increased motility of the intestines). Option C is incorrect: Diarrhea associated with inflammatory bowel disease is related to hypermotility.

40. *Answer:* C
Rationale: Grade 3 is experiencing more than seven stools per day or there is a need for parenteral support for dehydration. Option A is incorrect: Grade 1 is fewer than four stools per day over pretreatment. Option B is incorrect: Grade 2 is four to six stools per day or nocturnal stools. Option D is incorrect: Grade 4 has

physiologic consequences that require intensive care; possible hemodynamic collapse.

41. *Answer:* D
Rationale: Irrigation is appropriate for clients with sigmoid colostomies that are producing formed stool. The client must have a strong desire to learn the technique. Option A is incorrect: Irrigating is contraindicated if a client is receiving pelvic or abdominal radiation because of the risk of bowel perforation. Option B is incorrect: Irrigating a temporary colostomy can create bowel dependence and it may take a long time for the client to master the procedure. Option C is incorrect: Peristomal hernia irrigating is contraindicated. Clients frequently have delayed, prolonged, and incomplete evacuations. It can also increase the potential for bowel perforation.

42. *Answer:* A
Rationale: Senna is a laxative that chemically stimulates smooth muscles of the bowel and increases contractions. It is often ordered for clients receiving narcotics. Option B is incorrect: Methylcellulose is a bulk-forming laxative. Option C is incorrect: Docusate is an emollient and lubricant laxative that softens hardened stool. Option D is incorrect: Sodium phosphate does not stimulate smooth muscle.

43. *Answer:* B
Rationale: Sodium bicarbonate is frequently prescribed to alkalinize urine. Option A is incorrect. Leucovorin is generally administered after high-dose methotrexate to reduce the severity of drug-induced leukopenia. Option C is incorrect: Mesna is frequently given to reduce the severity and incidence of hemorrhagic cystitis. Option D is incorrect: Sodium thiosulfate is given before cisplatin to reduce the incidence of regimen-related nephrotoxicity.

44. *Answer:* C
Rationale: Observation of the client's technique in removing and applying the appliance will demonstrate the client's ability to carry out these procedures without causing trauma to the stoma. Option A is incorrect: A tight binder can cause trauma to the stoma mucosa and increase bleeding. Option B is incorrect: Stoma and peristomal skin should always be cleaned gently with warm water.

Option D is incorrect: Client should monitor the stoma and pouch for increased bleeding. Bleeding from a stoma is abnormal. There could be bleeding externally from the stoma mucosa or internally from the intestine, or the client could have a low platelet count.

45. *Answer:* A

Rationale: Nonsurgical adhesions are a cause of small bowel obstruction. Nonsurgical adhesions can occur at any time after an infection or completion of radiation therapy. Option B is incorrect: Volvulus causes large bowel obstruction. Option C is incorrect: Diverticulitis causes large bowel obstruction. Option D is incorrect: Gastrointestinal bleeding is not identified as a risk for small bowel obstruction.

46. *Answer:* D

Rationale: Bulking agents are most frequently prescribed to manage fecal incontinence. Option A is incorrect: Antispasmodics are prescribed for urinary incontinence. Option B is incorrect: Anticholinergics can cause urinary retention and overflow incontinence. Option C is incorrect: Calcium antagonists cause urinary retention.

BIBLIOGRAPHY

Agency for Health Care Policy and Research. (1996). *Managing acute and chronic incontinence: Quick reference guide for clinicians.* (AHCPR Publication No. 96-00686). Rockville, MD: U.S. Department of Health and Human Services.

Ahn, S.H., Mayo-Smith, W.W., Murphy, B.L., et al. (2002). Acute nontraumatic abdominal pain in adult patients: Abdominal radiography compared with CT evaluation. *Radiology* 225(1), 159-164.

Aviv, R.I., Shymalan, G., Watkinson, A., et al. (2002). Radiological palliation of malignant colonic obstruction. *Clinical Radiology* 57(5), 347-351.

Bliss, D., Jung, H.J., Savik, K., et al. (2001). Supplementation with dietary fiber improves fecal incontinence. *Nursing Research* 50(4), 203-213.

Bresalier, R. (2002). *Sleisinger and Fordtran's gastrointestinal and liver disease volume II* (7th ed.). Philadelphia: W. B. Saunders.

Carlson, K., & Nitti, V. (2001). Prevention and management of incontinence following radical prostatectomy. *Urologic Clinics of North America* 28(3), 595-609.

Carter, J., Valmadre, S., Dalyrmple, C., et al. (2002). Management of large bowel obstruction in advanced ovarian cancer with luminal stents. *Gynecological Oncology* 84(1), 176-179.

Colwell, J., Goldberg, M., & Carmel, J. (2001). The state of the standard diversion. *Journal of Wound, Ostomy, & Continence Nursing* 28(1), 6-17.

Doughty, D. (2002). When fiber is not enough: Current thinking on constipation management. *Ostomy, and Wound Management* 48(12), 30-41.

Flessir, A., & Blarvis, J. (2002). Evaluating incontinence in women. *Urologic Clinics of North America* 29(3), 515-526.

Floruta, C. (2001). Dietary choices of people with ostomies. *Journal of Wound, Ostomy, & Continence Nursing* 28(1), 28-31.

Gromley, E. (2002). Biofeedback and behavioral therapy for the management of female urinary incontinence. *Urologic Clinics of North America* 29(3), 551-558.

Kintzel, P. (2001). Anticancer drug-induced kidney disorders: Incidence, prevention, and management. *Drug Safety* 24(1), 19-38.

Krupski, T., & Theodorescu, D. (2001). Orthotopic neobladder following cystectomy: Indications, management, and outcomes. *Journal of Wound, Ostomy, & Continence Nursing* 28(1), 37-46.

Matsuoka, J., Takahara, T., Masaki, T., et al. (2002). Preoperative evaluation by magnetic resonance imaging in patients with bowel obstruction. *American Journal of Surgery* 183(6), 614-617.

Murphy, J., Stacey, D., Crook, J., et al. (2000). Testing control of radiation-induced diarrhea with a psyllium bulking agent: A pilot study. *Canadian Oncology Nursing Journal* 10(3), 96-100.

O'Rourke, M. (2000). Urinary incontinence as a factor in prostate cancer treatment selection. *Journal of Wound, Ostomy, & Continence Nursing* 27(5), 146-154.

Potter, K. (2000). Surgical oncology of the pelvis: Ostomy planning and management. *Journal of Surgical Oncology* 73(4), 237-242.

Robinson, J. (2000). Managing urinary incontinence following radical prostatectomy. *Journal of Wound, Ostomy, & Continence Nursing* 27(5), 138-145.

Schiller, K. (2002). *Sleisinger and Fordtran's gastrointestinal and liver disease volume I* (7th ed.). Philadelphia: Saunders.

Schoolwirth, A., & Gehr, T. (2000). *Textbook of critical care* (4th ed.). Philadelphia: W.B. Saunders.

Spratto, G.R., & Woods, A.I. (2004). *PDR nurse's drug handbook.* Clifton Park, NY: Thompson Delmar Learning.

Viele, C.S., Stern, J.M., Ippoliti, C., & Rosenoff, S.H. (2002). *Symptom management of chemotherapy-induced diarrhea: A multidisciplinary approach.* ONS 2002 Annual Congress Symposia Highlight, 17-20.

Waldman, A.R. (2001). Bowel obstruction. *Clinical Journal of Oncology Nursing* 5(6), 281-282, 286.

Wein, A., & Rovner, E. (2002). Pharmacologic management of urinary incontinence in women. *Urologic Clinics of North America* 29(3), 537-550.

Yarbo, C.H, Frogge, M., H., Goodman, M., & Groenwald, S.L (2002). *Cancer nursing: Principles and practices* (5th ed.). Sudbury, MA: Jones and Bartlett Publishers.

Yasko, J.M. (2002). *Nursing management of symptoms associated with chemotherapy*. West Conshohocken, PA: Meniscus Healthcare Communications.

PART FOUR

CARDIOPULMONARY FUNCTION

16 Alterations in Ventilation

CYNTHIA CHERNECKY

1. Abnormal accumulation of air within the pleural space is known as
    A. empyema.
    B. pneumothorax.
    C. hemothorax.
    D. pleural effusion.

2. Mr. J. is scheduled for surgery as a result of being diagnosed with non–small cell lung cancer. He tells you that the doctor explained the surgery to him as having his "whole left lung taken out" in surgery tomorrow morning. You know that this surgical procedure is called a
    A. wedge resection.
    B. segmental resection.
    C. lobectomy.
    D. pneumonectomy.

3. Which client has the highest number of risk factors for alterations in ventilation? Client with
    A. tuberculosis, treatment with isoniazid (INH) and vitamin B$_6$ for 6 months, smoker, cholecystectomy 3 months ago, and productive cough with yellow sputum.
    B. non–small cell lung cancer diagnosis, history of left upper lobe lung removal, history of chronic obstructive pulmonary disease (COPD), and atherosclerotic heart disease.
    C. ovarian cancer with total hysterectomy 2 weeks ago, type 2 diabetes mellitus

for 5 years, history of latex allergies, and history of asthma.
    D. cardiac stents placed 3 months ago, prostate cancer diagnosed 2 months ago, currently receiving radiation therapy for his prostate cancer, history of abdominal aortic aneurysm (AAA) repair 12 years ago.

4. You are doing a physical examination on Mrs. K. and note she has a "whistling sound" upon auscultation of the lungs. You would document this in the progress notes as
    A. dyspnea.
    B. tachypnea.
    C. egophony.
    D. wheezing.

5. Your client has just been given the diagnosis of empyema. You should anticipate what to be prescribed for the client?
    A. Radiation therapy to the lung field(s) involved.
    B. Systemic antibiotics.
    C. Subcutaneous epinephrine 1:100 solution.
    D. Oxygen at 30% face mask.

6. Your client had a right-sided cerebral vascular accident 8 months ago and requires an assistive device for activities of daily living. He has only minimal left leg weakness as a result of his stroke. Which assistive device would be

best to assist the client in activities of daily living and will increase ventilation?

A. Walker with wheels.
B. Cane.
C. Motorized three-wheel scooter.
D. Wheelchair.

7. Your client has been receiving radiation therapy and bleomycin (Blenoxane) chemotherapy for treating his cancer. He is at risk for which type of pulmonary toxicity:

A. Superior vena cava syndrome (SVCS).
B. Pulmonary empyema.
C. Pneumonitis.
D. Pleural effusion.

8. Your client is being treated with glucocorticoids for her radiation-induced pneumonitis. Her symptoms have begun to improve by 50%. The physician states, "Stop the glucocorticoids, she is doing much better." You know that

A. the glucocorticoids can be discontinued as prescribed.
B. you should auscultate the client's lungs and review her complete blood cell count (CBC) results before you discontinue the glucocorticoids.
C. you will also need a prescription for a cough suppressant and antipyretic to counteract glucocorticoids' short-term effects.
D. abrupt discontinuation of glucocorticoids can flare up the pneumonitis.

9. Your client is receiving his first dose of gemcitabine (Gemzar) chemotherapy for treatment for pancreatic cancer. During treatment the client begins to have dyspnea, fever of 100.5° F (38.05° C), and a nonproductive cough. What should be your initial nursing intervention?

A. Get the code cart and prepare for intubation.
B. Stop the chemotherapy.
C. Obtain a STAT chest x-ray.
D. Administer oxygen at 2 L by nasal cannula, give epinephrine 1:1000 subcutaneously, and administer an acetaminophen (Tylenol) suppository.

10. Your client has just been given the diagnosis of a pulmonary toxicity as a result of radiation therapy and chemotherapy. What would you expect his ABG results to indicate?

A. Hyperoxygenation and hypercapnia.
B. Metabolic acidosis with an increased pH.
C. Hypoxia and hypocapnia.
D. High total lung residual capacity and a decreased forced expiratory volume at 1 second (FEV-1).

11. Which of the following conditions/diseases commonly have dyspnea as a symptom?

A. Hyperthyroidism, SVCS, hypertension.
B. Pancreatitis, thrombocytopenia, constipation.
C. Lung cancer, anemia, infection.
D. Asthma, hypertension, schizophrenia.

12. Which of the following classes of pharmacologic agents is used to decrease local inflammation in the client with dyspnea?

A. Bronchodilators.
B. Glucocorticoids.
C. Anxiolytics.
D. Diuretics.

13. Your client develops dyspnea after walking in the hall. You wish to determine the severity of his hypoxia. What is the best intervention to accomplish this? Obtain a STAT

A. white blood cell count (WBC).
B. pulse oximetry.
C. chest x-ray.
D. sputum culture.

14. Which of the following body positions would you recommend to your client who has dyspnea?

A. Lie flat and on your right side.
B. Lie in semi-Fowler's position at a 45-degree angle.
C. Sit upright with your legs crossed and your hands over your head.
D. Sit upright, lean forward with your elbows on a table.

15. Which of the following is a complementary therapy that can help decrease the sense of dyspnea and enhance psychosocial well-being?

A. Coffee ground enemas.
B. Prayer.

C. Intravenous morphine sulfate.

D. Use of incentive spirometer.

16. Your client has just had a thoracentesis for treatment of a pleural effusion. You know that he may present with decreased oncotic pressure in the microvasculature, as a result of

    A. hypoproteinemia.

    B. heart failure.

    C. atelectasis.

    D. acute pain.

17. Your client comes in for her 3-month postoperative chemotherapy visit for breast cancer, and you note on your physical examination that she has tachypnea, dullness to percussion in the right lower lobe (RLL) of the lung, absent breath sounds in the RLL, egophany on the right side of the chest, and a slight fever. This client most likely has a(n)

    A. AAA.

    B. severe anemia.

C. pulmonary fibrosis.

D. pleural effusion.

18. Which two pharmacologic agents used to treat seizure disorders can cause anemia?

    A. Estrogen and valproic acid (Depakote).

    B. Furosemide (Lasix) and hydrochlorothiazide (HCTZ).

    C. Phenobarbital (Luminal) and phenytoin (Dilantin).

    D. Diazepam (Valium) and somatropin (Genotropin).

19. What cardiovascular effects can appear on physical examination of the client with anemia?

    A. Dry skin and decreased ejection fraction.

    B. Increased hematocrit and bradycardia.

    C. Tachycardia and systolic murmurs.

    D. Hepatomegaly and hypertension.

NOTES

ANSWERS

1. *Answer:* B
Rationale: A pneumothorax is air in the pleural space. An empyema is an abnormal accumulation of infected fluid or pus in the pleural space. A hemothorax is blood in the pleural space. A pleural effusion is the presence of abnormal amounts of fluid in the pleural space.

2. *Answer:* D
Rationale: A pneumonectomy is removal of the entire lung. A wedge resection is the removal of a small wedge-shaped area near the lung surface. A segmental resection is the removal of one or more segments of a lung lobe. A lobectomy is the removal of a lobe of a lung.

3. *Answer:* B
Rationale: A history of lung cancer, surgery, COPD, heart disease, cardiac stents, and asthma are all risk factors for alterations in ventilation. Tuberculosis, treatment for tuberculosis, cholecystectomy, diabetes, and latex allergies are not risk factors

4. *Answer:* D
Rationale: Wheezing is a musical or whistling sound heard in the lungs when a client has difficulty breathing. Dyspnea is shortness of breath. Tachypnea is abnormal rapid respirations. Egophony is an abnormal change in tone, like a bleat of a goat, heard during auscultation of the lungs.

5. *Answer:* B
Rationale: An empyema is an abnormal accumulation of infected fluid or pus in the pleural space. Systemic antibiotics are used to treat infection. Radiation therapy is done to reduce obstructions caused by lung tumors. Epinephrine is used to treat anaphylaxis. Oxygen is used to treat anaphylaxis or the anoxic client.

6. *Answer:* B
Rationale: A cane would increase his walking, which would increase ventilation and minimize interference with activities of daily living. Because he has only minimal leg weakness, a walker with wheels would restrict activities of daily living and therefore ventilation. A scooter or wheelchair would make him dependent and decrease activity, which would decrease ventilation.

7. *Answer:* C
Rationale: Bleomycin and radiation therapy are high-risk factors for pneumonitis. Radiation therapy should decrease SVCS, and SVCS is not a pulmonary toxicity. An empyema is pus in the pleural space and is not associated with radiation and chemotherapy listed. A pleural effusion is the presence of abnormal amounts of fluid in the pleural space and is not associated with bleomycin therapy.

8. *Answer:* D
Rationale: Tapering of glucocorticoids is necessary to avoid flare-up of pneumonitis. A CBC will not be helpful in the evaluation of pneumonitis. Cough suppressants and antipyretics are part of management for radiation-induced pneumonitis.

9. *Answer:* B
Rationale: Dyspnea, nonproductive cough, and a fever during the infusion are the cardinal signs of pulmonary toxicity of drug-induced pneumonitis, and you stop the chemotherapy immediately. A crash cart may become necessary but is not your immediate intervention. A chest x-ray is not immediate; however, arterial blood gas evaluation (ABG) would be included in near immediate care. Oxygen may be required, but stopping the chemotherapy is your primary and immediate intervention. Epinephrine is helpful in treating anaphylaxis, and a Tylenol suppository is not indicated immediately.

10. *Answer:* C
Rationale: You would expect the ABGs to show decreased oxygenation and respiratory alkalosis. Hypoxia and hypocapnia are expected. Option D includes the results of a pulmonary function test, not an ABG.

11. *Answer:* C
Rationale: Lung cancer, anemia, and infection commonly have dyspnea as a symptom, especially as severity increases. Dyspnea is common with SVCS but not with hypertension, schizophrenia, and hyperthyroidism.

12. *Answer:* B
Rationale: Glucocorticoids decrease local inflammation. Bronchodilators increase airflow to the lungs. Anxiolytics decrease anxiety. Diuretics decrease fluid overload.

13. *Answer:* B
Rationale: Pulse oximetry measures the severity of hypoxia. The WBC measures the risk for infection. A chest x-ray detects structural abnormalities. A sputum culture detects infectious organisms, and results take several days.

14. *Answer:* D
Rationale: Sitting upright and leaning forward with elbows on a table will increase ease of respiration and effectiveness of each breath. Lying down, lying in a semi-Fowler's position, or sitting with legs crossed increases respiratory effort.

15. *Answer:* B
Rationale: Prayer and meditation have been shown to be effective in decreasing the sense of dyspnea. The position needed to administer the enema will increase use of energy. Morphine is not a complementary therapy. Incentive spirometry is not a complementary therapy and will increase respiratory effort.

16. *Answer:* A
Rationale: Hypoproteinemia decreases oncotic pressure in the microvasculature. Heart failure increases hydrostatic pressure. Atelectasis increases negative pressure in the pleural space. Acute pain increases blood pressure and respirations.

17. *Answer:* D
Rationale: Tachypnea, dullness to percussion, absent breath sounds, egophany, and a slight fever are classic symptoms of a pleural effusion. Signs of an AAA are abdominal pain or flank pain, low back pain, and gastric fullness. Signs for anemia include dyspnea on exertion, fatigue, weakness, headache, decreased blood pressure, tachypnea, and tachycardia. Signs of a pleural effusion include moist rales, tachypnea, and dyspnea.

18. *Answer:* C
Rationale: Phenobarbital and phenytoin are used to treat seizures and can cause anemia. Estrogen, furosemide, hydrochlorothiazide, and somatropin are not used to treat seizures. Depakote and diazepam can be used in seizure disorders.

19. *Answer:* C
Rationale: Tachycardia occurs in anemia, as do systolic murmurs in severe anemia. Dry skin is a sign of the integumentary system, not the cardiovascular system, and a decreased ejection fraction cannot be determined by physical examination. Anemia results in a decreased hematocrit and tachycardia. There is hepatomegaly, but this is found in an abdominal exam, and hypotension will occur in anemia.

BIBLIOGRAPHY

Chernecky, C., & Berger, B. (2004). *Laboratory tests and diagnostic procedures* (4th ed.). St. Louis: Elsevier.

Chernecky, C., & Sarna, L. (2000). Pulmonary toxicities. *Critical Care Nursing Clinics of North America* 12, 281-295.

Cooley, M.E., Short, T.H., & Moriarty H.J. (2002). Patterns of symptom distress in adults receiving treatment for lung cancer. *Journal of Palliative Care* 18(3), 150-159.

Loney, M. & Chernecky, C. (2000). Anemia. *Oncology Nursing Forum* 27, 951-966.

Sarna, L., Cooley, M., & Danao, L. (2003). The global epidemic of tobacco and cancer. *Seminars in Oncology Nursing* 19, 233-243.

17 Alterations in Circulation

KRISTINE TURNER STORY

Select the best answer for each of the following questions:

1. Lymphedema is defined as
   A. obstruction of the lymphatic system that causes fluid overload in the interstitial space.
   B. accumulation of fluid in the interstitial space.
   C. fluid accumulation in the peritoneal cavity that causes lower limb swelling.
   D. edema of a limb with associated erythema.

2. Lymphedema can be worsened by which of the following?
   A. Application of an elastic sleeve to the affected limb.
   B. Administration of chemotherapy in the unaffected limb.
   C. Radiation therapy to the affected limb.
   D. Administration of intravenous fluids.

3. The malignancy most commonly associated with lymphedema is
   A. basal cell carcinoma.
   B. leukemia.
   C. renal cell carcinoma.
   D. breast cancer.

4. Stage 3 lymphedema is classified as
   A. a cool, pulseless limb.
   B. tight, shiny skin with pitting edema.
   C. unilateral erythema of the affected limb.
   D. an affected limb that is more than 5 cm in diameter than the unaffected limb.

5. Early detection and treatment of lymphedema involves
   A. regular measurement of extremities and application of elastic sleeves.
   B. massage therapy and vigorous weight lifting of the affected limb.
   C. weight lifting of the affected limb and antibiotic therapy.
   D. fluid restriction and immobility of the affected limb.

6. The assessment of a person with lymphedema includes which of the following?
   A. Daily weight.
   B. Arterial pulse of affected limb.
   C. Mobility and strength of affected limb.
   D. Loss of hair of affected limb.

7. Interventions aimed at preventing lymphedema include
   A. vigorous exercise of affected extremity.
   B. use of compression garments with activity.
   C. elevation of the affected limb.
   D. fluid restriction to decrease swelling.

8. The incidence of lymphedema may decrease in the future as a result of

A. use of less invasive breast surgery.
B. use of tamoxifen (Nolvadex).
C. use of trastuzumab (Herceptin).
D. use of sentinel lymph node dissection.

9. Which of the following conditions is usually related to cancer surgery?
A. Pericardial effusion.
B. Pleural effusion.
C. Lymphedema.
D. Local edema.

10. Risk factors associated with the development of lymphedema include
A. history of deep vein thrombosis (DVT).
B. infection of surgical extremity.
C. low-dose radiation therapy.
D. immobility of extremity.

11. Treatments for lymphedema include
A. oral diuretics.
B. keeping extremity dependent.
C. high-sodium diet.
D. manual lymph drainage.

12. A client calls stating her arm has become tight and red after a long plane trip. The most appropriate advice to give her is
A. keep the arm elevated and see her provider in 2 weeks.
B. don't worry — this is a normal response to travel.
C. arrange to see provider this day for probable antibiotics for cellulitis.
D. refer to physical therapy to start manual lymph drainage.

13. An appropriate client outcome for a client with lymphedema includes
A. client verbalizes acceptable level of pain control.
B. client reports weight gain of more than 2 lb per day
C. client reports absence of dyspnea.
D. client exhibits normal vital signs.

14. Abnormal leakage of fluid from blood and lymph vessels leading to an excessive accumulation of fluid in the interstitial space is defined as
A. lymphedema.
B. edema.

C. hematoma.
D. hepatoma.

15. Increased dietary sodium and inadequate dietary protein are examples of which type of risk factor for edema of cancer?
A. Iatrogenic.
B. Treatment-related.
C. Lifestyle-related.
D. Disease-related.

16. Venous obstruction resulting in edema may be caused by which of the following?
A. Thrombophlebitis.
B. Cellulitis.
C. Peritonitis.
D. Pleurisy.

17. Objective findings related to edema of cancer include
A. presence of S_2 heart sound.
B. decreased blood pressure and heart rate.
C. increased jugular venous pressure.
D. increased peripheral pulses.

18. The incidence of edema associated with cancer is
A. unknown as a result of underreporting.
B. decreasing as a result of longer survival.
C. increasing as a result of more aggressive treatments.
D. universal in all clients with cancer and metastatic disease.

19. Abnormal laboratory/diagnostic findings associated with edema of cancer include
A. decreased blood urea nitrogen (BUN) and creatinine.
B. decreased serum albumin and protein.
C. decreased size of heart shadow on chest x-ray film.
D. increased ejection fraction on echocardiogram.

20. An appropriate client outcome for a person with edema of cancer would be
A. client reports weight gain of more than 2 lb per day.
B. client verbalizes warm, dry extremities.

C. client requires assistance with bathing and hygiene.

D. client reports normal bowel status.

21. Which of the following statements regarding malignant pericardial effusions is true?
   A. Many are asymptomatic.
   B. Testicular cancer is a common cause.
   C. It is an oncologic emergency.
   D. It is always associated with pleural effusions.

22. Tumors commonly associated with malignant pericardial effusions include
   A. melanoma.
   B. lung cancer.
   C. renal cell carcinoma.
   D. leukemia.

23. Risk factors associated with malignant pericardial effusion include
   A. low fraction size of radiation therapy.
   B. diabetes mellitus.
   C. history of DVT.
   D. preexisting cardiac disease.

24. Subjective findings associated with malignant pericardial effusion include
   A. sharp, positional chest pain.
   B. jugular venous distention.
   C. productive cough.
   D. dyspnea on exertion.

25. High-dose cyclophosphamide (Cytoxan) is associated with which cardiac toxicity?
   A. Asymptomatic bradycardia.
   B. Coronary artery spasm.
   C. Cardiomyopathy.
   D. Myocardial necrosis caused by endothelial damage.

26. Which of the following is the definitive test for diagnosing malignant pericardial effusion?
   A. Electrocardiography.
   B. Computed tomography (CT) scan of chest.
   C. Cardiac catheterization.
   D. Echocardiography.

27. The nurse is caring for a client with malignant pericardial effusion. The following intervention should be implemented:

   A. Keep head of bed flat.
   B. Administer diuretics.
   C. Increase activity level.
   D. Administer no intervention if asymptomatic.

28. The nurse is preparing a client for a pericardial window. The indication for this procedure is
   A. short-term emergent removal of slow or rapidly developing effusions.
   B. palliative management of recurrent effusions with limited life expectancy.
   C. chronic, severe effusions in clients with otherwise good performance status.
   D. life-threatening cardiac tamponade with moderate to large effusion when an open procedure is not feasible.

29. An appropriate client outcome for a client with malignant pericardial effusion is
   A. client reports ability to perform activities of daily living.
   B. client maintains oxygen saturation below 90%.
   C. client reports palpitations.
   D. client verbalizes understanding of high cure rate.

30. Cardiovascular toxicity in a client receiving treatment for cancer is defined as
   A. alteration in cardiac conduction and function caused by treatment.
   B. increased risk of myocardial infarction caused by treatment-induced hypertension.
   C. bilateral lower limb edema caused by DVT.
   D. asymptomatic bradycardia caused by radiation therapy to the chest.

31. Asymptomatic bradycardia is related to which of the following chemotherapy agents?
   A. Daunorubicin (Cerubidine, DaunoXome).
   B. Methotrexate.
   C. Paclitaxel (Paxene, Taxol).
   D. High-dose 5-fluorouracil (5-FU).

32. Cardiac toxicities that begin several weeks after chemotherapy administration are most likely
   A. chronic.
   B. subacute.

C. acute.

D. irreversible.

33. The most common chronic cardiac toxicity associated with cancer treatment is

    A. cardiomyopathy.

    B. asymptomatic bradycardia.

    C. hemorrhagic myocardial necrosis.

    D. coronary artery spasm.

34. Factors that are associated with increased risk of cardiotoxicity from chemotherapy include

    A. high-dose cyclophosphamide, radiation therapy to the chest, and multiple cardiotoxic drugs.

    B. standard dose cyclophosphamide, advanced age, and history of smoking.

    C. history of smoking, bony metastasis, and history of lung cancer.

    D. high-dose cyclophosphamide, radiation therapy to the chest, and history of breast cancer.

35. The administration schedules of chemotherapy that increase the risk of cardiotoxicity include

    A. high doses of drug over short periods of time.

    B. low doses of drug administered rapidly.

    C. 24-hour administration of drug.

    D. combination administration of drugs.

36. Abnormalities of which of the following can interfere with cardiac function?

    A. Sodium and calcium.

    B. Potassium and chloride.

    C. Potassium and calcium.

    D. Sodium and chloride.

37. Tachycardia, shortness of breath, and neck vein distention are signs and symptoms of which of the following:

    A. Lung cancer.

    B. Congestive heart failure.

    C. Cardiomegaly.

    D. Pleural effusion.

38. An appropriate client outcome for clients with cardiac toxicity related to cancer treatment is

    A. client is able to complete activities of daily living.

    B. client verbalizes absence of pain.

    C. client reports weight gain or more than 2 lb per day.

    D. client reports normal urinary elimination.

39. Prevention of doxorubicin (Adriamycin)-related cardiomyopathy includes

    A. exercise and smoking.

    B. smoking cessation and oxygen therapy.

    C. exercise and use of dexrazoxane (Zinecard).

    D. oxygen therapy and low-fat diet.

40. When the ejection fraction is less than 45%, the nurse should expect the following:

    A. Increase in the chemotherapy dose.

    B. Decrease in the chemotherapy dose.

    C. Monitoring electrocardiogram.

    D. Increase in intravenous fluids.

41. A client is admitted with congestive heart failure. Records indicate a history of breast cancer treated with chemotherapy and radiation therapy. The most likely late effect of this treatment is

    A. pulmonary fibrosis.

    B. pleural effusion.

    C. cardiomyopathy caused by anthracycline therapy.

    D. coronary artery disease.

42. Cardiotoxicity with doxorubicin can be minimized by the administration of which of the following cardioprotective agents?

    A. Intravenous steroids.

    B. Amifostine.

    C. Calcium gluconate.

    D. Dexrazoxane.

43. Risk factors for thrombotic events include

    A. thrombocytopenia.

    B. anemia.

    C. disseminated intravascular coagulation (DIC).

    D. neutropenia.

44. Thrombotic events are more common in which of the following malignancies:

    A. Ovarian and endometrial cancer.

    B. Renal cell and prostate cancer.

C. Leukemia and lymphoma.
D. Melanoma and basal cell carcinoma.

45. Symptoms associated with pulmonary embolism include
   A. chest pain.
   B. palpitations.
   C. abdominal pain.
   D. paroxysmal nocturnal dyspnea.

46. A client with an arterial embolus may complain of which of the following symptoms?
   A. A dull ache in the calf.
   B. Coolness of the affected extremity.
   C. Easy bruising of the affected extremity.
   D. A palpable venous cord.

47. The nurse caring for a client with DVT should implement which of the following interventions:
   A. High vitamin K diet.
   B. Increase activity level.
   C. Use of elastic stockings.
   D. Keep legs dependent.

48. The management of long-term indwelling central venous catheters to prevent thrombotic events includes
   A. weekly flushing with tissue plasminogen activator.
   B. daily low-dose warfarin.
   C. daily high-dose aspirin.
   D. low-dose subcutaneous heparin.

49. Diagnostic tests used to diagnose pulmonary embolism include
   A. chest x-ray.
   B. echocardiography.
   C. spiral chest CT.
   D. venous duplex scan.

50. Laboratory findings in DVT include
   A. thrombocytopenia.
   B. a positive D-dimer test.
   C. leukocytosis.
   D. anemia.

51. Risk factors for DVT include
   A. tamoxifen use.
   B. malnutrition.
   C. young age.
   D. family history of DVT.

52. An appropriate client outcome for the client with DVT includes
   A. client reports cool extremities.
   B. client maintains intact skin.
   C. client reports increased blood pressure.
   D. client reports increased fatigue.

NOTES

ANSWERS

1. *Answer:* A
Rationale: Lymphedema is caused by an obstruction of the lymphatic system that results in an overload of lymph fluid in the interstitial spaces. Accumulation of fluid in the interstitial space is defined as edema. Fluid accumulation in the peritoneal cavity would not cause lower limb swelling. Edema with erythema is suggestive of infection.

2. *Answer:* C
Rationale: Radiation therapy worsens lymphedema by causing fibrosis and scarring in a limb where lymph flow is already impaired by surgery. Intravenous fluids would not contribute to lymphedema, because the fluid is in the vascular space. The remaining options are interventions to prevent lymphedema.

3. *Answer:* D
Rationale: Breast cancer is most closely associated with lymphedema caused by axillary lymph node dissection. The other malignancies typically do not require node dissection.

4. *Answer:* D
Rationale: Comparison of the affected and nonaffected limb is used to determine the stage of lymphedema. Stage 1 is less than 3-cm difference. Stage 2 is 3- to 5-cm. difference. Stage 3 is greater than 5 cm. A cool, pulseless limb indicates arterial occlusion. Pitting edema is typically seen in edema. Unilateral erythema could indicate DVT or cellulitis.

5. *Answer:* A
Rationale: Regular measurement of the extremities allows early detection of lymphedema and early application of elastic sleeves. Massage therapy is also helpful, but lifting weights can worsen lymphedema. Fluid restriction has no effect on lymphedema.

6. *Answer:* C
Rationale: Impaired mobility of the affected extremity can worsen lymphedema and also indicate worsening condition, there-fore assessment of mobility is important. The client's daily weight is not affected by lymphedema. Arterial pulse and assessment of hair growth are more indicative of arterial abnormalities.

7. *Answer:* C
Rationale: Elevation of the affected limb will reduce dependent edema and lymphedema. Regular exercise is important, but vigorous exercise could be detrimental. Compression garments should be worn continuously, not just with exercise. Fluid intake has little impact on degree of lymphedema.

8. *Answer:* D
Rationale: Sentinel lymph node dissection limits the number of nodes removed, thus minimizing the disruption of lymphatic flow. Less invasive breast surgery still requires lymph node dissection for staging. Chemotherapy and targeted therapies do not appear to affect lymphedema development.

9. *Answer:* C
Rationale: Lymphedema development is closely tied to lymph node dissection. The other conditions may be caused by primary or metastatic disease or by other comorbidities.

10. *Answer:* B
Rationale: An infection of the affected limb increases risk of lymphedema. High-dose radiation therapy is more likely to result in lymphedema. Overuse of a limb is a greater risk factor than immobility. There does not appear to be a relationship between DVT and lymphedema.

11. *Answer:* D
Rationale: Manual lymph drainage is an important treatment for lymphedema. Diuretics have no role. The affected limb should be kept elevated and the client placed on a low-sodium diet.

12. *Answer:* C
Rationale: Redness may indicate infection and requires prompt intervention. The other

options result in delay of treatment of the underlying problem.

13. *Answer:* A
Rationale: A client should expect a reasonable degree of comfort after treatment for lymphedema. Weight, vital signs, and dyspnea are not important factors related to lymphedema.

14. *Answer:* B
Rationale: Edema is accumulation of fluid in the interstitial space. Lymphedema is the abnormal collection of lymph fluid in the interstitial space. Hematoma is an abnormal collection of blood in the tissues. Hepatoma is a type of malignant liver tumor.

15. *Answer:* C
Rationale: Dietary factors are considered lifestyle changes over which clients have some control.

16. *Answer:* A
Rationale: Mechanical obstruction by a thrombus changes the pressure gradient so that fluid remains in peripheral tissues.

17. *Answer:* C
Rationale: Jugular venous distension occurs with edema as fluid backs up in the heart. An S_2 heart sound is normal; blood pressure and pulse usually increase with edema; peripheral pulses usually diminish as a result of poor cardiac output.

18. *Answer:* A
Rationale: Edema is not a commonly reported condition and may be blamed on other comorbidities.

19. *Answer:* B
Rationale: Hypoproteinemia contributes to edema by shifting fluids into the interstitial space. BUN and creatinine are often increased as a result of nephrotic syndrome; heart size may enlarge as a result of congestive failure; ejection fraction often declines as a result of congestive failure.

20. *Answer:* B
Rationale: Warm, dry extremities indicate adequate tissue perfusion. Weight gain indicates fluid retention; clients should be independent in activities of daily living; bowel status is unrelated to this diagnosis.

21. *Answer:* A
Rationale: The majority of clients with pericardial effusions are asymptomatic. Testicular cancer is rarely associated with pleural effusion. Cardiac tamponade is an emergency, not effusion, unless the client has symptoms, which is unusual and associated with rapidly developing effusions. Pleural and pericardial effusions can occur independently.

22. *Answer:* B
Rationale: Lung cancer is much more likely to result in pericardial effusion caused by intrathoracic metastasis and direct extension to the myocardium.

23. *Answer:* D
Rationale: Preexisting heart disease increases the risk because of a compromised cardiac status. High fractions of radiation therapy are more likely to cause effusions. Diabetes and DVT do not increase the risk.

24. *Answer:* D
Rationale: Dyspnea (both at rest and with exertion) is reported by the client with a pericardial effusion. Chest pain is usually dull; jugular venous distention is unlikely; cough is usually nonproductive.

25. *Answer:* D
Rationale: High-dose cyclophosphamide damages cardiac endothelium, which can lead to myocardial necrosis and death. Paclitaxel may cause asymptomatic bradycardia; 5-fluorouracil can cause coronary artery spasm; anthracyclines cause cardiomyopathy.

26. *Answer:* D
Rationale: Echocardiography allows measurement of volume of an effusion. Electrocardiography and cardiac catheterization may be used to rule out other cardiac causes of chest pain. Chest CT may be helpful in a large tumor burden but is not definitive for fluid in the pericardium.

27. *Answer:* D
Rationale: Many clients do not have symptoms, and no intervention may be chosen depending on performance status. The head of bed should be elevated; diuretics are not helpful; clients should be taught energy-conserving measures.

28. *Answer:* C
Rationale: A window is reserved for persons with chronic effusions with a good performance status and expected longer term survival.

29. *Answer:* A
Rationale: Subjective reports from the client of satisfactory performance of ADLs demonstrate an approximate outcome. Oxygen saturation should be maintained at more than 90%; palpitations are not a common finding with pericardial effusion and are not an appropriate outcome; cure rates are low and the presence of pericardial effusion is associated with poor survival.

30. *Answer:* A
Rationale: Cancer therapies affect cardiac function and conduction.

31. *Answer:* C
Rationale: Paclitaxel is associated with asymptomatic bradycardia. Daunorubicin causes cardiomyopathy, methotrexate has no cardiac toxicities, and high-dose 5-fluorouracil can cause coronary artery spasm.

32. *Answer:* B
Rationale: Subacute toxicities occur within 4 to 5 weeks after therapy and are usually reversible. Acute changes occur within 24 hours of drug administration. Chronic changes are not reversible.

33. *Answer:* A
Rationale: Anthracycline-related cardiotoxicity occurs in up to 40% of clients depending on the cumulative dose administered.

34. *Answer:* A
Rationale: Although a history of smoking and old age is associated with an increased risk of cardiotoxicity, standard-dose cyclophos-phamide, bone metastases, and lung and breast cancer are not.

35. *Answer:* A
Rationale: High doses of drug administered quickly expose tissues to high levels of agents, thus increasing risk of toxicity. Lower doses of drugs and 24-hour infusions are not as strongly associated with toxicity.

36. *Answer:* C
Rationale: Potassium and calcium, when abnormal, are associated with muscle weakness and cramping, cardiac abnormalities, and cardiac arrest.

37. *Answer:* B
Rationale: During heart failure, cardiac output decreases, thus causing congestion in the lungs and neck veins because cardiac output cannot equal venous return to the heart.

38. *Answer:* A
Rationale: Subjective reports from the client of satisfactory performance of ADLs demonstrate an appropriate outcome. The complete absence of pain may be an unrealistic outcome; weight gain may indicate fluid overload, a complication of cardiomyopathy; urinary elimination is not important to this diagnosis.

39. *Answer:* C
Rationale: Exercise strengthens cardiac muscle, thus increasing function. Dexrazoxane protects cardiac muscle against the effects of doxorubicin.

40. *Answer:* B
Rationale: A normal ejection fraction is more than 60%. A decrease of more than 5% over baseline or an ejection fraction of less than 45% requires dose reduction.

41. *Answer:* C
Rationale: Most treatment regimens for breast cancer include an anthracycline, which is a risk factor for cardiomyopathy.

42. *Answer:* D
Rationale: Dexrazoxane is a cardioprotectant that protects cardiac muscle against the

effects of doxorubicin. The other agents have no role as cardioprotectants.

43. *Answer:* C
Rationale: DIC is an abnormality of the clotting cascade that causes coagulopathies.

44. *Answer:* C
Rationale: Leukemia and lymphoma are much more likely to be associated with coagulopathies than the other malignancies listed.

45. *Answer:* A
Rationale: A pulmonary embolism usually causes a sharp, stabbing chest pain. The other symptoms are not associated with pulmonary embolism. Paroxysmal nocturnal dyspnea is defined as acute dyspnea occurring at night, waking the client after 1 to 2 hours of sleep, and is associated with pulmonary congestion caused by congestive heart failure.

46. *Answer:* B
Rationale: An arterial embolus obstructs arterial flow, causing cool or cold extremities. A dull ache in the calf and palpable venous cord are more characteristic of DVT. Bruising is not a symptom of embolus.

47. *Answer:* C
Rationale: Elastic leg stocking provide venous support, improve circulation, and help reduce edema. A low vitamin K diet is indicated with warfarin (Coumadin), a common treatment for DVT. Activity level should be curtailed and legs kept elevated during initial treatment of DVT.

48. *Answer:* B
Rationale: The American College of Chest Physicians recommends 1 mg of warfarin daily to maintain patency of central venous catheters.

49. *Answer:* C
Rationale: A spiral CT scan is used to diagnose pulmonary emboli. Chest x-ray and echocardiography do not detect pulmonary emboli. A venous duplex scan is used to diagnose DVT.

50. *Answer:* B
Rationale: A positive D-dimer test has a high predictive value for DVT, but does not exclude DVT in clients with cancer. The other laboratory abnormalities are not associated with DVT.

51. *Answer:* A
Rationale: Tamoxifen is associated with clot formation. The other risk factors are not.

52. *Answer:* B
Rationale: Intact skin integrity indicates adequate perfusion; clients should have warm extremities; blood pressure and fatigue are unassociated with DVT.

BIBLIOGRAPHY

Camp-Sorrell, D. (2000). Chemotherapy: Toxicity management – cardiotoxicity. In C.H. Yarbro, M.H. Frogge, M. Goodman, & S. L. Groenwald (Eds.). *Cancer nursing: Principles and practice* (5th ed.). Sudbury, MA: Jones and Bartlett Publishers, pp. 472-474.

Chapman, D.D., & Goodman, M. (2000). Breast cancer – chronic lymphedema. In C.H. Yarbro, M.H. Frogge, M. Goodman, & S.L. Groenwald (Eds.). *Cancer nursing: Principles and practice* (5th ed.). Sudbury, MA: Jones and Bartlett Publishers, pp. 1038-1039.

Cope, D.G. (2000). Lymphedema. In D. Camp-Sorrell, & R.A. Hawkins. (Eds.). *Clinical manual for the oncology advanced practice nurse*. Pittsburgh: Oncology Nursing Society, pp. 649-652.

Dell, D.D. (2002). Deep vein thrombosis in the patient with cancer. *Clinical Journal of Oncology Nursing 6*, 43-46.

Martin, V. (2000). Ovarian cancer – lymphedema. In C.H. Yarbro, M.H. Frogge, M. Goodman, & S.L. Groenwald (Eds.). *Cancer nursing: Principles and practice* (5th ed.). Sudbury, MA: Jones and Bartlett Publishers, pp. 1390-1391.

National Lymphedema Network (2002). *Lymphedema: A brief overview*. Retrieved on February 3, 2003, from http://www.lymphnet.org/prevention. html.

National Lymphedema Network. (2001). *Prevention*. Retrieved on February 3, 2003, from http://www.lymphnet.org/prevention.html.

Ridner, S.H. (2002). Breast cancer lymphedema: Pathophysiology and risk reduction guidelines. *Oncology Nursing Forum 29*, 1285-1293.

Ryan, M., Stainton, M.C., Jaconelli, C., et al. (2003). The experience of lower limb lymphedema for women after treatment for gynecologic cancer. *Oncology Nursing Forum 30*, 417-423.

Shelton, B.K. (2000). Pericarditis/pericardial effusion/cardiac tamponade. In D. Camp-Sorrell D, & R.A. Hawkins (Eds.). *Clinical manual for the oncology advanced practice nurse.* Pittsburgh: Oncology Nursing Society, pp. 307-316.

Story, K.T. (2000). Deep vein thrombosis. In D. Camp-Sorrell & R.A. Hawkins (Eds.). *Clinical manual for the oncology advanced practice nurse.* Pittsburgh: Oncology Nursing Society, pp. 235-243.

Viale, P.H. (1999). Management of thromboembolism in patients with cancer. *Oncology Nursing Forum 26,* 1625-1632.

Winokur, M.A. (2000). Peripheral edema. In D. Camp-Sorrell & R.A. Hawkins (Eds.). *Clinical manual for the oncology advanced practice nurse.* Pittsburgh: Oncology Nursing Society, pp. 215-220.

Works, C., & Maxwell, M.B. (2000). Malignant effusions and edemas. In C.H. Yarbro, M.H. Frogge, M. Goodman, & S.L. Groenwald (Eds.). *Cancer nursing: Principles and practice* (5th ed.). Sudbury, MA: Jones and Bartlett Publishers, pp. 813-830.

NOTES

PART FIVE

ONCOLOGIC EMERGENCIES

18 Metabolic Emergencies

BARBARA HOLMES GOBEL

Select the best answer for each of the following questions:

1. Which of the following is a risk factor for the development of disseminated intravascular coagulation (DIC)?
   A. Dehydration.
   B. Hyperkalemia.
   C. Hypercalcemia.
   D. Gram-negative infection.

2. DIC is a clotting disorder frequently seen in what malignancy?
   A. Leukemia.
   B. Breast cancer.
   C. Ovarian cancer.
   D. Multiple myeloma.

3. On day 4 of chemotherapy for the treatment of acute myelogenous leukemia, a client develops a fever of 101.5° F (38.6° C), complains of shortness of breath with associated hypoxia, and develops blood in the urine. The nurse suspects what process is occurring?
   A. DIC.
   B. Sepsis.
   C. Hypercalcemia.
   D. Syndrome of inappropriate antidiuretic hormone (SIADH).

4. DIC represents an imbalance of normal coagulation. Which of the following statements best summarizes the characteristics of this condition?
   A. Failure of the fibrinolytic system.
   B. Blocked internal pathway of clotting.
   C. Excessive amounts of clotting factors.
   D. Accelerated coagulation and the formation of excessive thrombin.

5. Of the following tests that may be done to help determine the diagnosis of DIC, what tests are specific and sensitive for DIC?
   A. D-dimer assay and fibrinogen degradation products (FDP) titer.
   B. Platelet count and fibrinogen level.
   C. Antithrombin III level and fibrinopeptide A level.
   D. Plasminogen level and plasmin α-2-antiplasmin complex levels.

6. What is the primary management strategy for treating clients with DIC?
   A. Treat the bleeding.
   B. Administer chemotherapy.
   C. Treat the underlying cause.
   D. Treat the intravascular clotting.

7. The client in question #3 is suspected of experiencing DIC. In addition to antibiotic therapy, what treatment strategies will likely be undertaken next in the treatment of DIC?
   A. Vasopressors.
   B. Fibrinolytic therapy.

C. Mechanical ventilation.

D. Low-dose heparin therapy.

8. When assessing the client for DIC, the nurse should be particularly concerned about

A. bradycardia.

B. mottled extremities.

C. decreased bowel sounds.

D. elevated specific gravity.

9. A 26-year-old disoriented and irritable man with Hodgkin's disease and diabetes is admitted to the hospital. His temperature is 100° F (37.7° C), pulse 110, blood pressure 90/40, respiratory rate 30, white blood cell (WBC) count 500/mm^3, and platelets 150,000/mm^3. Urine output is normal and positive for glucose (blood sugar is 190 mg/dl). Which condition would the nurse most likely suspect in this client?

A. DIC.

B. Septic shock.

C. Hypocalcemia.

D. Diabetic shock.

10. The most common cause of sepsis is

A. fungi.

B. viruses.

C. gram-positive bacteria.

D. gram-negative bacteria.

11. What is the single most important risk factor for the development of sepsis?

A. Fever.

B. Diabetes.

C. Inadequate nutritional intake.

D. Duration of granulocytopenia.

12. Early signs and symptoms of sepsis in a client with granulocytopenia include

A. fever and chills.

B. lethargy and disorientation.

C. purulent drainage from venous access site.

D. hypotension and narrowing pulse pressure.

13. Septic shock is differentiated from sepsis by which of the following parameters?

A. Fever.

B. Tachypnea.

C. Tachycardia.

D. Hypotension.

14. Which absolute granulocyte count places a client with cancer at the greatest risk for development of septic shock?

A. Less than 500/mm^3.

B. Less than 1000/mm^3.

C. Less than 2500/mm^3.

D. Less than 4000/mm^3.

15. What is one of the most important strategies to prevent infections in clients with low WBC counts?

A. Adequate mobility.

B. Adequate oral intake.

C. Control of blood sugar.

D. Hand hygiene of the clients and health care team.

16. Early intervention in a client suspected of experiencing septic shock includes

A. intravenous fluids and hemodynamic monitoring.

B. intravenous fluids, hemodynamic monitoring, and empiric antibiotics.

C. intravenous fluids, hemodynamic monitoring, and antineoplastic therapy.

D. intravenous fluids, hemodynamic monitoring, and antiendotoxin therapy.

17. Tumor lysis syndrome (TLS) occurs most commonly in persons with what cancer?

A. Breast cancer.

B. Pancreatic cancer.

C. Renal cell carcinoma.

D. High-grade lymphoma.

18. Which of the following is an electrolyte abnormality associated with TLS?

A. Hypokalemia.

B. Hypercalcemia.

C. Hyperuricemia.

D. Hypophosphatemia.

19. A client is admitted to the hospital for chemotherapy and biotherapy because of a diagnosis of Hodgkin's lymphoma, with an associated large bulky mediastinal tumor. The client is short of breath, which has contributed to her dehydration over the past week. What metabolic oncologic emergency does the nurse suspect that this client may experience?

A. Hypercalcemia.

B. TLS.

C. DIC.

D. SIADH.

20. TLS is a complication of cancer therapy. TLS occurs most commonly in tumors that are
   A. large and rapidly dividing.
   B. small and rapidly dividing.
   C. slow growing and radiosensitive.
   D. slow growing and chemosensitive.

21. Treatment of hyperkalemia associated with TLS includes which treatment strategy?
   A. Antibiotic therapy.
   B. Hypertonic glucose and insulin.
   C. Phosphate-binding, aluminum-containing antacids.
   D. Exchange resins such as sodium polysterene sulfonate (Kayexalate)

22. Which of the following medications is given for TLS to decrease deposits of uric acid in the kidneys?
   A. Mannitol (Osmitrol).
   B. Allopurinol (Zyloprim, Aloprim).
   C. Rasburicase (Elitek).
   D. Loop diuretic (e.g., furosemide [Lasix]).

23. A possible complication of TLS is
   A. acute sepsis.
   B. hypokalemia.
   C. bowel obstruction.
   D. acute renal failure.

24. Which of the following is an appropriate client/family teaching strategy to help prevent TLS in a client starting outpatient treatment for a diagnosis of non-Hodgkin's lymphoma?
   A. Initiate and explain the need for fluid restriction.
   B. Explain the need for increased activity during treatment.
   C. Discuss the need for increased intake of foods high in potassium and phosphorus.
   D. Review of medications before treatment to minimize exogenous intake of potassium and phosphorus.

25. A 70-year-old client with a diagnosis of small cell lung cancer is admitted to the hospital with mental status changes. Upon review of the client's electrolytes, you find that the client has a serum calcium of 14 mg/dl, a potassium of 3.0 mEq/L, and a phosphorus of 7 mg/dl. What metabolic oncologic emergency are you concerned that this client may be experiencing?
   A. Hypercalcemia.
   B. TLS.
   C. DIC.
   D. SIADH.

26. The client most at risk for the development of hypercalcemia has a diagnosis of
   A. glioblastoma.
   B. ovarian cancer.
   C. promyelocytic leukemia.
   D. breast cancer with skeletal metastasis.

27. J.D. is a 59-year-old woman with breast cancer. Her serum calcium is 12.5 mg/dl. She is alert and oriented with good urine output. The most appropriate intervention to aid in decreasing the serum calcium concentration is to
   A. encourage her to ambulate.
   B. order a footboard for the bed.
   C. assist her to stand at the bedside.
   D. perform active range-of-motion exercises.

28. L.B. is a 62-year-old man with a diagnosis of lung cancer with metastasis to his right hip. He is admitted to the hospital with a serum calcium level of 16 mg/dl. His wife explains to you that he has been "acting very funny" and has not been eating or drinking well for 3 days. He complains of significant nausea. The most appropriate intervention to aid in decreasing the serum calcium concentration is to
   A. hydrate the client.
   B. encourage the client to ambulate.
   C. administer bisphosphonate therapy.
   D. administer chemotherapy right away.

29. Which of the following is considered to be a contributing factor for the development of hypercalcemia?
   A. Male sex.
   B. Young age.
   C. Immobility.
   D. Fluid overload.

30. The cancer that is most often associated with the development of SIADH is
    A. leukemia.
    B. breast cancer.
    C. prostate cancer.
    D. small cell lung cancer.

31. The nurse should explain to the client that the initial treatment for mild hyponatremia (serum sodium of 125 to 134 mEq/L) would include
    A. medication management.
    B. ambulation of the client.
    C. fluid restriction of free water to 500 to 1000 ml/day.
    D. fluid restriction of free water to 1500 to 2000 ml/day.

32. Emergency treatment of SIADH may be required if
    A. the serum sodium is 125 mEq/L.
    B. the serum sodium is 135 mEq/L.
    C. cardiopulmonary changes are present.
    D. significant neurologic changes are present.

33. Which of the following clients is most at risk for the development of SIADH?
    A. A client with colon cancer undergoing a colon resection.
    B. A client with non–small cell lung cancer receiving weekly paclitaxel (Taxol) and carboplatin (Paraplatin).
    C. A client with acute myelogenous leukemia receiving induction therapy with cytarabine (Cytosar) and idarubicin (Idamycin).
    D. A client with small cell lung cancer who is admitted to the hospital for pneumonia and is taking morphine for pain control.

34. Signs and symptoms of SIADH include
    A. rales, wheezes, and dyspnea.
    B. pallor, petechiae, and ecchymosis.
    C. headache, vomiting, and confusion.
    D. polyuria, polydipsia, and dehydration.

35. A client with a diagnosis of non–small cell lung cancer is admitted to the hospital with vomiting and altered mental status. His serum sodium is 118 mEq/L, urine sodium is 30 mEq/L, and potassium is 3.0 mEq/L. What is the most appropriate immediate nursing intervention with this client?
    A. Medicate the client for pain.
    B. Implement seizure precautions.
    C. Encourage the client to do frequent mouth care.
    D. Encourage the client to increase his fluid intake.

36. During administration of L-asparaginase (Elspar), a client complains of "feeling funny" and being short of breath. The nurse hears wheezes in bilateral lung fields. What oncologic emergency does the nurse suspect is occurring in this client?
    A. TLS.
    B. Hypersensitivity/anaphylaxis.
    C. DIC.
    D. SIADH.

37. In the above question, what is the most appropriate immediate nursing intervention?
    A. Call a code.
    B. Stop the infusion.
    C. Intubate the client.
    D. Initiate cardiopulmonary resuscitation.

38. Signs and symptoms of anaphylaxis include
    A. feeling of fatigue.
    B. urticaria and angioedema.
    C. pain around an intravenous insertion site.
    D. itching around an intravenous insertion site.

39. Intradermal skin tests are undertaken when
    A. giving any new chemotherapy agent.
    B. clients have a history of multiple allergies.
    C. chemotherapy agents have a high risk of causing hypersensitivity reactions.
    D. giving chemotherapy agents that have already caused a hypersensitivity reaction in a client.

40. Prevention of anaphylaxis includes
    A. instructing the client to drink lots of fluids.

B. having emergency equipment available in a treatment area

C. premedication of the client with acetaminophen, famotidine (Pepcid), and diphenhydramine.

D. administering an intradermal skin test when a chemotherapy agent has a high risk of causing a hypersensitivity reaction.

41. A client with recurrent ovarian carcinoma has agreed to participate in a clinical trial involving a new agent with anaphylactic potential. What precautions should the nurse take the first time that the drug is given?

A. Premedicate the client with diazepam.

B. Reject the client as a candidate for the study.

C. Take vital signs before agent administration and every 4 hours thereafter.

D. Administer the agent only in an environment where emergency medications and equipment are available.

42. The client's risk for anaphylaxis increases when medications are

A. given at low doses.

B. given intravenously.

C. given as a single dose.

D. synthetically prepared.

NOTES

ANSWERS

1. *Answer:* D
   Rationale: Infection and sepsis are the most common causes of DIC in cancer, particularly infection with gram-negative bacteria. Dehydration, hyperkalemia, and hypercalcemia are not associated with DIC. They are metabolic abnormalities associated with metabolic oncologic emergencies.

2. *Answer:* A
   Rationale: The most common cancers associated with DIC are the acute leukemias and the mucin-producing adenocarcinomas. Of these, the most common cancer associated with DIC is acute promyelocytic leukemia. Breast cancer, ovarian cancer, and multiple myeloma do not carry a high incidence of DIC.

3. *Answer:* A
   Rationale: Early recognition of the signs and symptoms of DIC is critical to prompt intervention and treatment. Bleeding (from at least three unrelated sites), hypoxia, shortness of breath, and a fever are all signs and symptoms related to the diagnosis of DIC.

4. *Answer:* D
   Rationale: The pathophysiology of DIC involves extensive triggering of the coagulation system, which results in abnormal activation of thrombin formation. Clotting factors are depleted. Fibrinolysis and the clotting pathways continue at a rapid rate.

5. *Answer:* A
   Rationale: The D-dimer assay, often done in combination with the fibrinogen degradation product (FDP) titer, reflect the microangiopathy of DIC. These tests have been found to be sensitive, specific, and efficient in the diagnosis of DIC. The platelet count and fibrinogen level may be decreased in DIC, but they are not specific or sensitive tests for DIC. Option C are tests used to detect accelerated coagulation, and Option D are tests used to detect accelerated fibrinolysis, once the diagnosis of DIC has already been established.

6. *Answer:* C
   Rationale: The primary management strategy for treating clients with DIC is to treat the underlying cause of the DIC. Although other treatments such as treating the bleeding and the intravascular clotting may be necessary, they will only provide temporary relief of symptoms.

7. *Answer:* D
   Rationale: Heparin therapy interferes with thrombin production and is often given for the management of intravascular clotting. The goal of heparin therapy is to maintain a partial thromboplastin time (aPTT) at 1 to 2 times the normal levels. Low-dose heparin minimizes the risk of bleeding. Vasopressors may be used to treat an associated hypotension, which this client is not experiencing. Fibrinolytic therapy may be given after the heparin therapy. The client may require mechanical ventilation at some point, but not based on the current status of the client.

8. *Answer:* B
   Rationale: Acral cyanosis, or mottled extremities, is a hallmark of DIC. Heart rate is usually increased, not decreased. Specific gravity is not applicable in this condition. Bowel sounds may be decreased but are not a specific sign of DIC.

9. *Answer:* B
   Rationale: The signs and symptoms are early manifestations of septic shock. Sepsis usually presents with two or more of the following manifestations: temperature greater than 100.4° F (37.9° C), heart rate greater than 90 beats/min, respiratory rate greater than 20/min, and a WBC count greater than 12,000/mm^3 or less than 4000/mm^3. No mention is made of serum calcium or symptoms of hypocalcemia. No mention is made of signs and symptoms of bleeding as seen in DIC. The client's blood sugar is not significantly elevated as in diabetic shock.

10. *Answer:* D
    Rationale: Gram-negative bacteria are the most common cause of sepsis. The other organisms may also cause sepsis.

11. *Answer:* D

Rationale: Duration of granulocytopenia is the single most important risk factor for the development of sepsis. Fever is a sign of infection. Diabetes and inadequate nutritional intake may contribute to the development of infection but are not risk factors for sepsis.

12. *Answer:* A

Rationale: Fever and chills are early signs and symptoms of sepsis in a client with granulocytopenia. Purulent drainage from a venous access site may be absent because of the granulocytopenia. Options B and D are late signs of sepsis.

13. *Answer:* D

Rationale: Septic shock is manifested by hemodynamic instability, for example hypotension. Fever, tachypnea, and tachycardia can also be seen in sepsis.

14. *Answer:* A

Rationale: An absolute granulocyte count of less than $500/mm^3$ places the client at a higher risk for infection, which may progress to septic shock.

15. *Answer:* D

Rationale: Basic infection control precautions with any client with a low WBC count starts with hand hygiene of the client and health care team. Adequate mobility, adequate oral intake, and control of blood sugar can all help to maintain a client's immune system.

16. *Answer:* B

Rationale: Intravenous fluids, hemodynamic monitoring, and empiric antibiotics are all early interventions for septic shock. Antineoplastic therapy may be important for a client with cancer but would not be given during a period of suspicion for septic shock. Antiendotoxin therapy is experimental, not a first-line therapy for septic shock.

17. *Answer:* D

Rationale: Persons who have rapidly dividing cancers such as high-grade lymphoma are at risk for the development of TLS because of the large number of cells lysed during therapy. Breast, pancreatic, and renal cell carcinomas are not rapidly dividing cancers, and TLS is rare in clients with solid tumors.

18. *Answer:* C

Rationale: TLS is defined as a potentially life-threatening metabolic imbalance that occurs with the rapid release of intracellular potassium, phosphorus, and nucleic acid (uric acid) into the blood as a result of rapid tumor cell kill.

19. *Answer:* B

Rationale: The client is exhibiting risk factors for the development of TLS, including a diagnosis of non-Hodgkin's lymphoma, dehydration, and the plan to receive chemotherapy and biotherapy for a highly proliferative tumor. The other oncologic emergencies do not present this way.

20. *Answer:* A

Rationale: TLS most frequently occurs after chemotherapy administration in cancers with a rapidly dividing, large tumor burden.

21. *Answer:* B

Rationale: Intravenous hypertonic glucose and insulin will shift the excessive extracellular potassium concentrations back into the intracellular stores. Antibiotic therapy does not have a role in the management of TLS. Phosphate-binding antacids are used to help lower the phosphate level. Exchange resins may be used to manage mild hyperkalemia, because their effects are not immediate and may take up to 24 hours to be effective.

22. *Answer:* B

Rationale: Allopurinol (oral [Zyloprim] or injectable [Aloprim]) blocks the enzyme xanthine oxidase to decrease uric acid production and to decrease subsequent deposits of uric acid in the kidney. Mannitol and lasix are diuretics. Rasburicase is used to treat high uric acid levels in pediatric cases involving TLS.

23. *Answer:* D

Rationale: Acute renal failure is associated with TLS because of the precipitation of uric acid and phosphate salts in the kidneys. Acute sepsis and bowel obstruction are not seen with TLS. Hyperkalemia, not hypo-kalemia, is associated with TLS.

24. *Answer:* D
Rationale: Because of the risk of hyper-kalemia and hyperphosphatemia in TLS, it is important to review all medications the client is taking that may increase the serum potas-sium and phosphorus before initiating treat-ment. Prevention of TLS requires high fluid requirements. Increasing activity level is not critical with the prevention of TLS.

25. *Answer:* A
Rationale: Hypercalcemia is demon-strated by an elevated calcium level. Clients with a diagnosis of lung cancer or breast can-cer account for 80% of all clients in whom hypercalcemia develops. Mental status changes are one of the signs and symptoms of hypercalcemia.

26. *Answer:* D
Rationale: Clients with breast cancer and an associated skeletal metastasis account for the highest incidence of hypercalcemia. Hypercalcemia is not commonly seen in glioblastoma, ovarian cancer, or promyelcytic leukemia.

27. *Answer:* A
Rationale: Although all the interventions help to decrease serum calcium, ambulating the client is the action that will most likely encourage calcium to return to the bone, espe-cially because this client is awake, alert, and oriented.

28. *Answer:* C
Rationale: The nurse should anticipate administering a bisphosphonate, because they are the agent of choice to treat cancer-induced hypercalcemia. All of the other interventions will help to lower the calcium, but immediate action needs to be taken because the level of calcium puts the client at great risk of neuro-logic complications.

29. *Answer:* C
Rationale: Exercise and weight bearing are essential to maintaining bone mass; thus immobility contributes to the development of hypercalcemia. The other factors listed, male

sex, young age, and fluid overload, have not been found to be contributing factors for the development of hypercalcemia.

30. *Answer:* D
Rationale: Small cell lung cancer accounts for more than 75% of all tumors associated with SIADH. SIADH can occur in leukemia, breast cancer, and prostate cancer, although it is rare in these tumors.

31. *Answer:* C
Rationale: The initial treatment of choice for mild hyponatremia (serum sodium between 125 to 134 mEq/L) is fluid restriction of free water of 500 to 1000 ml/day. Medication management generally occurs if the client can-not maintain a fluid restriction. Although ambulation is good for most clients, it is not a treatment strategy for SIADH.

32. *Answer:* D
Rationale: Emergency treatment of SIADH may be required if the client experiences signifi-cant neurologic changes, because this can lead to an irreversible neurodegenerative disorder called central pontine myelinolysis.

33. *Answer:* D
Rationale: The client in Option D has three risk factors for the development of SIADH. Small cell lung cancer (SCLC) accounts for more than 75% of all tumors associated with SIADH. Other risk factors for SIADH include pneumo-nia and morphine/narcotic use. SIADH can occur in clients with non–small cell lung cancer and acute myelogenous leukemia, although not as frequently as with SCLC. SIADH is not usually seen in clients with colon cancer.

34. *Answer:* C
Rationale: Headache, vomiting, and con-fusion are all signs of moderate hyponatremia. Respiratory symptoms listed in Option A would not be apparent. Pallor, petechiae, and ecchymosis are all signs and symptoms of DIC. Polyuria, polydipsia, and dehydration can all be signs of hypercalcemia.

35. *Answer:* B
Rationale: The client is experiencing moder-ate hyponatremia with neurologic changes, which should alert the nurse to implement

seizure precautions immediately to ensure safety for the client. There is no indication that the client has complaints of pain. Encouraging good mouth care is essential for any client on a fluid restriction, but not an immediate nursing action in this case. This client would be placed on a fluid restriction based on his serum sodium level.

36. *Answer:* B
Rationale: Signs and symptoms of hypersensitivity reactions include client complaints of altered sensations, or "feeling funny," including a "feeling of impending doom." Other signs and symptoms include client complaints of shortness of breath and wheezing. This client was also at risk for the development of a hypersensitivity reaction, because she was receiving a chemotherapy agent with a known increased incidence of hypersensitivity reactions.

37. *Answer:* B
Rationale: The first thing that a nurse should do when a hypersensitivity reaction is suspected while infusing a medication is to stop the infusion of the offending agent. There is no indication in this scenario that any of the other actions—call a code, intubate the client, or initiate cardiopulmonary resuscitation—are necessary at this time.

38. *Answer:* B
Rationale: Signs and symptoms of anaphylaxis include urticaria and angioedema. Feelings of fatigue are common in clients with cancer but are not indicative of anaphylaxis. Options C and D are potential signs or symptoms of a localized hypersensitivity reaction.

39. *Answer:* C
Rationale: Intradermal skin tests are undertaken when chemotherapy agents have a high risk of causing hypersensitivity reactions, because a positive reaction helps to identify those clients who are at high risk of having a hypersensitivity reaction to the agent. If a client has a positive reaction to the intradermal skin test, that agent may be withheld from the treatment regimen.

40. *Answer:* C
Rationale: Commonly used medications for the prophylaxis of anaphylaxis include corticosteroids, histamine$_1$ receptor blockers (such as diphenhydramine), histamine$_2$ receptor blockers (such as Famotidine), and an antipyretic (such as acetaminophen). The other options provided will not help to prevent a hypersensitivity/anaphylactic reaction.

41. *Answer:* D
Rationale: Because an anaphylactic reaction may be a life-threatening emergency, appropriate emergency equipment and drugs should be readily available. Diazepam is not a normal premedication for preventing hypersensitivity reactions. Because every agent has the potential to cause anaphylaxis, clients are not rejected for studies for this reason alone. Premedications may be given as a precautionary measure. Vital signs usually are taken more often for a drug with anaphylactic potential, especially during the first hour.

42. *Answer:* B
Rationale: Intravenous administration of drugs increases the risk for anaphylaxis because of the rapid, systemic effect. Other factors associated with an increased risk of anaphylaxis are high dosages, naturally occurring agents, and intermittent administration (that delays the antibody formation to the antigen).

BIBLIOGRAPHY

Arkel, T.S. (2000). Thrombosis and cancer. *Seminars in Oncology 27*, 362-374.

Arnold, S.M, Patchell, R., Lowy, A.M., & Foon, K.A. (2001). Paraneoplastic syndromes. In V.T. DeVita, S.S. Hellman, & S.A. Rosenberg (Eds.). *Cancer: Principles and practice of oncology* (6th ed.). Philadelphia: Lippincott Williams & Wilkins, pp. 2511-2536.

Bayne, M.C., & Illidge, T.M. (2001). Hypercalcemia, parathyroid hormone-related protein and malignancy. *Clinical Oncology 13*, 372-377.

Bick, R.L. (2003). Disseminated intravascular coagulation current concepts of etiology, pathophysiology, diagnosis, and treatment. *Hematology Oncology Clinics of North America 17*(1), 149-176.

Body, J.J. Bartl, R., Burckhardt, P., et al. (1998). Current use of bisphosphonates in oncology. International Bone and Cancer Study Group. *Journal of Clinical Oncology 16*, 3890-3899.

Bone, R.C., Balk, R.A., Cerra, F.B., et al. (1992). Definition for sepsis and organ failure and guidelines for the use of innovative therapies in sepsis. *Chest 101*, 1644-1655.

Camp-Sorrell, D. (2000). Chemotherapy: Toxicity management. In C.H. Yarbro, M.H. Frogge,

M. Goodman, & S.L. Groenwald (Eds.). *Cancer nursing: Principles and practice* (5th ed.). Sudbury, MA: Jones and Bartlett Publishers, pp. 444-486.

Craig, S. (2001). Hyponatremia. *eMedicine.com*, Retrieved April 1, 2003, from http://www.emedicine.com/emerg/topic275.htm.

DeSancho, M.T., & Rand, J.H. (2001). Bleeding and thrombotic complications in critically ill patients with cancer. *Critical Care Clinics 17*, 599-622.

Doane, L. (2002). Overview of tumor lysis syndrome. *Seminars in Oncology Nursing 18* (Suppl 3), 2-5.

Drain, K.L., & Volcheck, G.W. (2001). Preventing and managing drug-induced anaphylaxis. *Drug Safety 24*, 843-853.

Ellerhorst-Ryan, J.M. (2000). Infection. In C.H. Yarbro, M.H. Frogge, M. Goodman, & S.L. Groenwald (Eds.). *Cancer nursing: Principles and practice* (5th ed.). Sudbury, MA: Jones and Bartlett Publishers, pp. 691-708.

Esbrit, P. (2001). Hypercalcemia of malignancy—new insights into an old syndrome. *Clinical Laboratory 47*, 67-71.

Flombaum, C.D. (2000). Metabolic emergencies in the cancer patient. *Seminars in Oncology 27*, 322-334.

Freeman, T.M. (1998). Anaphylaxis: Diagnosis and treatment. *Primary Care: Clinics in Office Practice 25*, 809-817.

Gobel, B.H. (2003). Disseminated intravascular coagulation. *Clinical Journal of Oncology Nursing 7*, 339-340.

Gobel, B.H. (2000). Disseminated intravascular coagulation. In C.H. Yarbro, M.H. Frogge, M. Goodman, & S.L. Groenwald (Eds.). *Cancer nursing: Principles and practice* (5th ed.). Sudbury, MA: Jones and Bartlett Publishers, pp. 869-875.

Gobel, B.H. (2002). Management of tumor lysis syndrome: Prevention and treatment. *Seminars in Oncology Nursing 18* (Suppl 3), 12-16.

Goldman, S.C., Holcenberg, J.S., Finklestein, J.Z., et al. (2001). A randomized comparison between rasburicase and allopurinol in children with lymphoma or leukemia at high risk for tumor lysis. *Blood 97*, 2998-3003.

Haapoja, I.S. (2000). Paraneoplastic syndromes. In C.H. Yarbro, M.H. Frogge, M. Goodman, & S.L. Groenwald (Eds.). *Cancer nursing: Principles and practice* (5th ed.). Sudbury, MA: Jones and Bartlett Publishers, pp. 792-811.

Heffner, M., & Polman, L.S. (1998). Hyperuricemia. In C.C. Chernecky & B.J. Berger (Eds.). *Advanced and critical care oncology nursing: Managing primary complications*. Philadelphia: W.B. Saunders, pp. 314-325.

Kaplow, R. (2002). Pathophysiology, signs, and symptoms of acute tumor lysis syndrome. *Seminars in Oncology Nursing 18* (Suppl 3), 6-11.

Kempin, S.J. (1997). Hemostatic defects in cancer patients. *Cancer Investigation 15*, 23-36.

Koscove, E.M. (1998). Sepsis and septic shock. In J.C. Brillman & R.W. Quenzer (Eds.). *Infectious disease in emergency medicine* (2nd ed.). Philadelphia: Lippincott-Raven, pp. 129-152.

Labovich, T.M. (1999). Hypersensitivity reactions to chemotherapy. *Seminars in Oncology Nursing 15*, 222-231.

Merck Manual of Geriatrics (3rd ed.). (2000). Whitehouse Station: Merck Research Laboratories.

Murphy-Ende, K. (1998). Disseminated intravascular coagulation. In C.C. Chernecky & B.J. Berger (Eds.). *Advanced and critical care oncology nursing: Managing primary complications*. Philadelphia: W.B. Saunders, pp. 119-139.

Peterson, J. (2000). Septic shock. In C.H. Yarbro, M.H. Frogge, M. Goodman, & S.L. Groenwald (Eds.). *Cancer nursing: Principles and practice* (5th ed.). Sudbury, MA: Jones and Bartlett Publishers, pp. 876-886.

Rangel-Frausto, M.S., & Wenzel, R.P. (1997). The epidemiology and natural history of sepsis. In A.M. Fein, E.M. Abraham, & R.A. Balk, et al. (Eds.). *Sepsis and multiorgan failure*. Baltimore: Williams & Wilkins, pp. 27-34.

Sachdeva, K., & O'Ballard. J.O. (2002). Granulocytopenia. *eMedicine.com*. Retrieved March 3, 2003 from http://www.emedicine.com/MED/topic927.htm.

Shanholtz, C. (2001). Acute life-threatening toxicity of cancer treatment. *Critical Care Clinics 17*, 483-502.

Smalley, R.V., Guaspari, A., Haase-Statz, S., et al. (2000). Allopurinol: Intravenous use for prevention and treatment of hyperuricemia in patients with leukemia or lymphoma. *Journal of Clinical Oncology 18*, 1758-1763.

Volker, D. (1998). Fever of unknown origin. *Nurse Practitioner Forum 9(3)* 170-176.

Wada, H., Sakuragawa, N., Mori, Y., et al. (1999). Hemostatic molecular markers before the onset of disseminated intravascular coagulation. *American Journal of Hematology 60*, 273-278.

Wickham, R.S. (2000). Hypercalcemia. In C.H. Yarbro, M.H. Frogge, M. Goodman, & S.L. Groenwald (Eds.). *Cancer nursing: Principles and practice* (5th ed.). Sudbury, MA: Jones and Bartlett Publishers, pp. 776-791.

Yu, M., Nardella, A., & Pechet, L. (2000). Screening tests of disseminated intravascular coagulation: Guidelines for rapid and specific diagnosis. *Critical Care Medicine 28*, 1777-1780.

Zanotti, K.M., & Markman, M. (2001). Prevention and management of antineoplastic-induced hypersensitivity reactions. *Drug Safety 24*, 767-779.

19 Structural Emergencies

JO ANN A. FLOUNDERS

Select the best answer for each of the following questions:

1. Superior vena cava syndrome (SVCS) occurs when
   A. excessive fluid in the pericardial space creates increased intrapericardiac pressure that compromises the heart's ability to fill and pump.
   B. excessive fluid in the pleural cavity causes dyspnea and tachycardia.
   C. the electrocardiogram (ECG) demonstrates tachycardia and atrial fibrillation.
   D. obstruction of the superior vena cava occurs as a result of extrinsic compression by tumor or enlarged lymph nodes or as a result of intrinsic obstruction by thrombosis or tumor.

2. The most common cause of SVCS is
   A. non-Hodgkin's lymphoma and advanced lung cancer.
   B. granulomatous infections caused by tuberculosis.
   C. radiation therapy-induced pneumonitis.
   D. mediastinal fibrosis caused by histoplasmosis.

3. The superior vena cava is a thin-walled blood vessel that is located
   A. in the pelvis.
   B. in the pleural cavity.
   C. within the thoracic cavity behind the sternum
   D. in the anterior cervical area.

4. Oncology nurses should recognize the following possible early signs of SVCS:
   A. Muffled heart rate of 100 beats/min, abdominal distention, and fever.
   B. Hypertension, bradycardia, widening pulse pressure, and abnormal respirations.
   C. Jugular vein distention and edema of the face, periorbital area, neck, upper thorax, breasts, and upper extremities.
   D. Hypotension and Cheyne-Stokes respirations.

5. Oncology nurses should recognize the following clinical manifestations of SVCS:
   A. Productive cough with green-yellow sputum.
   B. Dyspnea, facial plethora with ruddy complexion of face or cheek, and tachycardia.
   C. Bradycardia and diaphoresis.
   D. Fever, nausea, and vomiting.

6. The preferred diagnostic studies for SVCS are
   A. ECG and echocardiogram.
   B. magnetic resonance imaging (MRI) study and computed tomography (CT) scan.

C. chest x-ray (CXR) and barium swallow.
D. cervical spine x-rays and myelogram.

7. Medical treatment of a client with early clinical signs of SVCS includes
   A. instillation of tissue plasminogen activator (TPA) in central catheter that is patent.
   B. chemotherapy after diagnosis of lymphoma or small cell lung cancer is made.
   C. anticoagulation with heparin for all clients with SVCS.
   D. immediate chemotherapy before histologic diagnosis is obtained in clients with unknown cause of SVCS.

8. Nursing management of clients with cancer and SVCS includes
   A. attention to a client's inability to complete usual activities or button shirts.
   B. instructing the client to assume the supine position in bed.
   C. instructing clients to call the physician after temperature reaches 102° F (38° C).
   D. measurement of blood pressure in either upper extremity every 4 hours.

9. The oncology nurse should assess for side effects of treatment of SVCS, including
   A. hypoglycemia with corticosteroids.
   B. hypertension resulting from hypervolemia caused by diuretics.
   C. pancytopenia resulting from chemotherapy and/or radiation therapy.
   D. generalized rash caused by systemic antibiotics.

10. The principal cause of increased intracranial pressure (ICP) in clients with cancer is
    A. metabolic complications such as syndrome of inappropriate antidiuretic hormone (SIADH).
    B. side effects of treatment such as chemotherapy and radiation therapy.
    C. a space-occupying lesion such as a primary malignancy of the brain, or metastasis to brain tissue or skull from solid tumors.
    D. cerebral vascular accident or transient ischemic attack.

11. The clinical signs that indicate brain herniation, or shifting of intracranial contents, are
    A. hypotension, tachycardia, and rapid respirations.
    B. hypertension, bradycardia, widening pulse pressure, and abnormal respirations.
    C. hypotension and peripheral edema.
    D. hypotension, bradycardia, and peripheral edema.

12. The oncology nurse should recognize that the following clients with cancer have an increased risk of having increased ICP:
    A. Clients with basal cell carcinomas.
    B. Clients with adenocarcinoma of the cervix.
    C. All clients receiving radiation therapy.
    D. Clients with primary tumors of the brain or spinal cord, or solid tumors that metastasize.

13. A clinical manifestation of a client with cancer who has increased ICP may include
    A. round, equal pupils, ranging in size from 3 to 7 cm.
    B. pupils that respond briskly to light.
    C. sluggish or fixed pupils, in the absence of medications such as narcotics that may cause constriction.
    D. negative Romberg test.

14. The most definitive neuroimaging study to aid in the diagnosis of increased ICP is
    A. MRI study.
    B. lumbar puncture.
    C. arteriogram.
    D. carotid Doppler ultrasound.

15. Immediate medical treatment of increased ICP includes
    A. administration of calcium channel blockers and beta-blockers.
    B. administration of a nitroglycerin.
    C. administration of an osmotic diuretic such as mannitol (Osmitrol), and a corticosteroid.
    D. administration of a cardiac glycoside.

16. Nursing management of clients with cancer and increased ICP includes
    A. maintaining the client in a supine position without elevation of the head of the bed.

B. administration of stool softeners and laxatives to prevent constipation.

C. encouraging the client to do isometric muscle contractions and the Valsalva maneuver.

D. active range-of-motion exercises with 5 lb weights.

17. The oncology nurse should assess the client for side effects of medications used to control increased ICP such as

A. hypoglycemia with glucocorticoids.

B. hyperglycemia with glucocorticoids.

C. increased platelet count after chemotherapy.

D. hyperkalemia with furosemide.

18. Cardiac tamponade is defined as a life-threatening emergency that occurs when

A. a client experiences palpitations and premature ventricular contractions.

B. excessive fluid in the pericardial space creates increased pressure in the pericardial sac that decreases the heart's ability to fill and pump.

C. excessive fluid in the pleural cavity causes dyspnea and tachycardia.

D. the ECG demonstrates tachycardia and atrial fibrillation.

19. The most common cause of cardiac tamponade in many medical clients is

A. pericarditis caused by chemotherapy such as doxorubicin.

B. radiation therapy-induced pericarditis.

C. malignant disease that causes pericardial effusion.

D. diseases such as rheumatoid arthritis or systemic lupus erythematosus (SLE).

20. The pericardial space is located

A. between the visceral and parietal pericardial membranes.

B. inside the ventricles of the heart.

C. inside the atria of the heart.

D. between the visceral and parietal pleural membranes.

21. Pericardial effusion is defined as

A. excessive fluid in the peritoneal cavity.

B. excessive fluid that accumulates in the pericardial sac.

C. excessive fluid in the pleural space.

D. compression of the right atrium of the heart.

22. The pathophysiologic mechanisms that occur with pericardial effusions causing cardiac tamponade include

A. decreased ventricular filling during diastole, decreased cardiac output, and poor tissue perfusion.

B. increased ventricular filling during diastole, increased cardiac output, and adequate tissue perfusion.

C. increased fluid in the myocardium, causing increased ventricular filling during diastole, and improved perfusion.

D. increased ventricular filling during diastole, increased systemic perfusion.

23. Clients with the following diagnoses have the most risk for having cardiac tamponade:

A. Clients with stage I malignant melanoma.

B. Clients with stage I colon cancer.

C. Clients receiving systemic chemotherapy.

D. Clients with lymphoma.

24. Possible early signs of cardiac tamponade include

A. muffled heart rate of 100 beats/min, abdominal distention, fever, and edema.

B. hypertension, bradycardia, widening pulse pressure, and abnormal respirations.

C. hypotension and Cheyne-Stokes respirations.

D. hypotension, bradycardia, and peripheral edema.

25. The following symptoms are possible clinical manifestations of cardiac tamponade:

A. Productive cough with green-yellow sputum, dizziness, nausea, and vomiting.

B. Melena, hematochezia, and hematemesis.

C. Retrosternal chest pain causing the client to assume a forward-leaning position, progressive dyspnea, orthopnea, and restlessness.

D. Blood-tinged frothy sputum, periods of apnea, and frontal headache.

26. The most specific and sensitive test used to aid in the diagnosis of pericardial effusion is
    A. two-dimensional echocardiogram (2-D echo).
    B. ECG.
    C. CXR.
    D. CT scan.

27. Immediate medical treatment of a client with cardiac tamponade includes
    A. thoracentesis.
    B. administration of antibiotics.
    C. pericardiocentesis and administration of intravenous fluid, blood, and plasma.
    D. administration of systemic chemotherapy.

28. Spinal cord compression (SCC) is defined as
    A. compression of the spinal cord in the area of the medulla oblongata.
    B. compression of the superior vena cava by a malignant tumor.
    C. compression of the thecal sac by tumor in the epidural space of the spinal column.
    D. compression of the spinal cord in the level of the cerebrum and cerebellum.

29. The most common cause of spinal cord compression in clients with cancer is
    A. SIADH.
    B. herpes zoster infection.
    C. carcinomatous meningitis.
    D. metastatic tumor invasion.

30. Cauda equina describes
    A. the lobe of the brain in which the speech center is located.
    B. the area of the gluteus maximus in which radiation therapy is administered.
    C. spinal nerve roots at the tip of the spine that extend to the lumbar-sacral areas.
    D. the area of the spine in which the temperature and respiratory centers are located.

31. The meninges provide a protective covering for the brain and spinal cord and are layered in the following order, from outermost to innermost:
    A. Dura mater, arachnoid, pia mater.
    B. Pia mater, arachnoid, dura mater.
    C. Arachnoid, pia mater, dura mater.
    D. Dura mater, pia mater, arachnoid.

32. The most common location for malignant invasion of the spinal cord that causes SCC is
    A. intramedullary, or in the spinal cord itself.
    B. intradural, or in the meninges or nerve roots in the dura.
    C. extravertebral, or outside the vertebral column.
    D. extradural, or outside the spinal cord, as in bony metastasis to the vertebrae.

33. Because early detection of SCC is necessary for early intervention, the oncology nurse should know that the most common presenting symptom of SCC in clients with cancer is
    A. motor weakness and motor loss.
    B. sensory loss.
    C. neck or back pain.
    D. bowel and bladder incontinence.

34. An important distinction between pain caused by SCC and pain caused by herniated disk is
    A. pain caused by SCC worsens in the supine recumbent position and may be relieved in the sitting position, whereas the opposite is true for herniated disk.
    B. pain caused by SCC worsens in the sitting position and may be relieved in the supine recumbent position, whereas the opposite is true for herniated disk.
    C. pain caused by SCC causes severe frontal or occipital headache upon awakening in the morning, whereas herniated disk does not.
    D. pain caused by SCC is always localized to one area of the spinal column, whereas herniated disk is not.

35. The **least** important prognostic factor in clients with SCC is

A. neurologic status before the initiation of therapy.
B. the ability to "walk in" to the health care facility at the time of diagnosis, so as to "walk out" upon discharge.
C. ambulatory status at the time of diagnosis.
D. weight loss.

36. Physical examination of clients with SCC should include
A. a lumbar puncture.
B. vertebral palpation and percussion that may elicit client complaint of discomfort at the level of compression.
C. digital rectal examination to rule out rectal bleeding.
D. auscultation of the heart to detect any new or existing heart murmurs.

37. The following tests are diagnostic tests for SCC:
A. Plain x-ray films initially, then bone scan, MRI, CT scans, or myelography.
B. Myelography initially, followed by plain spine films.
C. Lumbar puncture at the onset of symptoms.
D. Myelography only.

NOTES

ANSWERS

1. *Answer:* D
   Rationale: The correct answer is Option D, obstruction of the superior vena cava. Tachycardia and atrial fibrillation may occur in clients with SVCS but are not defining characteristics of SVCS. Excessive fluid in the pericardial space is a pericardial effusion, causing pericardial tamponade. Excessive fluid in the pleural cavity is a pleural effusion.

2. *Answer:* A
   Rationale: Although other choices are possible causes of SVCS, the most common is Option A, non-Hodgkin's lymphoma and advanced lung cancer

3. *Answer:* C
   Rationale: The superior vena cava drains the blood from the upper extremities, upper thorax, head and neck, en route to the right atrium of the heart. The superior vena cava is located in the right anterior, superior mediastinum behind the sternum.

4. *Answer:* C
   Rationale: Obstruction of the superior vena cava causes jugular vein distention and edema of the face, neck, upper thorax, breasts, and upper extremities. Option A is incorrect because abdominal distention and fever are not diagnostic of SVCS. Option B is incorrect because tachycardia usually occurs. Cheyne-Stokes respirations are not diagnostic of SVCS.

5. *Answer:* B
   Rationale: Obstruction of the superior vena cava causes edema of the face, neck, and upper thorax as a result of decreased drainage of venous circulation. Plethora and ruddy complexion and dyspnea and tachycardia may result. Cough with yellow sputum is a symptom of an upper respiratory infection.

6. *Answer:* B
   Rationale: The best diagnostic studies to detect structural abnormalities are CT scans and MRI studies. ECG and echocardiograms can detect cardiac abnormalities that result from obstruction of the superior vena cava but not the obstruction itself. Barium swallow may detect esophageal obstruction but not SVC obstruction. Cervical spine x-rays and myelograms would not detect obstruction of the superior vena cava.

7. *Answer:* B
   Rationale: Treatment of SVCS includes treatment of the underlying disease that is causing SVCS. Administration of chemotherapy is the preferred treatment for clients with malignancy causing SVCS. Option A is incorrect because TPA is not instilled into a patent central catheter. Heparin use is controversial for clients with SVCS. Option D is incorrect because chemotherapy is not usually administered until a histologic diagnosis is obtained.

8. *Answer:* A
   Rationale: Close attention to subtle early symptoms is important in the early diagnosis of SVCS. The inability of clients to complete usual activities may be a sign of progressive dyspnea, and the inability to button shirts may be a sign of increased neck edema. Clients with obstruction of the superior vena cava usually have dyspnea in the supine position. Although fever is not diagnostic of SVCS, clients should be instructed to call physicians with fever above 100.5° (38° C). Clients with obstruction of the superior vena cava should avoid measurement of blood pressure in the affected extremity.

9. *Answer:* C
   Rationale: Treatment of SVCS includes treatment of the underlying disease that causes SVCS. Treatment of malignant causes of SVCS includes chemotherapy or radiation therapy. Therefore assessment for pancytopenia is necessary. Although corticosteroids may be used, a side effect of corticosteroid use is hyperglycemia, not hypoglycemia. Use of diuretics may cause hypotension due to volume depletion, not hypervolemia. Antibiotics are not used to treat SVCS.

10. *Answer:* C
    Rationale: Although clients with cerebral vascular accidents may have increased ICP, the

principal cause of increased ICP in clients with cancer is a space-occupying lesion . Metabolic complications are not principal causes of increased ICP. Chemotherapy and radiation therapy do not cause increased ICP. Other potential causes of increased ICP in clients with cancer include hemorrhage, venous sinus thrombosis, meningitis, head trauma, infarction, and abscess.

11. *Answer:* B
Rationale: The three clinical signs of hypertension, bradycardia, and abnormal respirations are known as Cushing's triad and indicate some shifting of intracranial contents, or herniation. The cerebral blood vessels dilate in response to accumulated carbon dioxide and lactic acid, causing increased blood volume and edema in the cranium. Increased sympathetic tone occurs in an effort to improve oxygenation, and the consequence is increased systolic blood pressure. Therefore hypotension, as listed in Options A, C, and D, does not usually occur with increased ICP.

12. *Answer:* D
Rationale: The principal cause of increased cranial pressure (ICP) in clients with cancer is a space-occupying lesion such as a primary malignancy of the brain, or metastasis to brain tissue or skull from solid tumors. Basal cell carcinomas do not usually metastasize. Although radiation therapy to the brain can cause increased ICP when inflammation and cerebral edema occur, increased ICP does not occur in all clients undergoing radiation therapy.

13. *Answer:* C
Rationale: Increased ICP will cause abnormal pupillary changes. Accurate assessment of pupils includes inspection of size, shape, and symmetry and evaluation of medications a person may be receiving that could cause pupillary constriction or dilation. Pupils should be round and equal, ranging from 3 to 7 cm, and should react briskly to light. Variations from normal include pupillary constriction, which occurs with narcotic analgesics, but may denote damage to the brainstem; pupillary dilation, which can occur with atropine-containing drugs, but can signify hypoxia; and unequal pupils, or anisocoria, which suggests possible brain herniation.

Clients with increased ICP may have a positive Romberg test (a test of coordination involving observation of a client standing with feet together and arms at sides, initially with eyes open, followed by eyes closed. The examiner assesses the client for loss of balance with eyes closed, which is called a positive Romberg sign.

14. *Answer:* A
Rationale: MRI is the more superior neuroimaging study and can better differentiate among solid tumor, edema, and fluid collection. A CT scan, without contrast, is usually completed initially to detect acute hemorrhage. After hemorrhage is ruled out, a CT with contrast enhancement is completed and can detect hydrocephalus or a mass with edema in the white matter. A lumbar puncture is contraindicated when increased ICP is suspected, because of the risk of herniation. Arteriograms and Doppler ultrasounds of the carotids are not performed to diagnose increased ICP.

15. *Answer:* C
Rationale: Immediate treatment of increased ICP includes administration of corticosteroids and osmotic diuretics to decrease cerebral edema. Administration of an osmotic diuretic such as mannitol, which is a hyperosmolar agent, causes hyperconcentration of the blood. The principle of water diffusion allows that water will flow from a hypoconcentrated solution to a hyperconcentrated solution to maintain equilibrium. Therefore when mannitol is administered intravenously, the blood becomes more concentrated than the edematous cerebral tissue, which is less concentrated because of edema. Water then crosses the semipermeable cell membrane and flows from the cerebral tissue into the blood, and cerebral edema is decreased. Calcium channel blockers, beta-blockers, nitroglycerin, and cardiac glycosides are not given to decrease intracranial pressure.

16. *Answer:* B
Rationale: Nurses should administer stool softeners to prevent constipation and antiemetics to prevent vomiting. Because ICP may increase with increased activity of a client, nursing interventions to prevent increases in

ICP resulting from activity include minimizing environmental stimuli and maintaining bed rest with head of bed elevated 15 to 30 degrees to promote venous drainage. The Valsalva maneuver should be avoided in clients with increased ICP. Therefore clients should be instructed to avoid any lifting and/or turning in bed.

17. *Answer:* B
    Rationale: Glucocorticoids may cause hyperglycemia, not hypoglycemia. Chemotherapy may cause decreased platelet count. Furosemide causes hypokalemia.

18. *Answer:* B
    Rationale: Cardiac tamponade occurs when excessive fluid in the pericardial space, called a pericardial effusion, creates increased pressure in the pericardial sac that decreases the heart's ability to fill and pump. Consequently, cardiac tamponade causes decreased cardiac output and decreased systemic perfusion. Clients with cardiac tamponade may exhibit palpitations, premature ventricular contractions (PVCs), dyspnea, tachycardia, and atrial fibrillation, but those clinical manifestations do not define cardiac tamponade.

19. *Answer:* C
    Rationale: Although the other choices include causes of cardiac tamponade in medical clients, malignant disease is the most common cause of cardiac tamponade in many medical clients.

20. *Answer:* A
    Rationale: The pericardial space cushions the myocardium and is located between the visceral and parietal pericardial membranes. It is not located inside the atria or ventricles of the heart. The pleural space is located between the visceral and parietal pleural membranes.

21. *Answer:* B
    Rationale: Pericardial effusion is the accumulation of fluid in the pericardial sac. Excessive fluid in the peritoneal cavity is ascites. Excessive fluid in the pleural space is a pleural effusion. The accumulation of fluid in the pericardial sac, or pericardial effusion, consequently causes compression of the chambers of the heart, ultimately causing decreased cardiac output and decreased systemic perfusion.

22. *Answer:* A
    Rationale: Pericardial effusion is the accumulation of fluid in the pericardial sac, resulting in compression of the chambers of the heart. Decreased ventricular filling occurs, causing decreased cardiac output and decreased systemic perfusion. Ultimately, compensatory mechanisms fail, causing circulatory collapse, shock, cardiac arrest, and death if not corrected.

23. *Answer:* D
    Rationale: Of the options provided, the client with lymphoma is most at risk. Lymphoma may involve the pericardium and may cause pericardial effusions with subsequent cardiac tamponade. Although malignancies can metastasize to the heart and pericardium, clients with stage I melanoma or stage I colon cancer do not have metastatic disease and therefore do not have pericardial effusions. Pericardial effusions and cardiac tamponade are not expected side effects of chemotherapy administration.

24. *Answer:* A
    Rationale: Physical examination of clients with cardiac tamponade includes the following early signs: muffled heart sounds, weak apical pulse, mild tachycardia, mild peripheral edema, mild abdominal distention, and fever. Clients do not usually exhibit hypertension, bradycardia, or Cheyne-Stokes respirations.

25. *Answer:* C
    Rationale: Clients with cardiac tamponade often assume a forward-leaning position to relieve retrosternal chest pain and dyspnea. Characteristic symptoms of cardiac tamponade do not include cough productive of yellow or blood-tinged sputum, or melena, hematochezia, or hematemesis.

26. *Answer:* A
    Rationale: While an EKG, CXR, or CT scan may identify a need for further evaluation, a 2-D echo is the most specific test for pericardial effusion. An echocardiogram uses ultrasound waves to reveal a picture of the heart and can reveal the collapse of the right

atrium and ventricle caused by the pressure of the increased pericardial fluid. An ECG can detect nonspecific changes such as tachycardia or premature ventricular contractions but cannot determine the cause of the changes. A CXR can demonstrate cardiac enlargement. In fact, a water bottle appearance of the heart may be seen on the CXRs of clients with pericardial effusions. However, CXR does not provide definite diagnosis of a pericardial effusion, because CXR can not differentiate the potential causes of cardiac enlargement.

27. *Answer:* C
Rationale: The goal of treatment of clients with cardiac tamponade is removal of pericardial fluid and restoration of hemodynamic stability. Immediate medical treatment of a client with cardiac tamponade includes pericardiocentesis and supportive treatment to maintain blood pressure and cardiac functioning. Pericardiocentesis is a drainage method in which a needle is inserted into the pericardial sac to drain the pericardial effusion, usually with guidance by either cardiac catheterization or echocardiogram. In addition, intravenous fluids, blood products, and plasma may be administered to expand circulatory volume and prevent circulatory collapse. Vasoactive drugs such as dopamine or isoproterenol may also be used to maintain tissue perfusion. Thoracentesis is a drainage technique to relieve pleural effusions, not pericardial effusions. Administration of antibiotics and systemic chemotherapy, while possibly simultaneously necessary, are not immediate specific medical interventions for cardiac tamponade.

28. *Answer:* C
Rationale: Spinal cord compression is defined as compression of the thecal sac by tumor in the epidural space. Malignant tumor compresses the spinal cord. Options A, B, and D are incorrect because the anatomic locations are not part of the spinal cord.

29. *Answer:* D
Rationale: The most common cause of spinal cord compression in clients with cancer is metastatic tumor invasion. The thoracic area of the spinal column is the most frequent site of metastasis that causes SCC. SIADH does not cause SCC. Herpes zoster infection and carcinomatous meningitis are not the most common causes of SCC.

30. *Answer:* C
Rationale: The spinal cord is approximately 10 inches shorter than the vertebral column. It arises from the medulla oblongata in the brain and extends to the first lumbar (L1) vertebrae. Therefore the lumbar-sacral spinal nerves extend from the distal lumbar spine to the lumbar-sacral areas. Because of the resemblance to a horse's tail, these long nerve roots are called cauda equina. Cauda equina is not located in the brain or gluteus maximus. Temperature and respiratory centers are not located in the spinal cord.

31. *Answer:* A
Rationale: There are three coverings, or meninges, that protect the brain and spinal cord. They are layered in the following order: dura mater, arachnoid membrane, and pia mater.

32. *Answer:* D
Rationale: The most common location for malignant invasion of the spinal cord that causes SCC is extradural, which occurs when a tumor arises outside the spinal cord. An example of extradural invasion is bony metastasis to the vertebrae.

33. *Answer:* C
Rationale: The most common presenting symptom of SCC is neck or back pain. Pain can actually occur before the actual compression of the spinal cord and before the development of any neurologic symptoms. The common progression of symptoms in SCC is pain, motor weakness, sensory loss, motor loss, and autonomic dysfunction.

34. *Answer:* A
Rationale: Pain caused by SCC may actually increase in the supine recumbent position and is usually relieved in the sitting position, whereas the opposite is true for pain caused by herniated disk. Pain caused by SCC may actually increase at night when lying down to sleep, whereas the opposite is true for degenerative disease of the spine.

35. *Answer:* D
Rationale: The neurologic status of clients with SCC is the most important prognostic indicator. Neurologic status includes ambulatory status. Weight loss, although an important prognostic indicator, is not the most important prognostic indicator in SCC.

36. *Answer:* B
Rationale: Physical examination should include vertebral palpation and percussion, which can elicit tenderness at the area of the SCC. Physical examination of clients with SCC does not usually include lumbar puncture or digital rectal examination. Although not diagnostic of SCC, physical examination of clients with cancer includes cardiac auscultation.

37. *Answer:* A
Rationale: Plain x-ray films are usually obtained initially and can identify up to 85% of vertebral lesions. Bone scans are more sensitive than x-rays in detecting vertebral abnormalities. MRI, CT, and myelography are used as definitive diagnostic tests for SCC. Because MRI is noninvasive, it has commonly replaced myelography. Lumbar puncture may be completed to assess cerebrospinal fluid but is not diagnostic of SCC.

BIBLIOGRAPHY

Beauchamp, K. (1998). Pericardial tamponade: An oncologic emergency. *Clinical Journal of Oncology Nursing* 2(3), 85-95.

Belford, K. (2000). Central nervous system cancers. In C.H. Yarbro, M.H. Frogge, M. Goodman, & S.L. Groenwald. (Eds.). *Cancer nursing: Principles and practice* (5th ed.). Sudbury, MA: Jones and Bartlett Publishers, pp. 1048-1096.

Bucholtz, J. (1999). Metastatic epidural spinal cord compression. *Seminars in Oncology Nursing 15*(3), 150-159.

DeMichele, A., & Glick, J. (2001). Cancer-related emergencies. In R. Lenhard, R. Osteen, T. Gansler (Eds.). Clinical oncology. Atlanta: American Cancer Society, Inc, pp. 733-764.

Haapoja, I., & Blendowki, C. (1999). Superior vena cava syndrome. *Seminars in Oncology Nursing 15*(3), 183-189.

Hunter, J.C. (2005). Structural emergencies. In J. Itano, & K. Taoka, (Eds.). *Core curriculum for oncology nursing* (4th ed.). St. Louis: Elsevier, pp. 422-439.

Keefe, D. (2000). Cardiovascular emergencies in the cancer patient. *Seminars in Oncology 27*(3), 244-255.

Knoop, T., & Willenberg, K. (1999). Cardiac tamponade. *Seminars in Oncology Nursing 15*(3), 168-173.

Myers, J.S. (2001). Oncologic complications. In S. Otto (Ed.) *Oncology Nursing* (4th ed.). St. Louis: Mosby, pp. 498-527.

Quinn, J., & DeAngelis, L. (2000). Neurologic emergencies in the cancer patient. *Seminars in Oncology 27*(3), 311-321.

Schafer, S. (1997). Oncologic complications. In S. Otto (Ed.). *Oncology nursing* (3rd ed.). St. Louis: Mosby Year Book, pp. 406-474.

Schrump, D.S., & Nguyen, D.M. (2001). Oncologic emergencies: Malignant pleural and pericardial effusions. In V.T. DeVita, S.A. Hellman, & S. Rosenberg (Eds.). *Cancer: Principles and practice of oncology*. Philadelphia: Lippincott Williams & Wilkins, pp. 2729-2752.

Wilkes, G.M. (2004). Symptoms of neurological disturbances. In C.H. Yarbro, M.H. Frogge, M. Goodman (Eds.). *Cancer symptom management* (3rd ed.). Sudbury, MA: Jones and Bartlett Publishers, pp. 331-399.

PART SIX

SCIENTIFIC BASIS FOR PRACTICE

20 Biology of Cancer and Carcinogenesis

DEBORAH L. VOLKER

Select the best answer for each of the following questions:

1. Cancer cells tend to live longer than normal cells because cancer cells have defects in
   A. apoptosis.
   B. initiation.
   C. promotion.
   D. pleomorphism.

2. Antiangiogenesis factors are of interest as potential treatments for cancer because they may
   A. damage cellular DNA.
   B. block production of tumor markers.
   C. inhibit the tumor's ability to metastasize.
   D. suppress cancer cells' ability to express oncogenes.

3. Mr. J., a client with small cell lung cancer, arrives for his clinic visit complaining of extreme thirst, headaches, and progressive weakness. His blood work reveals the following:
   Sodium: 120 mEq/L
   Potassium: 3.7 mEq/L
   Calcium: 10.1 mEq/L
   Chloride: 95 mEq/L
   Magnesium 1.6 mg/dl
   Phosphorus 3.4 mg/dl
   Uric acid: 5.0 mg/dl
   Glucose: 132 mg/dl
   Albumin: 3.9 g/dl

Which paraneoplastic syndrome would you suspect he has?
   A. Syndrome of inappropriate antidiuretic hormone (SIADH).
   B. Hypercalcemia.
   C. Cushing's syndrome.
   D. Tumor lysis syndrome.

4. A cancer that arises in glandular epithelial cells is termed a (an)
   A. liposarcoma.
   B. adenocarcinoma.
   C. chondrosarcoma.
   D. squamous cell carcinoma.

5. Mrs. J. is scheduled to receive chemotherapy before her surgery for breast cancer to control potential sites of metastases. This approach to chemotherapy is termed
   A. primary.
   B. adjuvant.
   C. neoadjuvant.
   D. prophylactic.

6. The purpose of evaluating CA 125 after treatment for ovarian cancer is to
   A. detect a primary tumor in another organ.
   B. monitor disease recurrence or progression.
   C. determine whether a cure has been achieved.

D. evaluate the genetic instability of any remaining cancer cells.

7. Which of the following is among the most common sites of metastasis?
   A. Kidney.
   B. Lung.
   C. Ovary.
   D. Spleen.

8. The nurse explains to the client that the tumor, node, metastasis (TNM) staging system is designed to
   A. evaluate extent of disease.
   B. predict the growth fraction of a tumor.
   C. decide whether the tumor is benign or malignant.
   D. determine the degree of differentiation of the malignant cells.

9. The nurse teaches the public to decrease risk of carcinogenesis by ultraviolet radiation by including a discussion of which risk factor?
   A. An increased amount of melanin in the skin.
   B. Exposure to known viral carcinogens.
   C. Concurrent use of tobacco.
   D. History of acute sunburn at an early age.

10. The difference between malignant and benign tumors is one of ability to
   A. cause death.
   B. produce pain.
   C. create metastases.
   D. impair functional status.

11. Proto-oncogenes are best described as genes that
   A. inhibit cell growth.
   B. repair damaged DNA.
   C. slow proliferation of cancer cells.
   D. regulate normal cell growth and repair.

12. The theory of immune surveillance against cancer may be useful to our understanding that
   A. cancer risk increases with age and immune senescence.
   B. cancers more often arise in immunocompetent individuals.
   C. chemical carcinogens are more vulnerable to immune surveillance.
   D. exposure to immunosuppressive agents is associated with a lesser risk of cancer.

13. The histologic term *dysplasia* refers to
   A. an increase in the number of cells in a tissue.
   B. a normal process that occurs in wound healing.
   C. variations in cell size, shape, and organization.
   D. replacement of one adult cell type by another adult cell type.

14. Which of the following represents a high-grade, poorly differentiated cancer?
   A. Grade I.
   B. Grade II.
   C. Grade III.
   D. Grade IV.

15. Because metastatic cells may be able to elicit necessary growth factors only in target organs,
   A. metastasis via lymphatic spread is enhanced.
   B. specific tumors tend to metastasize to specific organs.
   C. therapeutic levels of chemotherapy may not be achieved in target organs.
   D. target organs may become more genetically unstable and hospitable to metastatic cells.

ANSWERS

1. **Answer:** A
Rationale: Apoptosis refers to the induction of cell death in aging or damaged cells. Cancer cells resist the process of apoptosis. Options B and C are incorrect because they refer to processes by which normal cells become cancer cells but are not the source of abnormal cell longevity. Cancer cells do exhibit the property of pleomorphism (variability in cell size and shape), but this property does not account for increased longevity in cancer cells.

2. **Answer:** C
Rationale: Antiangiogenesis factors suppress a tumor's ability to stimulate growth of new blood vessels, thereby preventing an avenue for metastasis. Antiangiogenesis factors do not act via the other mechanisms described in Options A, B, and D.

3. **Answer:** A
Rationale: SIADH, hypercalcemia, and Cushing's syndrome are all potential paraneoplastic syndromes in persons with small cell lung cancer. However, only SIADH is correct in the case presented because of the client's low serum sodium level and symptoms associated with hyponatremia. Tumor lysis syndrome is not a paraneoplastic syndrome, nor are the client's electrolytes and uric acid consistent with tumor lysis syndrome.

4. **Answer:** B
Rationale: The correct choice is adenocarcinoma, because the prefix "Adeno-" refers to glandular tissue and because carcinomas arise in epithelial cells. Squamous cell carcinomas arise from squamous epithelium. Sarcomas originate in connective tissues.

5. **Answer:** C
Rationale: Neoadjuvant therapy is given before the primary treatment to control potential or known sites of metastasis. Adjuvant therapy is given after the primary treatment. Primary therapy refers to chemotherapy when it is the major modality used to treat a cancer, whereas prophylactic chemotherapy treatment is directed to a sanctuary site that is at high risk for developing cancer.

6. **Answer:** B
Rationale: CA 125 serves as a tumor marker in ovarian cancer for evaluation of response to treatment. The other options are incorrect because tumor markers are not useful for the purposes stated.

7. **Answer:** B
Rationale: The most common sites of metastatic disease include bone, liver, lung, and the central nervous system.

8. **Answer:** A
Rationale: The process of staging is done to determine disease extent via tumor size (T), lymph node involvement (N), and presence of metastasis (M). Options B, C, and D all refer to examination of the cellular characteristics of a tumor mass.

9. **Answer:** D
Rationale: The risk of developing melanoma as a result of sun exposure is associated with acute sunburn incurred at an early age. Increased skin pigmentation is protective against ultraviolet radiation. Options B and C are linked to increased risk of cancer resulting from exposure to viral and chemical carcinogens, respectively, but are not known to increase the risk of cancers induced by ultraviolet radiation.

10. **Answer:** C
Rationale: Option C is a defining characteristic of malignant growths, because benign tumors do not metastasize. Options A, B, and D are characteristics that both benign and malignant tumors may possess, because both may create physical pressure on vital structures and nerves.

11. **Answer:** D
Rationale: By definition, proto-oncogenes are normal genes that regulate cell growth and repair. Options A, B, and C refer to properties of various types of tumor suppressor genes.

12. *Answer:* A

Rationale: The theory of immune surveillance against cancer proposes that the immune system has the ability to recognize and destroy cancer cells. However, as the immune system ages and becomes less effective, this protective mechanism may fail. Some scientists believe that this provides support for the observation that cancers occur more frequently in older adults. Options B and D are incorrect because certain cancers arise more often in chronically immunosuppressed individuals. Option C is incorrect because the theory of immune surveillance is not specific to a particular classification of carcinogenic agents.

13. *Answer:* C

Rationale: Tissue dysplasia is defined as a loss of uniformity in the appearance and organization of cells. Options A and B are characteristics of tissue hyperplasia, whereas option D refers to tissue metaplasia.

14. *Answer:* D

Rationale: The term *grade* refers to the degree to which tumor cells resemble their normal counterparts. Grade I tumors most closely resemble their normal cellular counterparts and are termed low-grade, or well-differentiated cancers. Conversely, Grades II and III represent increasing dissimilarity, with grade IV characterized as the most poorly differentiated tumor and hence the "highest" grade.

15. *Answer:* B

Rationale: Option B reflects experimental study results that explain organ specificity of metastasis. The ability of metastatic cells to elicit growth factors in target organs is not linked to propensity to spread via metastasis (Option A), facilitate effectiveness of chemotherapy (Option C), or create genetic instability in target organs (Option D).

BIBLIOGRAPHY

DeVita, V.T., Hellman, & S., Rosenberg, S.A. (Eds.). (2001). *Cancer: Principles and practice of oncology* (6th ed.). Philadelphia: Lippincott Williams & Wilkins.

Lenhard, R.E., Osteen, R.T., & Gansler, T. (Eds.). (2001). *Clinical oncology.* Atlanta: American Cancer Society.

Pitot, H.C. (2002). *Fundamentals of oncology* (4th ed.). New York: Marcel Dekker, Inc.

Vogelstein, B., & Kinzler, K.W. (Eds.). (2002). *The genetic basis of human cancer* (2nd ed.). New York: McGraw-Hill.

Volker, D. L. (2005). Biology of cancer and carcinogenesis. In J. Itano & K. Taoka (Eds.). *Core curriculum for oncology nursing* (4th ed.). St. Louis: Elsevier, p. 443.

21 Immunology

JAMES C. PACE

Select the best answer for each of the following questions:

1. Which of the following key interactive functions of the immune system describes the body's ability to regulate, produce, and develop blood cells?
   - A. Self-recognition.
   - B. Hematopoiesis.
   - C. Homeostasis.
   - D. Immune surveillance.

2. The process of hematopoiesis begins with
   - A. polymorphonuclear neutrophils (PMNs).
   - B. noncommitted stem cells.
   - C. pluripotent stem cell.
   - D. B lymphocytes.

3. The myeloid cell line produces
   - A. B lymphocytes and natural killer (NK) cells.
   - B. monocytes and polymorphonuclear leukocytes.
   - C. T lymphocytes and associated antigens.
   - D. major histocompatibility complex (MHC) molecules.

4. Which of the following function as antigen-presenting cells for naïve T cells?
   - A. Null cells.
   - B. Auxiliary cells.
   - C. Dendritic cells.
   - D. NK cells.

5. Primary lymphoid organs
   - A. define the sites where foreign antigens encounter lymphocyte immune responses.
   - B. provide the major area for generating circulating blood cells in the adult.
   - C. allow for the maturation of lymphocytes including antigen receptors.
   - D. include Waldeyer's ring, spleen, and bone marrow.

6. Agglutination can best be described as
   - A. the ability of leukocytes to leak out of the vascular spaces into tissues.
   - B. a product of complement that encourages basophils to release histamines in the blood.
   - C. a result of the complement cascade that makes outer coatings of invading cells sticky.
   - D. an interactive network of serum and cell proteins combined in plasma.

7. In which of the four stages of inflammation would basophils, eosinophils, and mast cells release their vasoactive components?
   - A. Stage I—the vascular stage.
   - B. Stage II—cellular exudate stage.
   - C. Stage III—regeneration and repair.

D. Stage IV—increased bone marrow production of granulocytes and monocytes.

8. Humoral immunity refers to
   A. a cell-mediated response to foreign invaders.
   B. the recognition of peptide fragments bound to cell surface molecules.
   C. B-cell immunity that reflects antibody specificity.
   D. the ability of NK cells to directly attack foreign cells.

9. Which of the following best describes the monocyte/macrophage?
   A. Are distributed throughout tissue and capable of ingesting foreign cells/particles.
   B. Produce antibodies specific to antigen and are involved in the humoral response.
   C. Release histamine and chemotactic factors.
   D. Release a substance that triggers lysis of the cell.

10. Which of the following describes an organ of the immune system **rather** than a barrier to bacterial invasion?
    A. Mucous membranes.
    B. Lymphoid tissues.
    C. Saliva.
    D. Gastric secretions.

11. Which of the following type of phagocyte is particularly effective against large extracellular parasites?
    A. Type-2 T-helper cells (Th2).
    B. PMNs.
    C. Eosinophil polymorphs (eosinophils).
    D. Mononuclear phagocytes.

12. Which of the following components of the immune system serves to release inflammatory mediators through the process of thrombogenesis?
    A. Platelets.
    B. B cells.
    C. Large granular lymphocytes.
    D. Eosinophil polymorphs.

13. Which of the following cytokines limits the spread of certain viral infections, is produced early in response to infection, and offers the first line of viral resistance?
    A. Interferons (IFNs).
    B. Tumor necrosis factors (TNF-α or beta).
    C. Chemokines.
    D. Colony stimulating factors (CSFs).

14. Innate immunity differs from acquired or specific immunity in that
    A. innate immunity begins with an antigen presented to B or T lymphocytes.
    B. innate immunity is a cascade of mechanisms that occur before onset of infection.
    C. innate immunity involves epitopes that align themselves on molecules.
    D. innate immunity refers to B cell or humoral immunity.

15. The transfer of antibodies across the placenta from mother to infant is an example of
    A. acquired or specific immunity.
    B. innate immunity.
    C. passive immunity.
    D. T-cell-modulated immunity.

16. Tumor cells often evade immune system effector function by
    A. preserving immune competent T cells that are involved in immune surveillance.
    B. expressing antigens that ignite the immune response.
    C. losing the expression of antigens that target immune cell responses
    D. enabling class I MHC expression on tumor cells.

17. Which of the following is **not** a function of the helper T lymphocyte?
    A. Stimulate production and maturation of cytotoxic T cells.
    B. Activate macrophages.
    C. Inhibit production and maturation of suppressor T cells.
    D. Secrete lymphokines regulating immune function.

ANSWERS

1. *Answer:* B
Rationale: Hematopoiesis describes the body's ability to regulate, produce, and develop blood cells. Self-recognition is the body's ability to know self from non-self; homeostasis is the body's ability to maintain a balance of blood cell supply but does not entail the ability to produce and develop blood cells; and immune surveillance implies the recognition and destruction of malignant and/or altered cells.

2. *Answer:* C
Rationale: Blood cell development (hematopoiesis) begins with a single cell, the pluripotent stem cell. Option A is incorrect because blood cell development does not begin with PMNs. Option B is incorrect because the pluripotent stem cell divides to produce undifferentiated stem cells that are committed to one of two cell lineages (lymphoid or myeloid). Option D is incorrect because hematopoiesis describes that initial process that begins with a pluripotent stem cell and not a B cell, which develops later.

3. *Answer:* B
Rationale: The myeloid lineage produces monocytes, polymorphonuclear leukocytes (neutrophils, eosinophils, and basophils/mast cells), and platelets. Options A and C are incorrect because B lymphocytes and T lymphocytes arise from the lymphoid cell line (antigens are foreign substances that induce the immune response), and Option D is incorrect because MHC molecules are antigenic peptide fragments that bind to cell-surface molecules.

4. *Answer:* C
Rationale: The correct answer is dendritic cells. Null cells do not express T cell surface markers, and auxiliary cells are mediators of inflammation that play a pivotal role in attracting leukocytes toward a site of infection. NK cells' ultimate function is to identify and destroy virus-infected cells and certain tumor cells.

5. *Answer:* C
Rationale: Primary lymphoid organs allow for the maturation of lymphocytes including antigen receptors. Options A and D describe secondary lymphoid organs and tissues; Option B describes the bone marrow.

6. *Answer:* C
Rationale: Agglutination is the result of complement products that make the outer coatings of invading cells sticky; in the process, agglutination can change the structures of some viruses, making them nonvirulent. Options A, B, and D reflect additional aspects of the complement system but do not describe agglutination specifically.

7. *Answer:* A
Rationale: The release of vasoactive amines from basophils, eosinophils, and mast cells is a predominant feature of the first stage of the inflammatory response that prepares the way for the stages II-IV.

8. *Answer:* C
Rationale: Humoral immunity refers to the first type of acquired immunity that is associated with B cell activity. Options A, B, and D are all descriptive of T-cell (or cell-mediated) immunity (the second type of acquired immune response).

9. *Answer:* A
Rationale: The monocytes/phagocytes are distributed throughout the tissues and are capable of phagocytosis. Option B is incorrect because the B cell produces antibodies specific to antigen; Option C is incorrect because the mast cell or basophil releases histamine and chemotactic factors; and Option D is incorrect because the NK cell has the unique ability to release a substance that triggers lysis of the invading cell.

10. *Answer:* B
Rationale: Lymphoid tissues are considered to be an organ of the immune system rather than barriers to invasion. Other barriers include mucous membranes, saliva, gastric secretions, skin, tears, and perspiration.

11. *Answer:* C

Rationale: Option A, type-2 T-helper cells, is incorrect because a T cell is classified as a lymphocyte; although Options B and D describe differing types of phagocytes, it is Option C, the eosinophil, that is particularly aggressive against large extracellular parasites.

12. *Answer:* A

Rationale: The correct answer is Option A, platelets. Option B: cells multiply and further differentiate into plasma cells upon recognition of specific antigen; Option C: large granular lymphocytes damage cells that have recognized surface changes; and Option D: eosinophil polymorphs are specialized cells that target parasites.

13. *Answer:* A

Rationale: The correct answer is Option A, interferons. Option B, TNFs, mediate inflammation and cytotoxic reactions; Option C, chemokines, activate cells to perform specialized immunologic functions and guide movement of cells around the body between blood and tissues; and Option D, CSFs, guide and direct cell division and differentiation of bone marrow stem cells and leukocytes.

14. *Answer:* B

Rationale: Innate immunity differs from acquired or specific immunity in that innate immunity is a cascade of mechanisms that occur before onset of infection. Options A, C, and D all refer to acquired or specific immune functions and not to innate immunity.

15. *Answer:* C

Rationale: Passive immunization is defined as the transfer of antibodies from an immunized individual to a nonimmunized individual. The only option that fits this definition is C.

16. *Answer:* C

Rationale: The loss of the ability to express antigens on tumor cells allows for the rapid and uncontrolled growth of tumors because immune cell response is altered. Options A, B, and D all describe ways that tumor cells encounter (rather than evade) immune system effector function.

17. *Answer:* C

Rationale: Helper T cells stimulate the production and maturation of suppressor T cells. Options A, B, and D are all functions of the helper T-lymphocyte.

BIBLIOGRAPHY

Buchsel, P. (Ed.). (2000). *Cytokine Therapy: The GM & D factor*. Pittsburgh: Oncology Education Services.

Cotran, R.S., Kumar, V., & Collins, T. (1999). Acute and chronic inflammation. In *Pathologic basis of disease*. Philadelphia: W.B. Saunders, pp. 50-88.

DeMeyer, E.S., & Bayer, J. (2000). *Dendritic cells: The sentry cells of the hematopoietic cell line*. Pittsburgh: Oncology Education Services.

DeMeyer, E., & Schirmer, M. (2004). *The healing power of colony stimulating factors*. Pittsburgh: Oncology Education Services.

Janeway, C.A., Traver, M.W., Shlomchik, M. (2001). *Immunobiology: The immune system in health and disease* (5th ed.). New York: Garland Publishing.

Kirton, C.A. (2001). Clinical application of immunological and virological markers. In C.A. Kirton, D. Talolta, & K. Kwolski (Eds.). *Handbook of HIV/AIDS nursing*. St. Louis: Mosby, pp. 26-48.

Male, D. (1986). *Immunology: An illustrated outline*. St. Louis: Mosby.

Zwolski, K. (2001). HIV immunopathogenesis. In C.A. Kirton, D. Talolta, & K. Kwolski (Eds.). *Handbook of HIV/AIDS nursing*. St. Louis: Mosby, pp. 3-25.

22 Genetics

KATHLEEN A. CALZONE

Select the best answer for each of the following questions:

1. A gene is which of the following?
   A. A threadlike structure that contains genetic information.
   B. An individual unit of hereditary information.
   C. A sequence of amino acids.
   D. Two nucleotide chains running in opposite directions that are coiled around one another to form a double helix.

2. Many of the genes responsible for familial cancer syndromes appear to be
   A. proto-oncogenes.
   B. oncogenes.
   C. tumor suppressor genes.
   D. mismatch repair genes.

3. What is a gene with a change in its DNA pattern?
   A. Tumor suppressor gene.
   B. Proto-oncogene.
   C. Mismatch repair gene.
   D. Mutation.

4. In autosomal dominant inheritance, what is the risk of transmitting a gene mutation, expressed in percent, for a first-degree relative?
   A. 75%.
   B. 50%.
   C. 25%.
   D. 10%.

5. One critical component of informed consent for predisposition genetic testing for inherited cancer risk is
   A. confirmation of the family history for cancer.
   B. overview of the risks, benefits, and limitations of predisposition genetic testing.
   C. recommending an individualized cancer risk management plan before testing should the client be found to harbor an alteration in a cancer susceptibility gene.
   D. completion of a full history and physical to rule out any suspicion of cancer.

6. The primary role of the nurse in predisposition genetic testing includes
   A. establishing a cancer risk management plan.
   B. determining which members of a family should be tested for a genetic alteration.
   C. facilitating informed decision making without being directive.
   D. selecting the laboratory to perform the test.

7. Which of the following represents the complementary pairing of a purine and pyrimidine base pair of DNA?

A. Adenine (A) and guanine (G).
B. Cytosine (C) and uracil (U).
C. Thymine (T) and cytosine (C).
D. Guanine (G) and cytosine (C).

8. Penetrance of a gene is best described as which of the following?
 A. Record of an individual's ancestral history showing inheritance patterns for a given trait or traits.
 B. Whether an individual of a given genotype expresses the corresponding phenotype.
 C. Characteristics (of appearance and activity) of an organism that result from the interaction between that organism's genotype and the environment.
 D. The process whereby a gene produces a protein from its DNA- and mRNA-coding sequences.

9. Which of the following items represents one application of pharmacogenetics in clinical practice?
 A. Drugs aimed at the genetic change and/or altered protein product.
 B. Introduction of a functioning gene into cells to replace missing function.
 C. Introduction of a functioning gene into the egg or sperm to prevent transmission of a gene mutation.
 D. Measurement of the structure, composition, and function of proteins that are made from genes.

10. Mutations in which gene have been correlated with an increased risk for both breast and ovarian cancer?
 A. *p53.*
 B. *PTEN.*
 C. *BRCA1.*
 D. *APC.*

11. Which of the following is a clinical feature of hereditary cancer?
 A. Older age of cancer onset.
 B. Telomerase.
 C. Metastatic cancer.
 D. Multiple primary cancers in a single individual.

12. What type of mutation adds or deletes one or more bases from the normal gene sequence ?
 A. Frameshift.
 B. Missense.
 C. Splicing.
 D. Translocation.

13. What is the risk for colon cancer in an individual who has never been diagnosed with cancer and has tested negative for a known colon cancer susceptibility gene mutation in the family?
 A. Colon cancer risk cannot be established.
 B. Colon cancer risk at least equivalent to general population.
 C. Colon cancer risk is eliminated.
 D. Colon cancer risk still elevated.

14. Which of the following is true about mismatch repair genes?
 A. Activate a program that leads to cell death.
 B. Maintain the ends of the chromosomes.
 C. Correct DNA replication errors.
 D. Control normal cell growth.

15. Mutations in *MSH2* have been associated with an increased risk for which form of cancer?
 A. Sarcoma.
 B. Ovary.
 C. Lung.
 D. Thyroid.

ANSWERS

1. *Answer:* B
Rationale: Genes are individual units of hereditary information located at a specific position on a chromosome and consist of a sequence of DNA that code for a specific protein. Option A refers to chromosomes; Option C: genes code for a sequence of amino acids resulting in a protein that has a specific function. Option D: DNA is two nucleotide chains, running in opposite directions that are coiled around one another to form a double helix.

2. *Answer:* C
Rationale: Tumor suppressor genes function as regulators of cell growth. Some tumor suppressor genes appear to play a role in cell cycle regulation, whereas others have a role in DNA repair. Many of the genes responsible for familial cancer syndromes appear to be tumor suppressor genes. Proto-oncogenes are essential for normal cell growth and regulation. Alterations occurring in proto-oncogenes result in oncogene activation, which can result in uncontrolled cell growth. Mismatch repair genes correct DNA replication errors. Although all of these genes appear to play a role in the development of cancer, familial cancer syndromes most often appear to be associated with tumor suppressor genes.

3. *Answer:* D
Rationale: Mutations are variations in the sequence of DNA. Tumor suppressor genes, proto-oncogenes, and mismatch repair genes are different types of regulatory genes that control cell growth and proliferation. When functioning normally without the presence of a pathologic mutation, all of these genes appear to prevent the development of cancer.

4. *Answer:* B
Rationale: Autosomal dominant inheritance requires only one altered copy of a gene to result in cancer susceptibility. The risk of transmission to a first-degree relative is 50%; 75% does not represent the risk of transmission to a first-degree relative for any mendelian pattern of inheritance; 25% risk represents the risk in autosomal recessive inheritance, which requires two altered copies of a gene, one from each parent, to result in cancer susceptibility. The principles of autosomal dominant inheritance indicate that genetic alterations can be transmitted equally between men and women. However, the specific cancer risks for men and women may differ.

5. *Answer:* B
Rationale: The decision whether to undergo predisposition genetic testing is hinged on the adequacy of the information provided to the individual regarding the risks, benefits, and limitations of testing. Confirmation of the family history of cancer is a critical component of determining eligibility for predisposition genetic testing but is not part of the informed consent process. Insufficient data exist regarding the benefits and limitations of all cancer risk management strategies in individuals at high risk for cancer because of an alteration in a cancer susceptibility gene. The health care provider should outline the potential alternatives and limitations of cancer risk management as part of the informed consent process but should not recommend a particular strategy. Informed consent for predisposition genetic testing does not depend on the client's personal health status. However, current health status established by a history and physical is an essential component of cancer risk counseling.

6. *Answer:* C
Rationale: The primary role of the nurse in predisposition genetic testing should be to provide the information necessary for an informed decision without being directive regarding the testing decision. Also, the nurse should be sure that the client understands that testing is completely voluntary and will not prejudice their future health care. The nurse should outline the potential alternatives and limitations of cancer risk management as part of the informed consent process but should not recommend a particular strategy. The nurse can play a role in identifying family members who are eligible for testing, but testing is completely voluntary, and no health care provider

should dictate who should be tested. In addition, this should not be considered a primary role for the nurse. Laboratories where predisposition genetic testing is performed should be Clinical Laboratory Improvement Act (CLIA) approved. However, the primary role of the nurse is to facilitate informed decision making.

7. *Answer:* D
Rationale: DNA base pairs are complementary; adenine (A) attaches to thymine (T), and guanine (G) attaches to cytosine (C). Adenine does not attach to guanine but instead attaches to thymine. In the DNA, cytosine does not attach to uracil. Thymine does not attach to cytosine but instead attaches to adenine.

8. *Answer:* B
Rationale: Penetrance refers to the cancer risks associated with a specific genetic mutation. Ancestral heritage is an important component of pedigree construction to assess for the presence of a founder effect. However, this does not reflect the definition of penetrance. The complex interaction between genes and the environment may affect the penetrance of a specific gene, but gene/environment interactions do not reflect the meaning of penetrance. The process whereby a gene produces a protein from its DNA and mRNA coding sequences is termed translation.

9. *Answer:* A
Rationale: Pharmacogenetics refers to drugs designed specifically for the genetic characteristics of the tumor. Introduction of a functioning gene into the somatic cells to replace missing or defective genes or to provide a new cellular function is somatic gene therapy. Introduction of a functioning gene into the egg or sperm to prevent transmission of a genetic mutation is germline gene therapy. The analysis of the structure, composition, and function of proteins is proteomics.

10. *Answer:* C
Rationale: Deleterious mutations in *BRCA1* are associated with an increased risk of breast, ovarian, colon, and other cancers. Deleterious mutations in *p53* are associated with an increased risk for cancers of the breast and brain as well as leukemias, sarcomas, and adrenal cortical tumors. Deleterious mutations in *PTEN* are associated with an increased risk for cancers of the breast, thyroid (most often follicular type), and endometrium as well as benign skin lesions. Deleterious mutations in *APC* are associated with an increased risk for colon and rectal cancer, colon polyposis (adenomas), and other desmoid tumors.

11. *Answer:* D
Rationale: Multiple primary cancers in one individual are a hallmark sign of hereditary cancer. One key feature of hereditary cancer is early age of cancer diagnosis, not later age of cancer diagnosis. Telomerase plays a role in cellular aging through the telomeres, which are the ends of the chromosomes and can be involved in carcinogenesis. But telomerase is not a clinical feature of the hereditary susceptibility. The presence of metastasis is not indicative of a hereditary susceptibility to cancer. Somatic mutations in genes are involved in the tumor developing the capacity to metastasize.

12. *Answer:* A
Rationale: Frameshift mutations occur when one or more bases are added or deleted from the normal sequence, resulting in an altered form of the protein. Missense mutations are single-base pair changes that result in the substitution of one amino acid for another in the protein being constructed. Some of the substituted amino acids may be critical to the function of the protein. Splicing mutations occur when DNA that should be removed from the coding sequence is retained, or DNA that should not be added is spliced in. Translocations are segments of one chromosome that break off and attach themselves to other chromosomes, resulting in altered protein production.

13. *Answer:* B
Rationale: A negative test result for a known genetic mutation in a family indicates that the client is within the general population risk of cancer associated with that branch of the family. However, family history from the other parent and other personal risk factors still influence the risk of developing cancer.

14. *Answer:* C
Rationale: Mismatch repair genes correct errors that occur during the process of DNA

replication. The activation of a program that leads to cell death refers to apoptosis. Telomerase maintains the ends of the chromosomes. Oncogenes control normal cell growth.

15. *Answer:* B

Rationale: The cancer risks associated with deleterious mutations in *MSH2* include increases in risk for the colon, ovary, and endometrium. Sarcoma is associated with germline mutations in *p53*. Lung cancer has not been seen with mutations in *MSH2*. Thyroid cancer in combination with breast cancer is associated with mutations in *PTEN*.

BIBLIOGRAPHY

American Society of Clinical Oncology. (2003). American Society of Clinical Oncology policy statement update: Genetic testing for cancer susceptibility. *Journal of Clinical Oncology 21,* 2397-2406.

American Society of Human Genetics. (1996). Statement on informed consent for genetic research. *American Journal of Human Genetics 59,* 471–474.

Geller, G., Botkin, J.R., Green, M.J., et al. (1997). Genetic testing for susceptibility to adult onset cancer: The process and content of informed consent. *Journal of the American Medical Association 277,* 1467–1474.

Innocenti, F., & Ratain, M.J. (2002). Update on pharmacogenetics in cancer chemotherapy. *European Journal of Cancer 38,* 639-644.

International Society of Nurses in Genetics (ISONG). (2000). Informed decision-making and consent: The role of nursing. Retrieved March 1, 2003 from International Society of Nurses in Genetics Web site: http://www.globalreferrals.com/consent.htm.

Lindor, N.M., & Greene, M.H. (1998). The concise handbook of family cancer syndromes. Mayo Familial Cancer Program. *Journal of the National Cancer Institute 90,* 1039-1071.

Loud, J.T., Peters, J.A., Fraser, M., & Jenkins, J. (2002). Applications of advances in molecular biology and genomics to clinical cancer care. *Cancer Nursing 25,* 110-122.

Patterson, S.D., & Aebersold, R.H. (2003). Proteomics: The first decade and beyond. *Nature Genetics 33* (Suppl.), 311-323.

Rieger, P., & Pentz, R. (1999). Genetic testing and informed consent. *Seminars in Oncology Nursing 15,* 104-115.

Scanlon, C., & Fibison, W. (1995). *Managing genetic information: Implications for nursing education.* Washington, D.C.: American Nurses Association.

Schnieder, K.A. (2002). *Counseling about cancer: Strategies for genetic counselors* (2nd ed.). Dennisport: Massachusetts Graphic Illusions.

Strauss-Tranin, A. (Ed.). (1997). Genetics and cancer. *Seminars in Oncology Nursing 12,* 67–144.

Tranin, A.S., Masny, A., & Jenkins, J. (Eds.). (2003). *Genetics in oncology practice: Cancer risk assessment.* Pittsburgh: Oncology Nursing Society.

23 Nursing Care of the Client with Breast Cancer

DIANE G. COPE

Select the best answer for each of the following questions:

1. Breast cancer hormone receptor assay test results may be used for
    A. determining the breast cancer stage.
    B. determining whether lymph node dissection needs to be performed.
    C. deciding on adjuvant treatment options.
    D. deciding between breast conservation or mastectomy.

2. Compared with mastectomy, breast conservation surgery results in
    A. equivalent lymphedema incidence rates.
    B. greater lymphedema incidence rates.
    C. equivalent 5-year survival rates.
    D. greater 5-year survival rates.

3. Which of the following is a known risk factor for breast cancer because of the increased exposure to estrogen and/or progesterone?
    A. Early first-term pregnancy.
    B. Lactation.
    C. Physical activity.
    D. Late menopause.

4. To decrease the risk of lymphedema after a sentinel lymph node biopsy or lymph node dissection, a woman should be instructed to
    A. elevate the affected arm above the level of the heart at all times.
    B. use a compression sleeve on the affected arm when taking airline trips.
    C. perform exercises such as golf or tennis with the affected arm.
    D. have blood pressures checked in the affected arm.

5. Which of the following is a **less** common clinical manifestation in the diagnostic assessment of early-stage breast cancer?
    A. Breast pain.
    B. Skin dimpling.
    C. Nipple inversion.
    D. Bloody nipple discharge.

6. Modified radical mastectomy may be indicated for women who have a
    A. bone metastasis.
    B. large tumor.
    C. positive lymph nodes.
    D. family history of breast cancer.

7. Mrs. K. is a 42-year-old premenopausal woman with stage II breast cancer who just completed four cycles of cyclophosphamide (Cytoxan)/doxorubicin (Adriamycin) and is experiencing hot flashes. The nurse may assist Mrs. K. by instructing her to
    A. consume a high-protein diet.
    B. begin a regular exercise program.
    C. dress in loose-fitting clothes.
    D. begin estrogen replacement therapy.

8. A woman with breast cancer who received adjuvant chemotherapy is at risk for
   A. acute leukemia.
   B. diabetes mellitus.
   C. hypertension.
   D. osteoporosis.

9. The most common site of metastases with breast cancer is
   A. bone.
   B. contralateral breast.
   C. endometrium.
   D. ovary.

10. Bisphosphonates are indicated for women with breast cancer that has metastasized to the bone to
   A. improve anemia.
   B. enhance bone demineralization.
   C. prevent hypocalcium.
   D. reduce bone pain.

11. Which of the following is a possible adverse effect of anastrozole (Arimidex) therapy?
   A. Decreased bone density.
   B. Endometrial cancer.
   C. Thrombosis.
   D. Weight gain.

12. Ten days after a cycle of Cytoxan/Adriamycin, Mrs. C.'s nadir blood counts are
WBC $1.0 \times 1000/mm^3$ Absolute neutrophil
Hemoglobin   count $0.4 \times 1000/mm^3$
   10.5 g/dl   Hematocrit 30.1%
Platelets 246,000/mm^3

The nurse should instruct Mrs. C. to
   A. avoid heavy lifting.
   B. discontinue the use of a straight-edge razor when shaving.
   C. avoid eating fresh green leafy vegetables.
   D. use a soft toothbrush.

13. Mrs. T. will be receiving radiation after her lumpectomy. Which of the following is a common side effect of breast irradiation?
   A. Chest pain.
   B. Dyspnea.
   C. Esophagitis.
   D. Fatigue.

14. Which of the following racial and ethnic groups have the highest breast cancer mortality rates?
   A. African Americans.
   B. American Indians.
   C. Asian and Pacific Islanders.
   D. Hispanics.

15. According to the American Cancer Society's recommendations for early cancer detection, at what age should a woman begin mammography screening?
   A. 30.
   B. 35.
   C. 40.
   D. 45.

ANSWERS

1. *Answer:* C
    Rationale: Hormone receptor assay results provide independent prognostic information and therefore can aid in decision making regarding treatment options. The tests have no bearing on decisions regarding the type of surgery, lymph node dissection, or breast cancer stage.

2. *Answer:* C
    Rationale: Breast conservation surgery has equivalent 5-year survival rates compared with mastectomy. Lymphedema occurs as a result of lymph node biopsies or axillary radiation, and therefore the type of breast surgery has no correlation with the incidence of lymphedema.

3. *Answer:* D
    Rationale: Early first-term pregnancy, lactation, and physical activity all decrease exposure to estrogen and progesterone, whereas late menopause increases exposure.

4. *Answer:* B
    Rationale: A compression sleeve should be worn while flying to decrease change in pressure. Repetitious activities against resistance and blood pressures in the affected arm may lead to increased pressure on the lymphatic system and cause lymphedema.

5. *Answer:* A
    Rationale: Pain is not common but may be present in advanced disease. Skin dimpling, nipple inversion, and bloody nipple discharge may be seen in early-stage breast cancer.

6. *Answer:* B
    Rationale: Women with a large breast tumor may require a mastectomy to remove all diseased breast tissue. A family history of breast cancer, bone metastases, or positive lymph nodes are not specific indications for a mastectomy.

7. *Answer:* C
    Rationale: Dressing in loose-fitting clothes will allow the skin to cool. A high-protein diet and regular exercise programs have not been shown to decrease hot flashes. Estrogen replacement therapy is contraindicated in women with breast cancer.

8. *Answer:* D
    Rationale: Women with breast cancer are at risk for osteoporosis related to chemotherapy and estrogen replacement therapy is contraindicated. Acute leukemia, diabetes mellitus, and hypertension are unrelated disorders.

9. *Answer:* A
    Rationale: The most common site of breast metastases is bone. Other sites may include lung (69%), liver (65%), and brain (20%).

10. *Answer:* D
    Rationale: Bisphosphonates are used to prevent hypercalcemia, inhibit bone demineralization, and reduce bone pain. There is no effect on anemia.

11. *Answer:* A
    Rationale: Decreased bone density is a possible adverse effect of Arimidex, and therefore women should be monitored for the development of osteoporosis. Thrombosis and endometrial cancer are possible side effects of tamoxifen (Nolvadex) therapy. Weight gain is not a documented side effect of anastrozole (Arimidex).

12. *Answer:* C
    Rationale: Mrs. C. is neutropenic and should avoid fresh fruits and vegetables. The client is not thrombocytopenic and therefore may use a regular toothbrush and razor.

13. *Answer:* D
    Rationale: Fatigue is a common side effect with radiation. The other side effects are not related to breast irradiation.

14. *Answer:* A
    Rationale: Overall, African Americans have the highest breast cancer incidence

and mortality rates, followed by Caucasians, Hispanic/Latinos, American Indian and Alaskan Natives, and Asian American and Pacific Islanders.

15. *Answer:* C

Rationale: The American Cancer Society recommends that annual screening mammograms begin at age 40. Breast self-examinations should be performed monthly at the age of 20, and annual clinical breast examinations should begin at age 40.

BIBLIOGRAPHY

American Cancer Soceity. (2004). Cancer Facts and Figures. 2004. Atlanta: Author.

Bonnadonna, G., Hortobagyi, G., & Gianni, A.M. (Eds.). (1998). *Textbook of breast cancer: A clinical guide to therapy.* London: Martin Dunitz Ltd.

Harris, J.R., Lippman, M.E., Morrow, M., & Osborne, C.K. (Eds.). (2000). *Diseases of the breast* (2nd ed.). Philadelphia: Lippincott Williams & Wilkins.

Smith, R. A., Saslow, D., Sawyer, K. A., et al. (2003). American Cancer Society guidelines for breast cancer screening: Update 2003. *CA: A Cancer Journal for Clinicians 53,* 141-169.

Wilkes, G.M., Ingwersen, K., & Barton-Burke, M. (Eds.). (2002). *Oncology nursing drug handbook.* Sudbury, MA: Jones and Bartlett Publishers.

Yarbro, C.H., Frogge, M.H., & Goodman, M. (Eds.). (2002). *Clinical guide to cancer nursing* (5th ed.). Sudbury, MA: Jones and Bartlett Publishers.

24 Nursing Care of the Client with Lung Cancer

MARIE FLANNERY

1. The identification of gene expression patterns for individuals with lung cancer
   A. has already been mapped.
   B. is standard practice as part of histopathology.
   C. determines treatment selection.
   D. is a high research priority.

2. The histopathologic diagnosis of small cell lung cancer (SCLC) as distinct from non-small lung cancer (NSCLC) is important because
   A. only clients with SCLC are at risk for metabolic emergencies.
   B. clients with SCLC cancer are not at risk for metabolic emergencies.
   C. clients with SCLC tend to have a more aggressive course than clients with NSCLC.
   D. clients with SCLC tend to have a less aggressive course than clients with NSCLC.

3. Common early signs and symptoms of lung cancer include
   A. nagging cough.
   B. pain.
   C. shortness of breath.
   D. no specific symptoms.

4. In the Unites States lung cancer rates
   A. are steadily rising for white men.
   B. are decreasing for the entire population.
   C. are increasing for the entire population.
   D. are rising for women.

5. Which of the following is true regarding the incidence of lung cancer in the United States?
   A. Lung cancer has the highest cancer incidence for men and women.
   B. Lung cancer has the highest mortality for men and women.
   C. Lung cancer has the highest mortality and incidence for men.
   D. Lung cancer has the highest mortality and incidence for women.

6. The most significant risk factor for developing lung cancer is
   A. smoking.
   B. asbestos exposure.
   C. radon exposure.
   D. pollution.

7. The subtype of lung cancer associated with asbestos exposure is
   A. squamous cell.
   B. small cell.
   C. mesothelioma.
   D. adenocarcinoma.

8. Recommended screening for the early detection of lung cancer includes
   A. chest x-ray annually at age 50 and older.

B. chest x-ray for individuals at high risk only.

C. spiral computed tomography (CT) and/or positron emission tomography (PET) scans for individuals at high risk.

D. no recommended screening.

9. The overall 5-year survival rate for lung cancer is

A. 5%.

B. 10%.

C. 15%.

D. 25%.

10. The median survival for clients treated for extensive stage SCLC is

A. 3 months.

B. 9 months.

C. 18 months.

D. 2 years.

11. If an individual is a candidate, surgery is the treatment of choice for lung cancer because

A. lung cancer is often a localized disease.

B. chemotherapy is ineffective for lung cancer.

C. surgery offers the only option for cure.

D. surgery has few complications and few side effects.

12. After the chest is opened for surgical resection, what percent of clients do not have resection, because metastases are found?

A. 10%.

B. 25%.

C. 50%.

D. 75%.

13. Prophylactic cranial irradiation (PCI) is used to prevent or delay the incidence of brain metastases for

A. individuals with early-stage NSCLC.

B. individuals with late-stage NSCLC.

C. individuals with limited stage SCLC.

D. individuals with extensive stage SCLC.

14. Chemotherapy is now commonly used as adjuvant therapy in NSCLC because

A. multiple clinical trials demonstrated an advantage over best supportive care.

B. chemotherapy regimens are better tolerated with the introduction of growth factors.

C. response rates for NSCLC are approaching 60%.

D. similar response rates are found as for individuals with SCLC.

15. The standard of care for treatment of stage IIIB NSCLC in clients with good performance status is

A. lobectomy followed by radiation therapy (RT).

B. lobectomy followed with adjuvant chemotherapy.

C. single modality treatment of either RT or chemotherapy.

D. concurrent chemoradiation.

16. American Society of Clinical Oncology (ASCO) guidelines recommend the following chemotherapy for NSCLC:

A. Platinum-based combination.

B. Single-agent therapy.

C. Cisplatin (Platinol) and etoposide (VP-16).

D. Carboplatin (Paraplatin) and paclitaxel (Taxol).

17. A clinical trial should always be considered as a treatment option for an individual with lung cancer because

A. clinical trials are available for all individuals.

B. phase I clinical trials have a goal to cure.

C. standard treatment options are not available.

D. current treatment options do not have a high cure rate.

18. Individuals with advanced lung cancer often experience

A. low incidence and severity of symptoms.

B. low incidence but high severity of symptoms.

C. high incidence but low severity of symptoms.

D. high incidence and high severity of symptoms.

19. Smoking cessation for an individual diagnosed with lung cancer
    A. is not indicated because of increased anxiety.
    B. is indicated for symptom improvement.
    C. is indicated to decrease feelings of guilt.
    D. is indicated to immediately decrease the risk of developing a second cancer.

NOTES

ANSWERS

1. *Answer:* A
Rationale: The genetic expression of lung cancer has been mapped; however, it is not standard practice to evaluate in histopathologic examination, because the impact of genetic expression on treatment selection has not been determined.

2. *Answer:* C
Rationale: The diagnosis of SCLC is associated with a more aggressive course than NSCLC. Both SCLC and NSCLC are associated with increased risk for metabolic emergencies.

3. *Answer:* D
Rationale: Early-stage lung cancer is not frequently associated with specific signs and symptoms. This results in later detection for most clients with lung cancer.

4. *Answer:* D
Rationale: The increased incidence is often associated with increased smoking in women. Lung cancer incidence rates are rising for all subgroups except for white men, for whom the incidence is stable or declining.

5. *Answer:* B
Rationale: Lung cancer has the highest mortality rates for both men and women. For women, breast cancer is associated with the highest incidence rate, and for men, prostate cancer has the highest incidence rate.

6. *Answer:* A
Rationale: Tobacco smoking accounts for approximately 90% of all lung cancers and is by far the most significant and modifiable risk factor. Incidence rates for lung cancer are 10 to 20 times higher in smokers than non-smokers.

7. *Answer:* C
Rationale: Mesothelioma is usually associated with asbestos exposure.

8. *Answer:* D
Rationale: At present, there are no reliable or recommended screening tests for the early detection of lung cancer. Clinical trials are ongoing that examine spiral CT and PET imaging as screening modalities for individuals at high risk.

9. *Answer:* C
Rationale: The overall 5-year-survival rate for lung cancer is 15%.

10. *Answer:* B
Rationale: Despite responses to chemotherapy, duration of survival is generally short in clients treated for extensive stage SCLC. Most survive on average only 9 months.

11. *Answer:* C
Rationale: Despite side effects and the potential for serious complications, in early-stage lung cancer the only curative modality is surgery. Lung cancer is often detected at a stage with disseminated disease, and there are limited response rates for chemotherapeutic agents.

12. *Answer:* C
Rationale: Estimates are that 50% of clients with lung cancer do not undergo the planned resection.

13. *Answer:* C
Rationale: PCI is indicated in limited stage SCLC because of the high rate of brain metastases.

14. *Answer:* A
Rationale: Multiple clinical trials demonstrated an advantage for clients with NSCLC receiving chemotherapy over best supportive care. Response rates are approaching 40%.

15. *Answer:* D
Rationale: Chemotherapy with concurrent RT is the recommended standard treatment for clients with stage IIIB NSCLC and good performance status.

16. *Answer:* A
Rationale: The ASCO guidelines recommend a platinum-based combination regimen.

17. *Answer:* D

Rationale: Despite standards of care for treatment, a clinical trial is a viable option for individuals with lung cancer because of the low cure rate and poor survival ratio of the currently available regimens.

18. *Answer:* D

Rationale: Individuals with advanced lung cancer experience multiple symptoms with highly rated severity.

19. *Answer:* B

Rationale: Smoking cessation provides immediate benefits by improving respiratory symptoms. The long-term benefit of decreased risk of developing a tobacco-related cancer may take up to 5 years.

BIBLIOGRAPHY

American Cancer Society (ACS). (2004). *Cancer facts & figures 2004.* Atlanta: American Cancer Society.

American Society of Clinical Oncology (ASCO). (2003). American Society of Clinical Oncology treatment of unresectable non-small cell lung cancer guideline: Update 2003. *Journal of Clinical Oncology 22,* 330-353.

American Society of Clinical Oncology (ASCO). (1997). Clinical practice guidelines for the treatment of unresectable non-small-cell lung cancer. *Journal of Clinical Oncology 8,* 2996-3018.

Bach, P.B, Niewoehner, D.E, & Black, W.C. (2003). Screening for lung cancer: The guidelines. *Chest 123,* 83S-88S.

Belani, C. (2000a). Combined modality therapy for unresectable Stage III non-small cell lung cancer: New chemotherapy combinations. *Chest 117,* 127S-132S.

Belani, C. (2000b). Paclitaxel and docetaxel combinations in non-small cell lung cancer. *Chest 117,* 144S-151S.

Bunn, P., & Kelly, K. (2000). New combinations in the treatment of lung cancer: A time for optimism. *Chest 117,* 138S-143S.

Bunn, P., Soriano, A., Johnson, G., & Heasley, L. (2000). New therapeutic strategies for lung cancer: Biology and molecular biology come of age. *Chest 114,* 163S-168S.

Cooley, M. (2000). Symptoms in adults with lung cancer: A systematic research review. *Journal of Pain and Symptom Management 19,* 137-153.

Franklin, W. (2000). Diagnosis of lung cancer: Pathology of invasive and preinvasive neoplasia. *Chest 117,* 80S-89S.

Jemal, A., Tiwari, R.C., Murray, T., et al. (2004). Cancer statistics, 2004. *CA: A Cancer Journal for Clinicians 54,* 8-29.

Jett, J., Scott, W., Rivera, M., & Sause, W. (2003). Guidelines on treatment of Stage IIIB non-small cell lung cancer. *Chest 123,* 221S-225S.

Johnson, D. (2000). Evolution of cisplatin-based chemotherapy in non-small cell lung cancer: A historical perspective and the eastern cooperative group experience. *Chest 117,* 133S-137S.

Laskin, J., Sandler, A., & Johnson, D. (2003). An advance in small-cell lung cancer treatment — more or less [editorial]. *Journal of the National Cancer Institute 95,* 1099-1101.

Meyerson, M., Franklin, W., & Kelley, M. (2004). Molecular classification and molecular genetics of human lung cancers. *Seminars in Oncology 31*(Suppl.1), 4-19.

Sarna, L. (1998). Effectiveness of structured nursing assessment of symptom distress in advanced lung cancer. *Oncology Nursing Forum 25*(6), 1041-1048.

Sekido, Y., Fong, K., & Minna, J. (2001). Molecular biology of lung cancer. In V. DeVita, S. Hellman, & S. Rosenberg (Eds.). *Cancer: Principles and practice of oncology* (6th ed.). Philadelphia: Lippincott Williams & Wilkins, pp. 917-925.

Simon, G., & Wagner, H. (2003). Small cell lung cancer. *Chest 123,* 259S-271S.

Wagner, H. (2000). Postoperative adjuvant therapy for patients with resected non-small cell lung cancer: Still controversial after all these years. *Chest 117,* 110S-118S.

25 Nursing Care of the Client with Cancers of the Gastrointestinal Tract

BRIDGET O'BRIEN AND LISA STUCKY-MARSHALL

Select the best answer for each of the following questions:

1. Which of the following is **not** associated with increased risk of colorectal cancer?
   A. Family history.
   B. Advanced age.
   C. Adenomatous polyps.
   D. Irritable bowel syndrome.

2. A client may report symptoms of tenesmus and bright red blood in the stool if the tumor is located in which region of the colon?
   A. Transverse.
   B. Rectum.
   C. Sigmoid.
   D. Ascending.

3. Which tumor marker is commonly used as an indicator of tumor burden and for monitoring recurrence of colorectal cancer?
   A. CA 19-9.
   B. CA 27-29.
   C. Carcinoembrionic antigen (CEA).
   D. Alpha-fetoprotein (α-FP).

4. What is the most common side effect in clients receiving radiation therapy for rectal cancer?
   A. Intestinal obstruction.
   B. Diarrhea.
   C. Nausea.
   D. Bone marrow suppression.

5. Which of the following is considered a late symptom of colorectal cancer?
   A. Flatulence.
   B. Change in bowel habits.
   C. Blood in the stool.
   D. Weight loss.

6. What is the most common site of colorectal metastasis?
   A. Brain.
   B. Adrenal glands.
   C. Liver.
   D. Bone.

7. Which type of colorectal surgery is associated with a higher incidence of quality of life issues after surgery?
   A. Abdominoperineal resection.
   B. Right hemicolectomy.
   C. Subtotal colectomy.
   D. Low anterior resection.

8. What is the most common type of esophageal cancer?
   A. Lymphoma.
   B. Adenocarcinoma.
   C. Small cell carcinoma.
   D. Squamous cell carcinoma.

9. A 70-year-old man with a 40-pack-year history of smoking presents with dysphagia. His barium swallow is suspicious for esophageal cancer. The nurse should educate

him about which test to confirm the diagnosis?
- A. Magnetic resonance imaging (MRI).
- B. Computed tomography (CT) scan.
- C. Positron emission tomography (PET) scan.
- D. Endoscopy.

10. A client with esophageal cancer who is experiencing dysphagia is trying to maintain caloric intake. The nurse should provide education on which of the following?
- A. Instructions to maintain a clear liquid diet.
- B. Instructions to lie flat for 30 minutes after each meal.
- C. Instructions to eat small, frequent meals throughout the day.
- D. Instructions to limit meals to twice a day with high-calorie foods.

11. The most common presenting complaint of esophageal cancer is which of the following?
- A. Pain.
- B. Dysphagia.
- C. Hoarseness.
- D. Cough when swallowing.

12. What is the second most common malignancy of the gastrointestinal tract?
- A. Liver.
- B. Gastric.
- C. Pancreas.
- D. Esophageal.

13. The only risk factor that is definitively linked with the development of pancreatic cancer is which of the following?
- A. Coronary artery disease.
- B. Cigarette smoking.
- C. Ingestion of smoked foods.
- D. Hyperbilirubinemia in infants.

14. What is the most common presenting symptom of pancreatic cancer?
- A. Pain.
- B. Ascites.
- C. Fatigue.
- D. Nausea and vomiting.

15. Which is the initial best choice of treatment for pancreatic cancer?
- A. Surgery.
- B. Chemotherapy.

- C. Radiation therapy.
- D. Radio frequency ablation.

16. What is the most common pathology of malignant gastric tumors?
- A. Lymphoma.
- B. Carcinoid tumors.
- C. Adenocarcinoma.
- D. Squamous cell carcinoma.

17. Which of the following is considered to be a risk factor for gastric cancer?
- A. History of *H. pylori* infection.
- B. High carbohydrate diet.
- C. Low-fiber diet.
- D. Gastroesophageal reflux disease (GERD).

18. What is the **most common** presenting symptom of gastric cancer?
- A. Hematemesis.
- B. Weight loss.
- C. GERD.
- D. Lower extremity edema.

19. The family member of a client diagnosed with gastric cancer asks the nurse what nutritional factors are important in the prevention of gastric cancer. Which of the following is **not** included in the education?
- A. Avoidance of spicy foods.
- B. Avoidance of highly salted foods.
- C. Limiting the intake of smoked foods.
- D. Increasing fruits and vegetables in the diet.

20. Because clients are at risk for "dumping syndrome" after gastric resection, nursing education for the client should include which of the following?
- A. Increasing fluid intake with meals.
- B. Ingesting small, frequent meals.
- C. Recommending a high-carbohydrate, low-protein diet.
- D. Suggesting a high-fiber diet.

21. The nurse is taking care of a client who has a history of a gastric resection. Which laboratory value is not likely a direct result of the previous surgery?
- A. Low hemoglobin.
- B. Low vitamin B_{12}.
- C. Decreased folate level.
- D. Low white blood cell count.

22. Which is the most common presenting symptom of primary liver cancer?
    A. Anorexia.
    B. Ascites.
    C. Right upper quadrant pain.
    D. Anemia.

23. Which of the following risk factors is **not** associated with the development of primary liver cancer?
    A. Hepatitis B virus.
    B. Aflatoxin B exposure.
    C. Cirrhosis.
    D. Age.

24. What is the most definitive treatment option for primary liver cancer?
    A. Surgery.
    B. Radiation therapy.
    C. Percutaneous ethanol injection.
    D. Systemic chemotherapy.

25. What is the tumor marker used to screen individuals at high risk for primary liver cancer?
    A. Carcinoembrionic antigen (CEA).
    B. CA 19-9.

C. α-FP.
D. Human chorionic gonadotropic beta subunit (β-HCG).

26. What is a common symptom that is difficult to manage in clients with advanced primary liver cancer?
    A. Infection.
    B. Bleeding.
    C. Pain.
    D. Bone metastasis.

27. What is the most common presenting sign of anal cancer?
    A. Bleeding.
    B. Pruritus.
    C. Lymphadenopathy.
    D. Change in stool habits.

28. The preferred initial therapy for anal cancer is which of the following?
    A. Surgery.
    B. Radiation.
    C. Chemotherapy.
    D. Chemoradiation.

NOTES

ANSWERS

1. *Answer:* D
   Rationale: Irritable bowel syndrome is not considered a significant risk factor. Common risk factors for colorectal cancer include family history, advanced age (older than age 50), and adenomatous polyps (precursors to cancer).

2. *Answer:* B
   Rationale: Tenesmus and bright red blood in the stool are symptoms produced by tumors located in the rectum. Tenesmus is characterized by the need to pass stool, accompanied by pain, cramping, and straining. Despite the straining, very little stool is passed.

3. *Answer:* C
   Rationale: CEA can be elevated in clients with colorectal cancer. It is generally used to monitor efficacy of treatment and indication of disease recurrence. CA 19-9 is often used as a tumor marker for pancreatic cancer. CA 27-29 is used for breast cancer, and AFP is used for both testicular cancer and primary liver cancer.

4. *Answer:* B
   Rationale: Gastrointestinal cells have rapid mitotic rates and are therefore sensitive to radiation therapy. The local approach of this type of therapy can result in diarrhea.

5. *Answer:* D
   Rationale: Weight loss, anorexia, and anemia are often indicative of advanced disease. The other symptoms are usually early symptoms of colorectal cancer.

6. *Answer:* C
   Rationale: The most common site of metastases from colorectal cancer is the liver.

7. *Answer:* A
   Rationale: Complications of abdominoperineal resection are injury to the ureters, bladder dysfunction, stoma complications, wound infections, sexual dysfunction issues, and body image alterations. Any of these can present chronic physical and emotional challenges for the client.

8. *Answer:* B
   Rationale: Squamous cell carcinoma previously was the most common pathologic type, but with the increase in cancers of the gastroesophageal junction, adenocarcinoma is currently the most common.

9. *Answer:* D
   Rationale: The diagnosis can be confirmed truly by biopsy only, which can be obtained with endoscopy. The other tests are helpful in staging the client but do not result in any tissue samples.

10. *Answer:* C
    Rationale: Clients with dysphagia should eat small and more frequent meals. A clear liquid diet will not provide enough calories. The client should not lie flat after meals but instead be upright for at least 30 minutes. Limiting the client to any number of meals will be difficult to maintain calories and promotes eating larger meals, which is difficult with dysphagia.

11. *Answer:* B
    Rationale: Dysphagia is the hallmark sign of esophageal cancer, and the majority of clients will present with this symptom. The other symptoms are also warning signs, yet less common.

12. *Answer:* C
    Rationale: Pancreatic cancer is the second leading gastrointestinal malignancy after colorectal cancer.

13. *Answer:* B
    Rationale: Cigarette smoking is the only risk factor of these listed that has been scientifically proven to cause pancreatic cancer. None of these other variables have any known increased risk for the development of pancreatic cancer.

14. *Answer:* A
    Rationale: Pain is the hallmark sign of pancreatic cancer, whereas these other symptoms are less common.

15. *Answer:* A
    Rationale: Surgery should always be the first consideration for individuals with pancre-

atic cancer, because it is the only chance for cure. Even though many clients are not candidates for surgical resection based on the extent of their disease, it should always be considered first in the evaluation for treatment.

16. *Answer:* C
Rationale: Adenocarcinoma is the most common form of gastric cancer.

17. *Answer:* A
H. pylori infection and familial clustering of *H. pylori* are considered risk factors for gastric cancer. High-carbohydrate and/or low-fiber diet are not related to gastric cancer. GERD is a risk factor for esophageal cancer.

18. *Answer:* B
Rationale: The most common presenting sign of gastric cancer is weight loss, with 62% of clients presenting with this symptom. Ten percent to 15% of clients will present with hematemesis and 6% with lower extremity edema. GERD is not a common presenting symptom.

19. *Answer:* A
Rationale: Spicy foods are not indicated as risk factors for the development of gastric cancer. Salted foods, smoked foods, and a low intake of fruits and vegetables are all listed as risk factors for gastric cancer.

20. *Answer:* B
Rationale: Dumping syndrome is exacerbated by increased fluid with meals and high-fiber intake. Clients should be educated to eat small, frequent meals and low-carbohydrate, high-protein diets.

21. *Answer:* D
Rationale: Low white blood cell counts should not be seen in this population. Clients with gastric resection are at risk for anemia related to folate deficiency and vitamin B_{12} deficiency.

22. *Answer:* C
Rationale: Although early symptoms of primary liver cancer may be vague, the most common presenting symptom is right upper quadrant pain that can be dull or aching or very severe in nature.

23. *Answer:* D
Rationale: The development of primary liver cancer is not associated with age.

24. *Answer:* A
Rationale: Surgery is the most definitive treatment and offers the client the best chance for cure. Unfortunately, only 15% to 30% of clients are candidates for surgery.

25. *Answer:* C
Rationale: The tumor marker α-FP can be used to screen individuals considered at high risk for the development of primary liver cancer. CEA is used most with colorectal cancer, CA 19-9 with pancreas cancer, and βHCG for choriocarcinoma or for testicular cancer.

26. *Answer:* C
Rationale: Pain is the most common symptom experienced by clients with advanced primary liver cancer. The pain tends to be very severe and should be managed aggressively.

27. *Answer:* A
Rationale: Bleeding occurs in more than half of the clients presenting with anal cancer. The other symptoms can occur but are much less common.

28. *Answer:* D
Rationale: Chemoradiation is the preferred therapy for most clients. In the past, surgery was the first approach, but it is associated with significant quality of life issues and a high risk for local recurrence.

BIBLIOGRAPHY

Benson, A.B., Myerson, R.J., Hoffman, J., et al. (2003). Pancreatic, neuroendocrine GI, and adrenal cancers. In R. Pazdur, L.R. Coia, W.J. Hoskins, & L.D. Wagman (Eds.). *Cancer management: A multidisciplinary approach* (7th ed.). New York: The Oncology Group, pp. 273-302.

Bonin, S.R., Schwarz, R.E., & Blanke, C.D. (2003). Gastric cancer. In R. Pazdur, L.R. Coia, W.J. Hoskins, & L.D. Wagman (Eds.). *Cancer management: A multidisciplinary approach* (7th ed.). New York: The Oncology Group, pp. 259-272.

Bush, N.J. (2001). Colorectal cancer. In E. Muscari Lin (Ed.). *Advanced practice in oncology nursing: Case studies & review*. Philadelphia: W.B. Saunders, pp. 45-55.

Ellerhorn, J.D.I., Cullinane, C.A., Coia, L.R., & Alberts, S.R. (2003). Colorectal and anal cancer. In R. Pazdur, L.R. Coia, W.J. Hoskins, & L.D. Wagman (Eds.). *Cancer management: A multidisciplinary approach* (7th ed.). New York: The Oncology Group, pp. 241-258.

Paz, I.B., Suntharalingam, M., Hwang, J.J., & Marshall, J.L. (2003). Esophageal cancer. In R. Pazdur, L.R. Coia, W.J. Hoskins, & L.D. Wagman (Eds.). *Cancer management: A multidiscipli-nary approach* (7th ed.). New York: The Oncology Group, pp. 241-258.

Stucky-Marshall, L., & O'Brien, B.E. (2002). Gastrointestinal malignancies. In K. Jennings-Dozier & S.M. Mahon (Eds.). *Cancer prevention, detection, and control*. Pittsburgh: Oncology Nursing Society, pp. 445-538.

Yarbro, C.H., Frogge, M.H., & Goodman, M. (Eds.). (2002). *Clinical guide to cancer nursing* (5th ed.). Sudbury, MA: Jones and Bartlett Publishers.

NOTES

26 Nursing Care of the Client with Cancers of the Reproductive System

SUSAN VOGT TEMPLE, CYNTHIA H. UMSTEAD*, AND PAULA FOREST

1. The most common presenting symptom of endometrial cancer is
   A. acute abdominal pain.
   B. increased abdominal girth.
   C. abnormal vaginal bleeding.
   D. milky vaginal drainage.

2. A woman recently given the diagnosis of endometrial cancer says she does not understand how she can have cancer when her Papanicolaou (Pap) test was negative 8 months ago. Which of the following responses is most appropriate?
   A. Many Pap tests are not interpreted correctly.
   B. Endometrial cancer may develop in a short time.
   C. The Pap test may have been obtained incorrectly.
   D. Pap tests do not commonly detect endometrial cancer.

3. The wife of a client with testicular cancer stops you in the hall. Her husband is receiving his first cycle of chemotherapy. She tells you she doesn't know what she will do when he dies. In forming your response, you remember the prognosis for testicular cancer is
   A. highly variable depending on stage.
   B. highly variable depending on histology.

C. excellent and considered a curable disease.
D. less than a 70% survival rate.

4. Ms. A. is receiving paclitaxel (Taxol) and carboplatin (Paraplatin) for ovarian cancer. Her pretreatment nursing assessment would include assurance that
   A. premedications were taken.
   B. mesna (Mesnex) orders have been received.
   C. her ejection fraction is within normal limits.
   D. antihypertensive medications were stopped 24 hours before chemotherapy administration.

5. Ms. M. is referred to your office for colposcopy after an abnormal Pap test. Preprocedure education would include
   A. avoiding vaginal intercourse for 1 month before the colposcopy.
   B. expecting copious vaginal drainage after the colposcopy.
   C. expecting a swabbing of the cervix with acetic acid solution during the colposcopy.
   D. douching with a betadine solution every night for 1 week before colposcopy.

6. Ms. L. presents to your office with presumed endometrial cancer. Which of the following would increase Ms. Lynch's risk of endometrial cancer?
   A. A diet high in beta carotene and retinoic acid.
   B. A history of unopposed estrogen therapy.

*Susan V. Temple and Cynthia H. Umstead are full-time employees of GlaxoSmithKline (GSK). The views and opinions expressed herein are those of the authors/editors and do not necessarily reflect those of GSK.

C. Use of talc in the perineal area.
D. A family history of ulcerative colitis.

7. Which of the following tumor markers would you expect to be elevated in a client with newly diagnosed gestational trophoblastic neoplasia?
    A. MRNA.
    B. PSA.
    C. ATP.
    D. β-HCG .

8. Ms. L. will begin radiation therapy for locally advanced cervical cancer next week and is scheduled to receive concurrent chemotherapy. Your pretreatment education would include information on
    A. cisplatin (Platinol) as a radiosensitizer.
    B. paclitaxel as an antineoplastic agent.
    C. dexrazoxane (Zinecard) as a cytoprotectant
    D. mensa as a uroprotectant.

9. Which of the following gynecologic oncology diseases is staged clinically?
    A. Ovarian cancer.
    B. Endometrial cancer.
    C. Cervical cancer.
    D. Bladder cancer.

10. Which of the following statements should alert the nurse that further education is needed?
    A. A woman should have a Pap test 3 years after beginning vaginal intercourse or by the age of 21.
    B. A woman who has had a hysterectomy for cervical cancer no longer needs a Pap test or screening.
    C. A 30-year-old woman who has had three consecutive normal Pap tests can begin having pap tests every 2 to 3 years when using liquid-based testing.
    D. Pap tests are an effective screening tool for cervical cancer.

11. Mrs. T. is undergoing chemotherapy (paclitaxel and carboplatin) for newly diagnosed ovarian cancer. Your prechemotherapy education would include information on expected toxicities including

    A. pedal edema, jugular vein distention (JVD), shortness of breath (SOB), and weight gain.
    B. peripheral neuropathy, alopecia, and neutropenia.
    C. dysuria, central nervous system symptoms, and diarrhea.
    D. palmar plantar erythrodysesthesia, stomatitis, and constipation.

12. Which of the following statements regarding squamous cell cervical cancer is correct?
    A. Cervical cancer is a hereditary disease.
    B. Oral contraceptives are protective for cervical cancer.
    C. Cervical cancer is caused by the Epstein-Barr virus.
    D. Certain human papillomavirus (HPV) subtypes are known to be oncogenic.

13. Which of the following tumor markers would you expect to be elevated in 80% of clients with advanced epithelial ovarian cancer?
    A. CA 125.
    B. CEA.
    C. CA 19-9.
    D. CA 27-29.

14. The most common sign or symptom noticed by men with testicular cancer is
    A. a heavy feeling or mass in the scrotum.
    B. nonproductive cough.
    C. confusion.
    D. abdominal pain.

15. Which testicular cancer is most responsive to radiation therapy?
    A. Nonseminoma.
    B. Seminoma.

16. Tumor markers are important in the diagnosis and follow-up of clients with cancer. The tumor markers alpha-fetoprotein (α-FP) and beta-human chorionic gonadotropin (β-HCG) are used to monitor response to treatment in
    A. testes.
    B. kidney.
    C. bladder.
    D. prostate.

17. Fertility issues may be important to the male client diagnosed with testicular cancer. In talking to a young married couple, you realize that they wish to have a family eventually. If a couple is interested in sperm banking, when is the best time to make a sperm bank deposit?

A. Before chemotherapy treatment.
B. During chemotherapy treatment.
C. At completion of chemotherapy.
D. When the tumor markers are in the normal range.

NOTES

ANSWERS

1. *Answer:* C
Rationale: Most clients with endometrial cancer present with abnormal vaginal bleeding. Abdominal discomfort and increased girth are symptoms of ovarian cancer. Milky vaginal discharge may occur with cervical cancer.

2. *Answer:* D
Rationale: Exfoliated malignant cells from the endometrium are rarely detected on cervical sampling (the Pap test). A Pap test is a screening test for cervical intraepithelial neoplasia or cervical cancer.

3. *Answer:* C
Rationale: Testicular cancer is a model for a curable solid tumor. Studies show that the cure rate is over 90% in all stages combined. The 5-year survival rate for stage I is 99%. For stage II disease, the 5-year survival rate is 95%, and for stage III disease, it is 75%.

4. *Answer:* A
Rationale: Premedications for paclitaxel include dexamethasone, an H_2 blocker, and an antihistamine. Mesna is a cytoprotectant used with ifosfamide (Ifex) or cyclophamide (Cytoxan). Transient asymptomatic bradycardia is associated with paclitaxel, and MUGA scans are not indicated. Antihypertensives are recommended to be stopped 24 hours before amifostine (Ethyol) administration.

5. *Answer:* C
Rationale: The client can expect the practitioner to swab the cervix with an acetic acid solution during the procedure. Clients should not douche, use any vaginal creams, or have intercourse 2 days before the examination. Ideally, the client should not be menstruating.

6. *Answer:* B
Rationale: The use of unopposed estrogen increases a woman's risk of endometrial cancer. Talc has been implicated in the pathogenesis of ovarian cancer. A family history for breast, ovarian, endometrial, and colon cancers would be significant when evaluating for genetic linkages.

7. *Answer:* D
Rationale: The quantitative β-HCG is an extremely sensitive tumor marker for gestational trophoblastic disease. PSA is prostate-specific antigen and is used in screening for prostate cancer. MRNA is messenger RNA, and ATP is adenosine triphosphate.

8. *Answer:* A
Rationale: Cisplatin is used as a radiosensitizer for advanced cervical cancer. Paclitaxel is a chemotherapic agent used in treating a wide variety of malignancies; dexazoxane is a protective agent for doxorubicin (Adriamycin)-induced cardiotoxicity; and mesna is a cytoprotectant used to prevent hemorrhagic cystitis associated with ifosfamide and cyclophosphamide.

9. *Answer:* C
Rationale: Cervical cancer is staged by clinical examination. Ovarian and endometrial cancer are staged surgically; bladder cancer is not a gynecologic malignancy.

10. *Answer:* B
Rationale: Women with a history of cervical cancer should continue to be screened for recurrent disease. Pap smears are obtained every 3 months in the first year after radiation therapy/surgery; every 4 months in the second year, and every 6 months for 3 to 5 years. The American Cancer Society recommends cervical cancer screening should begin approximately 3 years after a woman begins having vaginal intercourse, but no later than 21 years of age. It should be done every year with regular Pap tests or every 2 years using liquid-based tests. At or after age 30, women who have had 3 or more consecutive annual normal tests may be screened every 2 to 3 years unless they have significant risk for developing cervical cancer.

11. *Answer:* B

Rationale: Initial treatment of ovarian cancer often includes paclitaxel and carboplatin. Expected toxicities would include peripheral neuropathy in a stocking-glove distribution, alopecia, and neutropenia. Pedal edema, JVD, SOB, and weight gain would be associated with congestive heart failure, and palmar-plantar erythrodysestheia would be associated with liposomal doxorubicin (Doxil), 5-fluorouracil (5 FU), and capecitabine (Xeloda).

12. *Answer:* D

Rationale: Certain subtypes of HPV are known to be oncogenic including (but not limited to) HPV 16, 18, 31, and 45. Epstein-Barr is implicated in other malignancies/disease states including Burkitt's lymphoma, Hodgkin's disease, and nasopharyngeal carcinoma. There are little data to suggest cervical cancer is hereditary or that oral contraceptives are protective for cervical cancer.

13. *Answer:* A

Rationale: CA 125 is a tumor marker in 80% of clients with advanced ovarian cancer. Carcinoembryonic antigen (CEA), CA 19-9, and CA 27-29 may be elevated in clients with ovarian cancer but are generally used to follow clients with other tumor types. CEA is often used as a marker in clients with cancers of the colon, rectum, pancreas, stomach, lung, and gallbladder. CEA may also be elevated in clients with breast, head and neck, melanoma, lymphoma, liver, thyroid, cervix, bladder, kidney, and ovarian cancer. CA 19-9 may be elevated in colorectal cancer, pancreatic, hepatobiliary, and gastric cancer, and CA 27-29 is found in the blood of most clients with breast cancer but may be elevated by cancers of the colon, stomach, kidney, ovary, pancreas, uterus, and liver.

14. *Answer:* A

Rationale: A heavy feeling or mass in the scrotum is the symptom most offered by male clients. The symptoms of cough, pain, and confusion may be signs of metastatic disease

15. *Answer:* B

Rationale: The standard therapy for seminoma testicular cancer is radiation.

16. *Answer:* A

Rationale: α-FP and β-HCG are standard tumor markers to assess response to therapy for testicular cancer. PSA is the tumor marker for prostate cancer. There is not a tumor marker for kidney and bladder cancer at this time.

17. *Answer:* A

Rationale: The cancer process often affects the sperm, and clients may be sterile or subfertile at diagnosis. The likelihood of a successful pregnancy using sperm during or after chemotherapy treatment is markedly decreased or absent.

BIBLIOGRAPHY

American Cancer Society. (2004). *Cancer facts and figures 2004*. Atlanta: Author.

American Cancer Society. What are the risk factors for cervical cancer? What are the risk factors for testicular cancer? Retrieved February 16, 2003 from the World Wide Web www.cancer.org.

Barakat, R., Grigsby, P., Sabbatini, P., & Zaino, R. (2001). Corpus: Epithelial tumors. In W.J. Hoskins, C.A. Perez, & R.C. Young (Eds.). *Principles and practice of gynecology oncology* (3rd ed.). Philadelphia: Lippincott Williams & Wilkins, pp. 919–960.

Berkowitz, R., & Goldstein, D. (2001). Gestational trophoblastic diseases. In W.J. Hoskins, C.A. Perez, & R.C. Young (Eds.). *Principles and practice of gynecology oncology* (3rd ed.). Philadelphia: Lippincott Williams & Wilkins, pp. 1117–1138.

DeVita, V.T., Hellman, S., Rosenberg, S.A. (Eds.). (2001). *Cancer: Principles and practice of oncology* (6th ed.). Philadelphia: Lippincott Williams & Wilkins.

DiSaia, P.J., & Creasman, W.T. (2002). *Clinical gynecologic oncology* (6th ed.). St. Louis: Mosby.

Door, A. (2002). Gestational trophoblastic disease. *Journal of Gynecologic Oncology Nursing 12*(2), 19-21.

Fischer, M. (2002). Cancer of the cervix. *Seminars in Oncology Nursing 18*(3), 193-199.

Liles, W., & Itano, J. (2003). Human papillomavirus and cervical cancer: Not just a sexually transmitted disease. *Clinical Journal of Oncology Nursing 7*(3), 271-276.

O'Rourke, J., & Mahon, S. (2003). A comprehensive look at the early detection of ovarian cancer. *Clinical Journal of Oncology Nursing 7*(1), 41-47.

Ozols, R. (2002). Update in the management of ovarian cancer. *Cancer Journal 8*(3) (Suppl. 1), S22-S30.

Ozols, R., Rubin, S., Thomas, G., & Robboy, S. (2001). Epithelial ovarian cancer. In W.J. Hoskins, C.A. Perez, & R.C. Young (Eds.). *Principles and practice of gynecology oncology* (3rd ed.). Philadelphia: Lippincott Williams & Wilkins, 981-1058.

Solomon, D., Davey, D., Kurman, R., et al. (2002). The 2001 Bethesda System. Terminology for reporting results of cervical cytology. *Journal of the American Medical Association 287*(16): 2114-2119.

Spinelli, A. (2002). Preinvasive disease of the cervix, vulva, and vagina. *Seminars in Oncology Nursing 18*(3), 184-192.

Stehman, F., Perez, C., Kurman, R., & Thigpen, J. (2001). Uterine cervix. In W.J. Hoskins, C.A. Perez, & R.C. Young, (Eds.). *Principles and practice of gynecology oncology* (3rd ed.). Philadelphia: Lippincott Williams & Wilkins, 841-918.

Wright, Jr., T.C., Cox, J., Massad, L., et al. (2002). 2001 Consensus Guidelines for the Management of Women with Cervical Cytological Abnormalities. *Journal of the American Medical Association 287*(16), 2120-2129.

NOTES

27 Nursing Care of the Client with Cancers of the Urinary System

PAULA FOREST

Select the best answer for each of the following questions:

1. Which one of the following statements best describes the growth and progression of renal cell cancer (RCC)?
    A. Once the disease has spread to the lymph node, the 5-year survival rate is approximately 65% to 70%.
    B. New advances in the diagnosis and treatment of renal cell carcinoma have improved the 5-year survival rate by 65% to 70%.
    C. Renal cell tumors primarily spread to the liver and brain with a 5-year survival rate of 10% to 50%.
    D. Thirty percent of renal cell cancers are advanced at time of diagnosis, with a 5-year survival rate of 10% to 50%.

2. Which of the following diagnostic tests is standard workup for diagnosing RCC?
    A. Kidney, ureter, and bladder (KUB) radiography.
    B. Head/brain computed tomography (CT) scan.
    C. Bone scan.
    D. Carcinoembryonic antigen (CEA).

3. RCC that is localized is most responsive to which of the following primary therapies?
    A. Radiotherapy.
    B. Biotherapy.
    C. Adjuvant chemotherapy.
    D. Radical nephrectomy.

4. The classic triad of symptoms for the diagnosis of RCC is
    A. pain, hematuria, and a flank mass.
    B. pain, hematuria, and a productive cough.
    C. hematuria, weight loss, and bone pain.
    D. pain, weight loss, and hematuria.

5. Based on the guidelines from the American Cancer Society (ACS) about prostate cancer, which of the following statements is true?
    A. Annual digital rectal examination (DRE) should begin at age 40.
    B. A DRE and a prostate-specific antigen (PSA) blood test should be drawn annually, beginning at age 50, in men who have a life expectancy of at least 10 years.
    C. There is no consensus on prostate cancer guidelines.
    D. Prostate cancer guidelines are developed by the client's physician.

6. Side effects of radical prostatectomy include
    A. incontinence, impotence, and postoperative hematuria.
    B. impotence, myelosuppression, and dysuria.
    C. cystitis, urethral strictures, diarrhea, and lower extremity edema.
    D. hot flashes, decreased libido, and elevated PSA levels.

7. National trends in the incidence of prostate cancer have
    A. continued to grow since the advent of prostate cancer testing in 1992.
    B. not changed since the advent of prostate cancer testing.

C. seen an increased incidence followed by a leveling off from 1995 to 1999.
D. dropped dramatically for men greater than 65 years of age.

8. The highest incidence rate of prostate cancer is found in men of
  A. Caucasian descent.
  B. African American descent.
  C. Hispanic descent.
  D. Latino descent.

9. Which of the following is the most frequent front-line treatment for advanced prostate cancer?
  A. Strontium.
  B. Medical castration (leuprolide [Lupron]/ goserelin [Zoladex]) or surgical castration (orchiectomy).
  C. Surgery.
  D. Total body irradiation.

10. Which one of the following is the most common symptom leading to the diagnosis of bladder cancer?
  A. Hematuria.
  B. Nonproductive cough.
  C. Abdominal mass.
  D. Lower extremity edema.

11. Cancer of the bladder occurs most frequently in
  A. men.
  B. women.
  C. 70- to 85-year-olds.
  D. 25- to 35-year-olds.

12. Which of the following diagnostic tests is indicated in the workup of bladder cancer?
  A. Intravenous pyelogram (IVP) and cystoscopy.
  B. Positron emission tomography (PET) scan.
  C. Chest CT scan.
  D. Bone scan.

NOTES

ANSWERS

1. *Answer:* D
Rationale: Option D is the correct answer because the disease is advanced (Stage IV) at diagnosis in approximately one third of all clients, and the 5-year survival rate is 5% to 10%. Once the disease has spread, the 5-year survival rate is 50% or less. Renal cell tumors spread to the lymph nodes and the bones. New advances in treatment have not made a dramatic improvement in survival.

2. *Answer:* A
Rationale: A KUB, pelvic/abdominal CT scan, and magnetic resonance imaging are considered part of the standard workup for RCC. At this time, there is not a specific tumor marker for RCC. RCC does not originate in the brain or bone, so bone scans and CT scans of the head are not indicated.

3. *Answer:* D
Rationale: Radical nephrectomy is the surgery for RCC that is contained and has not spread. Radiotherapy has not had positive results with RCC. Biotherapy, such as interleukin-2 and interferons, has shown a small response.

4. *Answer:* A
Rationale: Pain, hematuria, and a flank mass remain the classically seen symptoms. RCC symptoms are generally clinically occult until signs of metastasis prompt an evaluation. Symptoms of cough, weight loss, and bone pain may suggest metastatic disease.

5. *Answer:* B
Rationale: The ACS stresses that both the DRE and PSA need to be used together for annual screening. These should begin at age 50 in men of average risk. African American men and those with a significant family history of prostate cancer may want to speak with their health care provider about starting screening at age 40.

6. *Answer:* A
Rationale: The side effects of surgery include incontinence, impotence, and post-operative hematuria. Chemotherapy is usually not as effective in the treatment of prostate cancer; therefore myelosuppression is not seen. Hot flashes, decreased libido, and elevated PSA levels are more often seen in advanced stages of prostate cancer. Cystitis and urethral strictures may occur after the surgery but are not as common as Option A.

7. *Answer:* C
Rationale: The ACS reports that the initial peak after the advent of the PSA has dropped and leveled. This is because the public's initial response to the PSA test has normalized.

8. *Answer:* B
Rationale: An important risk factor for the development of prostate cancer is being of African American descent.

9. *Answer:* B
Rationale: Metastatic disease control is achieved by decreasing the male hormone testosterone through medical castration. Strontium is an intravenous radioisotope used to treat metastatic bone pain. Surgery is not indicated for advanced disease, and total body irradiation is not indicated for advanced prostate cancer.

10. *Answer:* A
Rationale: Hematuria is the most common symptom of early bladder cancer; the other symptoms may indicate metastatic disease.

11. *Answer:* A
Rationale: ACS states that the incidence of bladder cancer is in the ratio of 4:1 for men:women.

12. *Answer:* A
Rationale: IVP or excretory urogram allow visualization of the bladder and cystoscopy is necessary to obtain a biopsy. A CT of the pelvis will aid in determining the extent of disease. Bladder cancer does not commonly go to the bone. Bone scans will show metastatic disease to the bone.

BIBLIOGRAPHY

American Cancer Society. (2004). *Cancer facts and figures—2004*. Atlanta: Author.

American Joint Commission on Cancer. (2002). *AJCC cancer staging manual* (6th ed.). New York: Springer-Verlag.

Brawley, O.W., & Barnes, S. (2001). The epidemiology of prostate cancer in the United States. *Seminars in Oncology Nursing 17*(2), 72-77.

Dest, V.M., & Wallace, M. (2001). Prevalent issues in patient education. In M. Wallace & L.L. Powell (Eds.). *Prostate cancer: Nursing assessment, management, and care*. New York: Springer Publishing, pp. 140-152.

Griffin, A.S., & O'Rourke, M.E. (2001). Expectant management of prostate cancer. *Seminars in Oncology Nursing 17*(2), 101-107.

Held-Warmkessel, J. (2001). Treatment of advanced prostate cancer. *Seminars in Oncology Nursing 17*(2), 118-128.

Iwamoto, R., & Maher, K.E. (2001). Radiation therapy for prostate cancer. *Seminars in Oncology Nursing 17*(2), 90-100.

Jemal J., Murray, T., Samuels, A., et al. (2003). Cancer statistics 2003. *CA: A Cancer Journal for Clinicians 53*, 5-26.

O'Rourke, M.E. (2001). Genitourinary cancers. In S. Otto (Ed.). *Oncology Nursing*. St. Louis, Mosby, pp. 213-247.

Stoller, M.L., & Carroll, P.R. (2003). Urology. In L.M. Tierney, S.J. McPhee, & M.A. Papadakis (Eds.). *CMDT, Current medical diagnosis and treatment*. New York: Lange Medical Books/McGraw-Hill, pp. 903-945.

United States Preventive Services Task Force. (2002). Screening for prostate cancer: Recommendations and rationale. *Annals of Internal Medicine 137*, 915-916.

NOTES

28 Nursing Care of the Client with Skin Cancer

ALICE J. LONGMAN

Select the best answer for each of the following questions:

1. Which of the following is **most** important in the prevention of skin cancer?
    A. Length of exposure to the sun.
    B. Geographic area of residence or recreation.
    C. Protection from the sun's rays.
    D. Altitude or overcast weather conditions.

2. Of the following persons, who would be at the **highest** risk of having nonmelanoma skin cancers?
    A. A 35-year-old Caucasian ski instructor.
    B. A 60-year-old Caucasian grain farmer in the midwestern United States.
    C. A 40-year-old Mexican American ranch hand in the southwestern United States.
    D. A 62-year-old African American cotton farmer in the southern United States.

3. In presenting information on the early detection of nonmelanoma skin cancers, nurses should target
    A. mothers of infants and children.
    B. elderly persons.
    C. adolescents.
    D. factory workers.

4. Which of the following is the most important follow-up care for persons who have been treated for skin cancer?
    A. Weekly, systematic self-examination of the skin for suspicious lesions.
    B. Limiting sun exposure to 2 hours during the summer months.

C. Evaluation at regular intervals by a physician and/or nurse.
    D. Use of sunscreens and sunblocks when outside during the summer months.

5. Which of the following is the major reason for accurate assessment of a lesion suspicious of malignant melanoma?
    A. Microscopic examination is essential for determination of the exact type of malignant melanoma.
    B. The level of invasion and tumor thickness is best assessed by microstaging.
    C. Palliative treatment of malignant melanoma is best achieved by accurate assessment.
    D. Malignant melanoma has the ability to spread rapidly to other sites of the body.

6. Which of the following chemotherapeutic agents has had the most consistent results in the treatment of malignant melanoma?
    A. Methotrexate.
    B. Monoclonal antibodies.
    C. Hormonal agents.
    D. Dacarbazine (DTIC-Dome).

7. In the initial treatment of skin cancer, which of the standard therapies for the treatment of skin cancer is most effective?
    A. Surgical excision.
    B. Radiotherapy.
    C. Chemotherapy.
    D. Biochemotherapy.

8. Which of the following lesion types has the highest risk of recurrence?
    A. Basal cell carcinoma.
    B. Squamous cell carcinoma.

C. Nodular melanoma.

D. Superficial spreading melanoma.

9. In counseling clients and families about continued care after treatment for skin cancer, which self-care activity is the most important?

A. Monitoring the site where the lesion occurred.

B. Monthly self-examination of the skin.

C. Updating family history of skin cancers.

D. Collecting information about skin cancer from national cancer-related organizations.

10. In teaching about the prevention of skin cancer, the major areas to be included initially are

A. length of exposure to sunlight, use of sunscreen (SPF of 15 or more), use of protective clothing, and use of sunglasses.

B. time of day during sun exposure, time of year of sun exposure, weather conditions during sun exposure, and recreational activities.

C. skin type, genetic history, family pedigree about skin cancer, and use of tanning parlors.

D. skin assessment, effect of altitude during sun exposure, time of year during sun exposure, and time of day of sun exposure.

11. In presenting information on the risks associated with the development of malignant melanoma, nurses should target

A. senior citizens.

B. mothers of adolescents.

C. construction workers.

D. mothers of infants and young children.

12. When using sunscreen, which area(s) of the body are most frequently neglected?

A. The cheeks.

B. The hands.

C. The back of the legs.

D. The back of the neck.

13. Which of the following is the most useful in the prediction of prognosis and recurrence of malignant melanoma?

A. Clark's level.

B. Breslow index.

C. Dermascopy.

D. Total body photography.

14. The major purpose of teaching routine self-examination of the skin is the

A. enhancement of clients' responsibility for their own care.

B. identification of suspicious lesions in the skin.

C. assistance to families in maintaining their own health.

D. incorporation of healthy behaviors into one's own lifestyle.

15. Which of the following is the most critical in addressing the plan of care for clients with advanced metastatic melanoma?

A. Exploring community resources to assist clients and their families.

B. Assessing family resources for assistance in meeting clients' needs.

C. Allowing clients to clearly state their goals for care, thus allowing them control.

D. Investigating palliative care with assistance from the health care team.

ANSWERS

1. *Answer:* C
   Rationale: All of the known risks for skin cancer are related to the magnitude of exposure to ultraviolet radiation. Protection from the sun's rays plays a critical role in the prevention of skin cancer. Options A, B, and D are potential risk factors for skin cancer.

2. *Answer:* B
   Rationale: A history of chronic exposure to ultraviolet radiation is important in the assessment of persons presenting with non-melanoma skin cancers. Those at highest risk for the development of nonmelanoma skin cancers are Caucasians with a chronic exposure to ultraviolet radiation. A 60-year-old Caucasian grain farmer would have a longer cumulative exposure to ultraviolet radiation than a 35-year-old Caucasian ski instructor. The Mexican American and African American have significant cumulative ultraviolet radiation exposure but have a slightly reduced risk of having skin cancer because of their skin type.

3. *Answer:* B
   Rationale: Efforts at early detection should be aimed at those with highest risk. Elderly persons have a history of exposure to ultraviolet radiation, which is one of the risk factors in the development of nonmelanoma skin cancers, in which most of the lesions appear on the face, head, and neck. Nonmelanoma skin cancers respond well to early treatment. Efforts at skin cancer prevention should especially be targeted at mothers of infants and small children and adolescents. This would include information about ways to reduce ultraviolet exposure.

4. *Answer:* C
   Rationale: The importance of continued surveillance cannot be overemphasized. Systematic assessment of the skin at regular intervals by a physician or a nurse is important; however, monthly self-examination of the skin is taught and recommended for those who have had skin cancer. Option D is incor-

rect because protective clothing, sunscreen, and sunblocks are important year-round, not just during the warm, sunny, summer months.

5. *Answer:* D
   Rationale: Of all the skin cancers, malignant melanoma is the most aggressive and virulent. Those persons at risk for having malignant melanoma are cautioned to have regular and complete examinations of the skin to detect changes in suspicious lesions and have them removed promptly.

6. *Answer:* D
   Rationale: Treatment for malignant melanoma, other than surgery, remains elusive. Of the chemotherapeutic agents used to date, the agent with the most consistent activity is dacarbazine. The challenge has been to identify which combination of other agents will offer consistent improvement over dacarbazine alone.

7. *Answer:* A
   Rationale: Although all of the standard therapies may be used during the course of treatment for skin cancer, particularly malignant melanoma, surgical excision is used 90% of the time. In the treatment of malignant melanoma, it may be necessary to remove nearby lymph glands, although this is controversial. Wide, clean, surgical margins are suggested whenever possible.

8. *Answer:* C
   Rationale: The most important prognostic feature in malignant melanoma is the size of the lesion at the time of diagnosis. Nodular melanoma has the highest risk of recurrence and metastasis because of the ability to invade the dermis from the onset with no apparent horizontal growth. Equally high cure rates with either surgery or radiation can be achieved for basal cell and squamous cell carcinomas. Although a possibility of recurrence exists with either one, continued surveillance improves the ability to detect it quickly.

9. *Answer:* B

Rationale: Evaluation at regular intervals by a physician or nurse is important for those who have received treatment for skin cancer. Clients and families also are instructed to assume responsibility for their own care. One of the most important activities is a systematic, monthly self-examination of the skin.

10. *Answer:* A

Rationale: Exposure to ultraviolet radiation should be limited between 10 AM and 3 PM in high-intensity sun areas. Sunscreens (SPF of 15 or more) are recommended with frequent reapplications during prolonged sun exposure. Protective clothing and sunglasses are also recommended during prolonged sun exposure. All of these are important in teaching about the prevention of skin cancer. Options B, C, and D are related to risk assessment and early detection activities.

11. *Answer:* D

Rationale: There is a possible link between severe sunburn in childhood and the risk of malignant melanoma in later life. Children should be protected from traumatic sunburn, and it is advisable to keep infants out of the sun.

12. *Answer:* D

Rationale: Most people are conscientious in applying sunscreen to their faces. The one area that many forget is the back of the neck. Often, this area is exposed to ultraviolet radiation for long periods of time.

13. *Answer:* B

Rationale: The Breslow index is the most commonly reported in microstaging. It is more reproducible in predicting prognosis than other tools. The Breslow index measures the vertical thickness of the tumor in millimeters. Clark's level measures the level of invasion in relation to the anatomic structures of the skin. Dermascopy enhances visualization of microscopic structures in pigmented lesions by non-invasive means. Total body photography is used to document stability or instability of suspected lesions in people at high risk.

14. *Answer:* B.

Rationale: Early detection and treatment of skin cancer are critical. Engaging in self-care activities contributes to the maintenance of one's health. Skin self-examination can often result in the detection of early malignancies between professional examinations.

15. *Answer:* C

Rationale: It is important to allow those with advanced metastatic disease to make their desired wishes for continued care known. Often, options are presented for treatment alone, and other options may not be discussed.

BIBLIOGRAPHY

American Cancer Society. (2004). *Cancer facts and figures—2004.* Atlanta: Author.

Brenner, S., & Tamir, E. (2002). Early detection of melanoma: The best strategy for a favorable prognosis. *Clinics in Dermatology 20,* 203-211.

Fu, M.R., Anderson, C.M., McDaniel, R., & Armer, J. (2002). Patients' perceptions of fatigue in response to biochemotherapy for metastatic melanoma: A preliminary study. *Oncology Nursing Forum 29,* 961-966.

Jerant, A.F., Johnson, J.T., Sheridan, C.M., & Caffrey, T.J. (2000). Early detection and treatment of skin cancer. *American Family Physician 62,* 357-374.

Longman, A.J. (2000). Nursing care of the client with skin cancer. In J.K. Itano & K.N. Taoka (Eds.). *Core curriculum for oncology nursing* (4th ed.). St. Louis: Elsevier, pp. 615-623.

Rigel, D.D., & Carucci, J.A. (2000). Malignant melanoma: Prevention, early detection, and treatment in the 21st century. *CA: A Cancer Journal for Clinicians 50,* 215-236.

Saraiya, M., Hall, H.I., & Uhler, R.J. (2002). Sunburn prevalence among adults in the United States, 1999. *American Journal of Preventive Medicine 23,* 91-97.

Thompson, N., Bond, L.K., Vance, R.B., et al. (2001). Addressing treatment options in metastatic melanoma. *Cancer Practice 9,* 221-226.

29 Nursing Care of the Client with Head and Neck Cancer

ELLEN CARR

Select the best answer for each of the following questions:

1. A client with head and neck cancer is likely to be a
   A. a male of Asian descent, nonsmoker, age 30 to 50.
   B. a Swedish woman who smokes and has been diagnosed with breast cancer.
   C. a male smoker and user of alcohol, age 50 to 70.
   D. an American woman with recent dental work, nonsmoker, nondrinker.

2. Head and neck cancers are typically
   A. adenocarcinoma.
   B. squamous cell cancer.
   C. sarcomas.
   D. lymphoid cancers.

3. When swallowing a bolus of food,
   A. the vocal cords open, and the larynx moves back and forward.
   B. the vocal cords open, and the larynx moves upward and back.
   C. the vocal cords close, and the larynx moves upward and back.
   D. the vocal cords close, and the larynx moves upward and forward.

4. If a client with a history of head and neck cancer presents with a second, new primary cancer, the most likely location of the second primary is the
   A. esophagus.
   B. head and neck.
   C. lung.
   D. brain.

5. For those diagnosed with a form of head and neck cancer, the best 5-year survival rate (all stages) is for
   A. thyroid cancer.
   B. nasopharyngeal cancer.
   C. laryngeal cancer.
   D. oral cancer.

6. A symptom that is common to several head and neck cancer sites is
   A. neutropenia.
   B. difficulty swallowing.
   C. sleep apnea.
   D. vision changes.

7. For recurrent metastatic head and neck cancer, the primary treatment modality is
   A. chemotherapy.
   B. radiation therapy.
   C. surgery.
   D. biotherapy.

8. When a client with head and neck cancer is recovering from surgical treatment, a primary concern in the nursing care plan includes
   A. skin integrity, fatigue, pharyngitis, appetite.
   B. stomatitis, xerostomia, taste changes, infection.
   C. nausea and vomiting, alopecia, thrombocytopenia, weight loss.
   D. skin care, range of motion (ROM) exercises, supporting coping to accommodate physical changes.

9. During the first year after diagnosis and treatment for detection of recurrence or a second primary tumor, clients with head and neck cancer should be followed every
   A. month.
   B. 2 months.
   C. 3 months.
   D. 4 months.

10. When a postoperative client with a tracheostomy reports that his secretions are thick and copious, the nurse can recommend
   A. applying a thin layer of prescribed ointment around the stoma twice each day.
   B. increasing humidity in the client's environment.
   C. changing the tracheostomy tube to a laryngectomy tube.
   D. stopping instillation of normal saline into the trachea.

11. When doing oral care, a method to minimize drying mucosa is to use
   A. lemon glycerin swabs.
   B. commercially prepared mouthwashes.
   C. 1/2 strength peroxide/normal saline solution.
   D. positive-pressure room air.

12. Before surgery for clients with head and neck cancer, one of the primary areas of nursing assessment should include
   A. nutrition.
   B. bladder and bowel habits.
   C. lower extremity mobility.
   D. hearing.

13. A client who undergoes a total laryngectomy can lose his or her ability to speak. Therefore before surgery, establishing a way to communicate can include
   A. testing hearing.
   B. a visit with a physical therapist.
   C. ROM exercises.
   D. teaching about an artificial larynx.

14. Swallowing can be assessed with
   A. a neck computed tomography (CT) exam.
   B. a video barium swallow test.
   C. a neck magnetic resonance imaging (MRI) exam.
   D. chest x-ray.

15. A nursing diagnosis for clients with head and neck cancer associated with care after radiation therapy treatments includes
   A. urinary retention.
   B. impaired skin integrity.
   C. fluid volume deficit.
   D. alteration in cardiac circulation.

16. Stage II head and neck cancer is staged as
   A. T1, N0, M0.
   B. T1, N1, M0.
   C. T2, N0, M0.
   D. T2, N0, M1.

17. When assessing a client for oral mucositis, the nurse first is looking for signs of
   A. indentation.
   B. fungal infection.
   C. inflammation.
   D. allergic reaction.

18. A client with cancer can experience trismus (a restriction in opening the mouth), which can be a side effect from radiation treatment. Therefore a major complication from trismus is
   A. the ability to produce enough mucus.
   B. the ability to eat.
   C. the ability to digest food.
   D. the ability to cough.

19. A client with head and neck cancer reports that he feels "washed out" after completing 20 of 30 scheduled radiation treatments. A helpful response to this client would be:
   A. "This is very unlikely, considering your diagnosis and treatment regimen."
   B. "We need to increase your nutritional supplements."
   C. "You will start to feel better after your 25th treatment."
   D. "Fatigue is an expected side effect from radiation therapy. Let's look at how you can conserve your energy."

20. A client with a new tracheostomy reports that she does not venture outside of the home. As her nurse, an assessment of her reluctance to go out in public requires evaluation of
   A. her trach size.
   B. the client's perception of her altered body image.
   C. transportation options.
   D. her ability to see at night.

ANSWERS

1. *Answer:* C
   Rationale: Head and neck cancers are more likely to be diagnosed in men ages 50 to 70; recurrent head and neck cancer is more likely in those who currently smoke or drink or have a smoking and drinking history. Nasopharyngeal cancer has a higher incidence rate with Asians, particularly those of Chinese ancestry.

2. *Answer:* B
   Rationale: Cases of squamous cell cancer make up an estimated 90% of head and neck tumors.

3. *Answer:* D
   Rationale: When swallowing, the bolus moves through the pharynx and is propelled toward the esophagus; the vocal cords close, and the larynx moves upward and forward, preventing aspiration.

4. *Answer:* B
   Rationale: If a client diagnosed with a head and neck tumor has a new primary tumor site, clinical statistics indicate that the location is likely to be in the head and neck (40%), lung (30%), esophagus (9%), elsewhere (20%).

5. *Answer:* A
   Rationale: The 5-year relative survival rate for thyroid cancer is 95%, laryngeal cancer (all stages) 65%, oral cavity 40% to 70%, and nasopharynx cancer, 26%.

6. *Answer:* B
   Rationale: A common symptom of several head and neck cancer sites is difficulty swallowing.

7. *Answer:* A
   Rationale: Chemotherapy with or without radiation therapy is used for recurrent and metastatic disease. Surgery and radiation are the primary treatment modalities for managing malignant head and neck tumors.

8. *Answer:* D
   Rationale: Care after surgery for clients with head and neck cancer primarily includes skin care, ROM exercises, and supporting coping to accommodate physical changes. Care after radiation therapy includes a focus on skin integrity, fatigue, pharyngitis, and appetite. Care after radiation for oral cancer includes a focus on stomatitis, xerostomia, taste changes, and infection. After chemotherapy, nursing care usually focuses on nausea and vomiting, alopecia, thrombocytopenia, and weight loss.

9. *Answer:* A
   Rationale: During the rehabilitation phase (first year after diagnosis and treatment) for head/neck cancers, clinical evaluation is recommended every month.

10. *Answer:* B
    Rationale: Symptoms of inadequate humidity include thick, tenacious secretions that are difficult to expectorate. Stoma care includes applying a thin layer of prescribed ointment around the stoma twice each day. When a stoma begins to narrow, a strategy to maintain the airway is to change the tracheostomy tube to a laryngectomy tube. To precipitate coughing and mobilize secretions if needed, instill 2 to 5 ml of normal saline solution into the tracheostomy. The saline provides lavage and stimulates the trachea and bronchi.

11. *Answer:* C
    Rationale: To minimize drying of the mucosa when performing oral care, avoid lemon glycerin swabs and commercially prepared mouthwashes (that contain alcohol). To gently cleanse the cavity, use gravity lavage or a jet-spray dental cleansing system. A recommended solution for oral care is 1/2 strength peroxide/normal saline solution.

12. *Answer:* A
    Rationale: Before surgery, 60% of clients with head and neck cancer initially present with malnutrition. During treatment, greater than 10% body weight can be lost.

13. *Answer:* D
    Rationale: For clients with a total laryngectomy, options to optimize speech include

the use of an artificial larynx, use of esophageal speech, and use of a tracheoesophageal prosthesis. Clients' hearing is not affected by a laryngectomy. A speech therapist, not a physical therapist, helps the client with communication challenges. ROM exercises do not help with speech limitations.

14. *Answer:* B
Rationale: A barium swallow study can show the stages of a swallow based on the movement of barium. The CT and MRI of the neck are static tests. A chest x-ray does not show the swallow function.

15. *Answer:* B
Rationale: A primary nursing diagnosis for clients undergoing postradiation therapy is impaired skin integrity. Urinary retention, fluid volume deficit, and alteration in cardiac circulation may affect the client, but they are not primary diagnoses.

16. *Answer:* C
Rationale: Stage 1: T1, N0, M0; stage II: T2, N0, M0; stage III: T3, N0, M0; T1, T2, or T3 with N1, M0; stage IV: T4a or b, N0 or N1, M0, any T, N2 or N3, M0, any T, any N, M1.

17. *Answer:* C
Rationale: Oral mucositis (also called stomatitis) is an inflammation of the mouth and throat lining, a frequent side effect of radiation treatment in clients with head and neck cancer (and of some chemotherapy treatments.) Inflammation appears as redness and swelling, with the client reporting pain. Indentation in the mouth, although causing redness or inflammation, is a mechanical trauma to the oral mucosa. Fungal infections typically appear as a white film on the mucosal layer. Allergic reactions are typically systemic or regional, not localized to the oral cavity.

18. *Answer:* B
Rationale: Trismus physically restricts the ability to open the mouth, which can affect speech, swallowing, mastication, and adequate oral hygiene. Although a client with trismus may have difficulty producing mucus and coughing, the main complication of trismus is the inability to open the mouth to eat.

19. *Answer:* D
Rationale: Radiation therapy as a treatment for head and neck cancers brings on profound fatigue as clients progress through their treatment regimens. That fatigue is not expected to wane until a few weeks after radiation treatments end. Clients reporting signs of fatigue are best supported by offering education about radiation treatment, its expected side effects, and how long those side effects may last.

20. *Answer:* B
Rationale: A client with a new tracheostomy is undergoing major body image changes. Assessment of body image can include trach hygiene and care, the ability of the client to communicate with others with her trach in place, and her overall capacity to cope with changes in her health and social functioning. The client's reluctance to interact socially is not unexpected but can be lessened by talking through issues with a knowledgeable and caring nurse.

BIBLIOGRAPHY

American Cancer Society. (2003). All about laryngeal and hypopharyngeal cancer. Retrieved February 19, 2003 from the ACS web site: *http://www.cancer.org/docroot/CRI/CRI_2x.asp?site area=CRI&dt=23.*

American Cancer Society. (2004). *Cancer facts and figures 2004.* Atlanta: Author.

American Cancer Society. (2003). Surgery for laryngectomy. Retrieved February 19, 2003 from the ACS web site: *http://www.cancer.org/ docroot/CRI/content/CRI_2_4_4X_Surgery_23.asp? sitearea.*

American Joint Commission on Cancer (AJCC). (2002). Head and neck sites. *In AJCC Cancer staging handbook* (6th ed). New York: Springer-Verlag, pp. 27-46.

Bauer, A.M. (2001). Current trends of surgical management of head and neck carcinomas. *Nursing Clinics of North America 36,* 501-506.

Cady, J. (2002). Laryngectomy: Beyond loss of voice—caring for the client as a whole. *Clinical Journal of Oncology Nursing 6,* 347-351.

Camp-Sorrell, D. (2000). Chemotherapy: Toxicity and management. In C.H. Yarbro, M.H. Frogge, M. Goodman, & S.L. Groenwald (Eds.). *Cancer nursing: Principles and practice* (5th ed.). Sudbury, MA: Jones and Bartlett Publishers, pp. 444-486.

Clarke, L.K. (2002). Pathways for head and neck surgery: A client-education tool. *Clinical Journal of Oncology Nursing 6*(2), 78-82.

Dropkin, M.J. (2001). Anxiety, coping strategies, and coping behaviors in clients undergoing head and neck cancer surgery. *Cancer Nursing 24,* 143-148.

Fang, B., & Forastiere, A. (2001). Head and neck cancer. In J. Abraham & C. Allegra (Eds.). *Bethesda handbook of clinical oncology.* New York: Lippincott, Williams & Wilkins, pp. 3-28.

Haggood, A.S. (2001). Head and neck cancers. In S. Otto (Ed.). *Oncology nursing* (4th ed.). St. Louis: Mosby, pp. 285-325.

Harris, L. (2000). Head and neck malignancies. In C.H. Yarbro, M.H. Frogge, M. Goodman, & S.L. Groenwald. (Eds.). *Cancer nursing: Principles and practice* (5th ed.). Sudbury, MA: Jones and Bartlett Publishers, pp. 1210-1243.

Maher, K. (2000). Radiation therapy: Toxicities and management. In C.H. Yarbro, M.H. Frogge, M. Goodman, & S.L. Groenwald (Eds.). *Cancer nursing: Principles and practice* (5th ed.). Sudbury, MA: Jones and Bartlett Publishers, pp. 323-351.

McGuire, J. (2000). Nutritional care of surgical oncology clients. *Seminars in Oncology Nursing 16,* 128-34.

Miller, S.D., & Sessions, R.B. (2001). Rehabilitation after treatment for head and neck cancer. In V.T. DeVita, S. Hellman, & S.A. Rosenberg (Eds.). *Cancer: Principles and practice of oncology* (6th ed). Philadelphia: Lippincott Williams & Wilkins, pp. 907-916.

NANDA. (2001). *Nursing diagnoses: Definitions and classification, 2001-2003.* Philadelphia: North American Nursing Diagnosis Association.

National Cancer Institute. (2002). Head and neck cancer: Questions and answers. Retrieved February 19, 2003, from Cancer Facts web site: http://cis.nci.nih.gov/fact/6_37.htm.

National Cancer Institute. (2002). Head and neck cancer: Treatment. Retrieved February 19, 2003, from CancerNet (PDQ) web sites for health professionals: http://www.nci.nih.gov/cancerinfo/treatment/head-and-neck.

National Cancer Institute. (2002). Hypopharyngeal cancer. Retrieved February 19, 2003, from CancerNet (PDQ) web sites for health professionals: http://www.nci.nih.gov/cancerinfo/pdq/treatment/hypopharyngeal/healthprofessional/.

National Cancer Institute. (2002). Nasopharyngeal cancer. Retrieved February 19, 2003, from CancerNet (PDQ) web sites for health professionals: http://www.nci.nih.gov/cancerinfo/pdq/treatment/nasopharyngeal/healthprofessional/.

Sidransky, D. (2001). Cancers of the head and neck. In V.T. DeVita, S. Hellman, & S.A. Rosenberg (Eds.). *Cancer: Principles and practice of Oncology* (6th ed). Philadelphia: Lippincott Williams & Wilkins, pp. 789-914.

Staiduhar, K.I., Neithercut, J., Chu, E., et al. (2000). Thyroid cancer: Clients' experiences of receiving iodine-131 therapy. *Oncology Nursing Forum 27,* 1213-1218.

Sweed, M.R., Schiech, L., Barsevick, A., et al. (2002). Quality of life after esophagectomy for cancer. *Oncology Nursing Forum 29,* 1127-1131.

30 Nursing Care of the Client with Cancers of the Neurologic System

SHIRLEY J. KERN

Select the best answer for each of the following questions:

1. Which of the following would be **unusual** for a nurse to see as a presenting symptom for clients with a brain tumor?
   - A. Seizure.
   - B. Unilateral headache.
   - C. Fever.
   - D. Hemiparesis.

2. Which of the following statements is true regarding high-grade astrocytomas?
   - A. They metastasize frequently to the liver or lungs or both.
   - B. They infiltrate into surrounding brain tissue.
   - C. They are usually encapsulated.
   - D. They respond well to standard chemotherapy.

3. The most common type of malignant brain tumors arises from
   - A. neurons.
   - B. astrocytes.
   - C. oligodendrocytes.
   - D. lymphatic tissues in the brain.

4. A client presents with a history of lung cancer and new onset of radicular pain of the left leg and spinal tenderness in the lower back. What nursing assessments are critical for this client?
   - A. Pupil checks.
   - B. Function of bowel and bladder.
   - C. Cranial nerve examination.
   - D. Upper extremity strength.

5. Which of the following functions is associated with the frontal lobe of the brain?
   - A. Mood and affect.
   - B. Pain.
   - C. Hearing.
   - D. Coordination.

6. Loss of balance, confusion, headache, and urinary incontinence are symptoms of
   - A. deep venous thrombosis (DVT).
   - B. dementia.
   - C. radiation necrosis.
   - D. hydrocephalus.

7. The client has a brain biopsy, and the final pathology report states that there are many abnormal and heterogeneous cells, in addition to areas of necrosis. Based on the pathology report, which of the following is the tumor grade?
   - A. Grade I.
   - B. Grade II.
   - C. Grade III.
   - D. Grade IV.

8. A recently approved oral, second-generation alkylating agent that can permeate the blood-brain barrier and is now frequently used in the treatment of malignant brain tumors is
   - A. carmustine (BCNU).
   - B. PCV3.
   - C. temozolomide (Temodar).
   - D. etoposide (VP-16).

9. Which of the following tumors arise from primitive neuroectodermal cells and is more common in children?
   A. Pinealblastoma.
   B. Glioblastoma multiforme.
   C. Oligodendroglioma.
   D. Anaplastic astrocytoma.

10. A client with a glioblastoma multiforme was diagnosed with a DVT 1 month ago and has been on daily warfarin (Coumadin) since that time. He calls the clinic stating that he has had a worsening headache over the last week that is not alleviated by acetaminophen (Tylenol). The nurse prepares the client to undergo which of the following initial tests?
    A. Magnetic resonance imaging (MRI).
    B. Noncontrast-enhanced computed tomography (CT).
    C. Ultrasound.
    D. Myelogram.

11. Which of the following primary sites would be more **unusual** to see as the source of spinal metastases?
    A. Breast.
    B. Lung.
    C. Colon.
    D. Prostate.

12. The client presents with a left visual field cut, and the MRI shows a brain tumor on the right. The nurse would expect which lobe of the brain to be affected?
    A. Parietal lobe.
    B. Frontal lobe.
    C. Temporal lobe.
    D. Occipital lobe.

13. Which of the following is the most appropriate nursing diagnosis for the client who has seizures related to his brain tumor?
    A. Risk for activity intolerance.
    B. Disturbed body image.
    C. Risk for injury.
    D. Risk for infection.

14. A client calls you, the nurse, reporting that she recently has been experiencing stomach irritation, depression, mood swings, sleep difficulties, and weight gain. Which of the following medications is most likely the culprit for the side effects that the client is experiencing?
    A. dexamethasone.
    B. phenytoin (Dilantin).
    C. carbamazepine (Tegretol).
    D. divalproex (Depakote).

15. Which of the following types of radiation therapy is delivered in a single high-dose fraction using a head frame?
    A. Standard conventional radiation.
    B. Brachytherapy.
    C. Stereotactic radiosurgery.
    D. Fractionated stereotactic radiotherapy.

ANSWERS

1. *Answer:* C
   Rationale: Seizure is the most common presenting symptom. Headaches and unilateral hemiparesis are also fairly common. Fever is not a common presenting symptom.

2. *Answer:* B
   Rationale: High-grade astrocytomas infiltrate surrounding brain tissue and usually are not encapsulated. They rarely metastasize outside the central nervous system. Most chemotherapy agents given intravenously or orally do not cross the blood-brain barrier.

3. *Answer:* B
   Rationale: Almost half of all malignant brain tumors arise from astrocytes. Malignant tumors arising from neurons are rare. Oligodendrogliomas account for only about 5% of malignant tumors. There are no lymphatic tissues in the brain.

4. *Answer:* B
   Rationale: Dysfunctions of bladder and bowel and deterioration of lower extremity motor and sensory function would indicate spinal cord compression and require emergency intervention. The other nursing measures would not assess this potential problem.

5. *Answer:* A
   Rationale: Mood and affect are functions of the frontal lobe. Pain is a function of the parietal lobe. Hearing is a function of the temporal lobe. Coordination is a function of the cerebellum.

6. *Answer:* D
   Rationale: Hydrocephalus can result from blockage of cerebrospinal fluid (CSF) pathways caused by tumor growth and/or edema. Symptoms of hydrocephalus include headache, loss of balance, memory loss, confusion, and urinary incontinence.

7. *Answer:* D
   Rationale: The World Health Organization (WHO) Classification System identifies a grade IV tumor as one with rapid reproduction with many abnormal and heterogeneous cells seen under the microscope. There are also areas of necrosis. Grade IV tumors are extremely infiltrative into normal brain tissue.

8. *Answer:* C
   Rationale: Temozolomide was approved by the Food and Drug Administration in 1999 for the treatment of grade III anaplastic astrocytoma tumors but not for glioblastomas. However, temozolomide is frequently used for glioblastomas, anaplastic astrocytomas, and anaplastic oligodendrogliomas across the United States and in Europe.

9. *Answer:* A
   Rationale: The pinealblastoma is an example of a primitive neuroectodermal tumor (PNET) and frequently occurs in young children. The glioblastoma multiforme arises from the astrocytes and is most common in the fifth to seventh decade. The anaplastic astrocytoma also arises from astrocytes and occurs more often in younger adults. The oligodendroglioma is a tumor that arises from the oligodendrocyte cells and usually occurs in adults ages 40 to 50.

10. *Answer:* B
    Rationale: Because the client was recently placed on warfarin, an anticoagulant, and is complaining of a worsening headache, it is possible that he has experienced a cerebral hemorrhage. The noncontrast-enhanced CT is most frequently used to evaluate for hemorrhage. Blood is high in density on the CT throughout the acute phase and can quickly be picked up on CT.

11. *Answer:* C
    Rationale: Colon cancer rarely metastasizes to the spine. The most frequent spinal metastases are from the following primary sites: breast, lung, and prostate.

12. *Answer:* D
    Rationale: The function of the occipital lobe includes sight and visual identification of

objects. The parietal lobe controls sensory input such as pain, temperature, pinprick, light touch, proprioception, stereognosis, and graphesthesia. The frontal lobe controls personality, intellect, judgment, abstract thinking, mood and affect, and some memory. The temporal lobe controls hearing, memory, and receptive speech.

13. *Answer:* C

Rationale: Seizures can be manifested in various ways including convulsions, unusual sensations, and loss of consciousness. Clients who are experiencing a seizure are at increased risk for injury because they may not be able to use proper judgment to protect themselves while the seizure activity is occurring.

14. *Answer:* A

Rationale: Dexamethasone, one example of a steroid, can have side effects. Some of the most common side effects include mood fluctuations, increased appetite and water retention, upset stomach, and sleep difficulties. The other medications are examples of anticonvulsants and have other side effects.

15. *Answer:* C

Rationale: Stereotactic radiosurgery (SRS) uses the same type of head frame that is used for stereotactic biopsy. This head frame allows the radiation to be focused on the tumor. The radiation is delivered in several arcs so that the tumor receives the full dose but normal tissues are spared. Standard conventional radiation is generally given over 6 to 7 weeks. Brachytherapy involves implantation of radioactive seeds into the tumor bed, and these are left in place for 3 to 4 days. Fractionated stereotactic radiotherapy uses a relocatable stereotactic frame so that several focused fractions can be delivered over several days.

BIBLIOGRAPHY

Blake, L.C., & Maravilla, K. R. (1999). Computed tomography. In M.S. Berger & C.B. Wilson (Eds.). *The gliomas*. Philadelphia: W.B. Saunders, pp. 242-274.

Kern, S.J. (2005). Nursing care of the client with cancers of the neurologic system. In J.K. Itano & K.N. Taoka (Eds.). *Core curriculum for oncology nursing* (4th ed.). St. Louis: Elsevier, pp. 656–675.

Kondziolka, D., Flickinger, J.C., & Lunsford, L.D. (2000). Stereotactic radiosurgery and radiation therapy. In M. Bernstein & M.S. Berger (Eds.). *Neuro-oncology: The essentials*. New York: Thieme Medical Publishers, Inc., pp. 183-197.

Macdonald, D.R. (2001). Temozolomide for recurrent high-grade glioma. *Seminars in Oncology* 28(4, Suppl. 13), 3-12.

Segal, G. (1998). *A primer of brain tumors: A patient's reference manual*. Chicago: American Brain Tumor Association.

31 Nursing Care of the Client with Leukemia

MOLLY J. MORAN

Select the best answer for each of the following questions:

1. Cerebellar toxicity and acral erythema are both associated with what chemotherapeutic agent?
   - A. Arsenic trioxide (Trisenox).
   - B. 5-fluorouracil (5-FU).
   - C. Any anthracycline.
   - D. High-dose cytarabine (Ara-C).

2. The bone marrow produces which of the following cells?
   - A. Osteoblasts.
   - B. Osteoclasts.
   - C. White blood cells.
   - D. Islet of Langerhans cells.

3. According to the American Cancer Society, there will be how many new cases of leukemia diagnosed annually?
   - A. 15,300.
   - B. 33,440.
   - C. 45,900.
   - D. 61,200.

4. Which chemotherapy agent has been approved by the Food and Drug Administration (FDA) to treat clients with CD33 positive acute myelogenous leukemia (AML) in first relapse who are 60 years of age and older and are not candidates for cytotoxic chemotherapy?

   - A. All-trans-retinoic acid (ATRA).
   - B. High-dose cytosine arabinoside (Cytosar).
   - C. Gemtuzumab ozogamicin (Mylotarg).
   - D. Rituximab (Rituxan).

5. Chronic phase, accelerated phase, and blast crisis are associated with which leukemia?
   - A. Acute lymphocytic leukemia (ALL).
   - B. Chronic lymphocytic leukemia (CLL).
   - C. AML.
   - D. Chronic myelogenous leukemia (CML).

6. Central nervous system (CNS) disease is most common in what type of leukemia?
   - A. ALL.
   - B. CLL.
   - C. AML.
   - D. CML.

7. The most common type of leukemia in children is
   - A. ALL.
   - B. AML.
   - C. CLL.
   - D. CML.

8. ATRA is being used as initial treatment for
   - A. AML.
   - B. APL.
   - C. CML.
   - D. AML.

9. Which fact is true about nonmyeloablative transplant?
   A. Uses more toxic preparation regimen.
   B. Graft-versus-host disease plays a role in intended effect.
   C. Offered to very young clients.
   D. Offered to clients with low risk factors.

10. A positive Philadelphia chromosome is most commonly associated with
   A. AML.
   B. hairy cell leukemia.
   C. CML.
   D. ALL.

11. The central nervous system and testes are common sanctuary sites for which type of leukemia?
   A. ALL.
   B. CLL.
   C. Hairy cell leukemia.
   D. AML.

12. Which is the best tool to assess for cerebellar toxicity?
   A. Finger to nose.
   B. Writing name.
   C. Stating date (year, month, and day).
   D. Hopping up and down on one foot.

13. Induction treatment for AML usually consists of
   A. one single antineoplastic agent.
   B. a plant alkaloid agent with prednisone.
   C. diet therapy.
   D. cytarabine plus an anthracycline.

14. Etiologic factors being considered as causes of leukemia include which of the following:
   A. Sun exposure.
   B. Exposure to high altitudes.
   C. Previous treatment with alkylating agents.
   D. Diet.

15. A 40-year old woman was referred to a hematologist with a tentative diagnosis of AML. The client's only complaint was fatigue. Which of the following diagnostic tests would the hematologist most likely order first?
   A. Liver function tests.
   B. Uric acid.
   C. Lumbar puncture.
   D. Bone marrow aspirate and biopsy with special stains and immunophenotyping.

NOTES

ANSWERS

1. *Answer:* D
   Rationale: Of the possible options, only high-dose cytarabine is known to cause both cerebellar toxicity and acral erythema. Doxorubicin (Adriamycin), an anthracycline; arsenic trioxide; 5 FU; high-dose cytarabine; and several other chemotherapy agents can cause acral erythema.

2. *Answer:* C
   Rationale: The pluripotent stem cell originates in the bone marrow. This cell is capable of self-replication, proliferation, and differentiation. White blood cells are one of the cell lines that it produces. Osteoblasts are involved in the production of bone. Osteoclasts are involved in the absorption of bone. Islet of Langerhans cells are found in the pancreas and have endocrine and exocrine function.

3. *Answer:* B
   Rationale: The American Cancer Society's *Cancer Facts and Figures 2004* estimates that there will be 33,440 new cases in 2004.

4. *Answer:* C
   Rationale: Gemtuzumab (Mylotarg) binds specifically to the CD33 antigen. All-trans retinoic acid (ATRA) route promyelocytic leukemia is used in the initial treatment of acute promyelocytic leukemia (APL). Cytosine arabinoside is used most commonly in the treatment of AML. Rituximab is used in the treatment of non-Hodgkin's lymphoma.

5. *Answer:* D
   Rationale: It is CML that has three distinct phases of the disease process.

6. *Answer:* A
   Rationale: The CNS is a sanctuary for leukemic cells in ALL. CNS treatment for disease or as prophylaxis can include intrathecal chemotherapy and/or high-dose systemic chemotherapy and possibly cranial radiation.

7. *Answer:* A
   Rationale: Landier's article on "Childhood Acute Lymphoblastic Leukemia: Current Perspectives" in the June 2001 issue of the *Oncology Nursing Forum* reports that ALL is the most common childhood malignancy and comprises 76% of the leukemias in children under the age of 15.

8. *Answer:* B
   Rationale: ATRA is used for treatment of promyelocytic leukemia to enhance differentiation rather than to cause cytotoxicity. The other three types of leukemia mentioned in this question are treated initially with cytotoxic drugs.

9. *Answer:* B
   Rationale: With nonmyeloablataive transplant, the intent is for the immune cells of the transplanted marrow to make antibodies against the client's tissues with graft-versus-tumor effect to destroy the disease. Nonmyeloablative transplant is a less toxic preparation regimen and is offered to elderly clients and clients with high risk factors.

10. *Answer:* C
    Rationale: Approximately 95% of clients with CML are Philadelphia chromosome-positive. This represents a translocation of the long arms of chromosomes 9 and 22. Clients who are Philadelphia chromosome-positive usually have a better response to treatment and a longer survival rate than Philadelphia chromosome-negative clients.

11. *Answer:* A
    Rationale: Lymphoblasts have a tendency to hide in the central nervous system and the testes. Even after remission has been obtained, leukemia cells can be found in these sites. Therefore the CNS is treated to prevent relapse of the disease at this site.

12. *Answer:* B
    Rationale: Having the client write his or her name is the most consistent assessment tool. Having the client put finger to nose is acceptable; however, as shifts change, each nurse may not perceive the task the same way. Having the client write his or her name allows documenta-

tion for the client's medical record. A baseline neurologic assessment should be performed before the client receives any therapy.

13. *Answer:* D

Rationale: Cytarabine, which is cell cycle-specific, is used with an anthracycline, which is not cell cycle-specific. The thought is that the anthracycline will entice the proliferating cells to enter the cell cycles.

14. *Answer:* C

Rationale: Leukemia is considered the most frequent second malignancy after aggressive chemotherapy treatment for a previous malignancy. The leukemia is associated with the use of alkylating agents and more recently with the administration of etoposide and topoisomerase II inhibitors.

15. *Answer:* D

Rationale: A bone marrow biopsy and aspirate with special stains is done. These tests show the cellularity of the marrow and will denote the presence of Auer rods, which are diagnostic of AML. Special stains such as Sudan Black and peroxidase are used to diagnose AML. The presence of leukemic cells in the CNS is more common in ALL rather than AML. Uric acid and lactic dehydrogenase levels may be elevated

BIBLIOGRAPHY

American Cancer Society. (2004). *Cancer facts and figures – 2004.* Atlanta: American Cancer Society.

Carell, A.M. & Giralt, S. (2000). Novel preparative regimens II: Non-myeloablative regimens. In J.M. Rowe, H.M. Lazarus, & A.M. Carella (Eds.). *Handbook of bone marrow transplantation.* Malden, MA: Blackwell Science, Inc.

Coyle, C., & Wenhold, V. (2001). Painful blistered hands and feet. *Clinical Journal of Oncology Nursing 5*(5), 219-230.

Landier, W. (2001). Childhood acute lymphoblastic leukemia: Current perspectives. *Oncology Nursing Forum 28*(5): 823-833.

Landier, W. (2002). Myeloid diseases. In C.R. Baggott, K.P. Kelly, D. Fochtman, & G.V. Foley (Eds.). *Nursing care of children and adolescents with cancer* (3rd. ed.). Philadelphia: W.B. Saunders, pp. 491-502.

Shannon-Dorcy, K. (2002). Nursing implications of Mylotarg: A novel antibody-targeted chemotherapy for CD33+ acute myeloid leukemia in first relapse. *Oncology Nursing Forum 29*(4), 642.

Sorokin, P. (2000). Mylotarg approved for patients with CD33+ acute myelogenous leukemia. *Clinical Journal of Oncology Nursing 4*(6), 279-280.

Tennant, L. (2001). Clinical update: Chronic myelogenous leukemia: An overview. *Clinical Journal of Oncology Nursing 5*(5), 218-219.

Westlake, S.K., & Bertolone, K.L. (2002). Acute lymphoblastic leukemia. In C.R. Baggott, K. P. Kelly, D. Fochtman, & G.V. Foley (Eds.). *Nursing care of children and adolescents with cancer* (3rd ed.). Philadelphia: W. B. Saunders, pp. 466-490.

Wujcik, D. (2000). Leukemia. In C.H. Yarbro, M.H. Frogge, M. Goodman, & S.L. Groenwald (Eds.). *Cancer nursing: Principles and practice* (5th ed.). Sudbury, MA: Jones and Bartlett Publishers, pp. 1244-1268.

32 Nursing Care of the Client with Lymphoma or Multiple Myeloma

SUSAN EZZONE

Select the best answer for each of the following questions:

1. Mr. J. presents at his physician's office with enlarged lymph nodes and a history of night sweats. Although the physician suspects Hodgkin's disease, which of the following will be required to make a diagnosis of Hodgkin's disease?
  A. Fevers accompanying night sweats.
  B. A history of infections within 3 months of presentation with enlarged nodes.
  C. An excisional biopsy with Reed-Sternberg cells noted by the pathologist
  D. A chest x-ray film and computed tomography (CT) scans of the chest and abdomen.

2. Pain in a client with multiple myeloma commonly results from
  A. intestinal obstruction caused by enlarging soft-tissue mass.
  B. neural infiltration of plasma cells.
  C. lytic bone lesions.
  D. marrow infiltration.

3. Mr. S., a 17-year-old client, is scheduled to receive initial chemotherapy for Hodgkin's disease. After watching a video on chemotherapy, he makes the following comment to his nurse: "I guess taking chemotherapy means I will never have children." Which of the following is the most appropriate nursing intervention?
  A. The nurse states, "I wouldn't worry about it," and starts Mr. S.'s chemotherapy.
  B. The nurse tells the client that some people have problems but that he may not and offers to call the doctor to talk with him further if the client wishes. When the client does not make further comment, the nurse proceeds with chemotherapy.
  C. The nurse discusses sperm banking, provides the client with information, notifies the physician that the client has concerns, and delays the chemotherapy until the client can make a decision.
  D. The nurse documents in her notes that the client has concerns and may need a consultation for sperm banking after this admission and then proceeds with chemotherapy.

4. Mr. R. has a diagnosis of multiple myeloma and has been receiving oral melphalan (Alkeran) and prednisone over a period of several months. The nurse notes a weight loss of 10 pounds in the past month. The client states, "The doctor said my blood protein was high so I was trying to avoid protein in my diet." The best nursing intervention is to

A. tell the client that he is doing well to avoid protein and congratulate him on his weight loss.
B. explain to the client that the high blood protein is not a problem, but that he should avoid a high-fat diet.
C. explain to the client that the protein in his blood is from the myeloma, not his diet, and encourage a well-balanced diet.
D. give the client a pamphlet on the importance of nutrition for persons with cancer.

5. One week after Mr. Z.'s fifth cycle of doxorubicin (Adriamycin), bleomycin (Blenoxane), vinblastine (Velban), dacarbazine (DTIC-Dome, ABVD) chemotherapy for treatment of Hodgkin's disease, he complains of extreme fatigue, tiredness, and shortness of breath with exertion. Blood work reveals a hemoglobin of 9.3 g/dl, white blood count of $1.4 \times 1000/mm^3$, and platelets of $67,000/mm^3$. Mr. Z. calls to ask why he feels so "bad" this time. The most appropriate response is

A. symptoms of fatigue, tiredness, and shortness of breath are most likely caused by the low hemoglobin and red blood cell count. Administration of darbepoetin alfa (Aranesp) or epoetin alfa (Procrit) may be appropriate to promote red blood cell recovery after chemotherapy.
B. these are common symptoms, and there is really nothing that can be done to help.
C. don't worry about these symptoms unless there are signs of bleeding.
D. call back if you develop a fever or upper respiratory tract infection symptoms.

6. Mr. T. is a 52-year-old who was diagnosed with an intermediate grade non-Hodgkin's lymphoma 2 years ago. He received six courses of cyclophosphasmide (Cytoxon), doxorubicin, vincristine (Oncovin), prednisone (CHOP) chemotherapy and achieved a complete remission. He presents to the outpatient clinic today for routine follow-up and complains of left leg swelling upon examination. Which action is most appropriate initially?

A. Recommend the client keep his leg elevated as much as possible and call if symptoms have not improved in 1 week.
B. Assess for lymphadenopathy in all lymph node regions with special attention to inguinal lymph nodes.
C. Discuss with the physician the need for Doppler studies to rule out deep venous thrombosis.
D. Determine a dietary history of sodium intake.

7. Upon examination, Mr. T. is found to have an enlarged left inguinal lymph node chain approximately 3×8 cm. Mr. T. is afebrile with stable vital signs. The physician will most likely order the following:

A. Reinitiate CHOP chemotherapy immediately.
B. Antibiotics, because enlarged lymph nodes may be a sign of infection.
C. Peripheral vascular physician consult to evaluate left leg swelling.
D. CT scans of abdomen, pelvis, and chest and a lymph node biopsy.

8. Mrs. S. was diagnosed recently with stage III multiple myeloma, immunoglobulin G (IgG) kappa light chain, and will receive the fourth cycle of vincristine, doxorubicin (Adriamycin), dexamethasone (VAD) chemotherapy today. She asks how the response to treatment will be monitored after completing chemotherapy. Which is the most appropriate response?

A. Response to treatment is best measured by a myeloma survey.
B. Quantitative immunoglobulins are checked only at the beginning of treatment.
C. A 24-hour urine is done to check creatinine clearance only.
D. Diagnostic studies may include quantitative immunoglobulins, serum protein immunoelectrophoresis (SPEP), C-reactive protein (CRP), beta 2 microglobulin, urea protein immunoelectrophoresis (UIEP), 24-hour urine for protein, creatinine, and a myeloma survey.

9. Mr. J. is a 55-year-old who presents to the emergency room complaining of shortness of breath, a lump under his arm, and extreme

fatigue. When obtaining the client history, which of the following is a priority for initial assessment?

    A. Aggravating or alleviating factors.
    B. Symptoms of fever, night sweats, or weight loss.
    C. Symptoms of nausea, vomiting, early satiety.
    D. All of the above.

10. A chest x-ray done in the emergency room reveals mediastinal widening. A chest CT is done, and a large mediastinal mass is detected. Upon axillary lymph node biopsy, a large cell follicular lymphoma is diagnosed. All of the following are necessary to determine treatment options **except**

    A. determine whether the lymph node biopsy is CD 20+.
    B. obtain a CT of the abdomen and pelvis.
    C. obtain a 24-hour urine.
    D. perform a bilateral bone marrow biopsy and aspirate.

11. Mr. J. is scheduled to receive CHOP chemotherapy plus rituximab. The nurse will provide client education on chemotherapy and common side effects to Mr. J. and his family. Which of the following topics is **incorrect?**

    A. Discuss the myelosuppressive effects of chemotherapy.
    B. Describe the gastrointestinal side effects commonly encountered.
    C. State that side effects to rituximab are uncommon.
    D. Review precautions to prevent infection.

12. In July, a client presents to the outpatient hematology clinic for a routine follow-up visit for Hodgkin's disease. The client complains of itching and open skin lesions. The most common etiology for itching in this client may be

    A. recurrence of Hodgkin's disease.
    B. poison ivy.
    C. contact dermatitis caused by soap allergy
    D. nervousness related to follow-up appointment.

13. The most helpful treatment of pruritus in a client with Hodgkin's disease may be

    A. calmoseptine lotion.
    B. antihistamines.
    C. chemotherapy and/or steroids.
    D. narcotics.

14. Mrs. C. is undergoing an autologous peripheral blood stem cell transplant for treatment of multiple myeloma. When getting out of bed this morning, she leans heavily on the side rail to get up. Suddenly she experiences pain in her forearm. The most likely cause of the pain may be

    A. just bruising caused by low platelet counts.
    B. fracture of the forearm.
    C. early morning aches and pains.
    D. pinched nerve.

15. Which of the following is an important medication that should be given to all clients diagnosed with multiple myeloma?

    A. Multivitamins.
    B. Bisphosphonates.
    C. Herbal supplements for bone strengthening.
    D. Aspirin to prevent blood clots.

ANSWERS

1. ***Answer:*** C
Rationale: The presence of Reed-Sternberg cells on biopsy is required to make a diagnosis of Hodgkin's disease. Fevers accompanying night sweats and frequent infections before diagnosis may be symptomatic of Hodgkin's disease but are not diagnostic. The chest radiograph and CT scans may be required for staging but not for diagnosis.

2. ***Answer:*** C
Rationale: Lytic bone lesions are the most common cause of pain in multiple myeloma. Although the marrow may be involved, this is not a common cause of pain. Neural infiltration and intestinal obstruction are not common in multiple myeloma.

3. ***Answer:*** C
Rationale: The client has raised an issue for which the nurse should provide more information. He will likely need some private time to make a decision or to call significant others for help with the decision. Sperm banking should be done before the first chemotherapy session if at all possible.

4. ***Answer:*** C
Rationale: The physician was referring to the myeloma (M) protein levels in the client's blood. The client needs a nutritious, well-balanced diet and should not be encouraged to lose weight during chemotherapy treatment. The nurse should clarify the misconception and then provide referral or information on a nutritious diet. Giving the client a pamphlet without clarifying issues would not be helpful.

5. ***Answer:*** A
Rationale: Fatigue, tiredness, and shortness of breath are common side effects of cancer treatment due to a decrease in hemoglobin. Darbepoetin alfa and epoetin alfa are used to promote recovery of hemoglobin after chemotherapy and may lessen the symptoms. The client should be instructed to call the physician if symptoms of infection occur.

6. ***Answer:*** B
Rationale: The client should be assessed for lymphadenopathy to evaluate disease status clinically. Enlarged lymph nodes may cause venous obstruction that may result in swelling. Other etiologies for leg swelling such as deep venous thrombosis should be considered in the absence of lymphadenopathy. Sodium dietary intake is unlikely the cause of unilateral leg swelling.

7. ***Answer:*** D
Rationale: CT scans and a lymph node biopsy should be done initially to restage the disease and determine the correct pathology. When recurrence of non-Hodgkin's lymphoma occurs, a lymph node biopsy is crucial to determine the type of lymphoma. Sometimes the cell type is different at the time of recurrence than the original diagnosis. The type of chemotherapy used will depend on the CT scan and lymph node biopsy results. Because Mr. T. is afebrile, infection is unlikely and a consult to peripheral vascular physicians is not indicated.

8. ***Answer:*** D
Rationale: Response to treatment for multiple myeloma is measured by obtaining a combination of blood and urine studies and a myeloma survey. Serum quantitative immunoglobulins are monitored to determine immunoglobulin levels for the specific type of myeloma such as IgG, IgA, or IgD. Serum and urine protein electrophoresis is done to detect presence of kappa or lambda light chains. A 24-hour urine is important to measure the protein and creatinine in the urine. The myeloma survey describes the presence of skeletal lesions throughout the body.

9. ***Answer:*** D
Rationale: Assessment of lymphadenopathy should include a review of systems. When assessing symptoms of enlarged lymph nodes, it is important to determine the timing of the development of lymphadenopathy and both alleviating and aggravating factors. Evaluation of other associated symptoms like

nausea and vomiting may lead to further physical assessment of abdominal lymphadenopathy. Fever, night sweats, and weight loss are considered "B" symptoms in staging of lymphoma that may indicate more systemic disease and poorer prognosis.

10. *Answer:* C
Rationale: To complete staging for non-Hodgkin's lymphoma, CT scans of the chest, abdomen, and pelvis must be completed. In addition, a bilateral bone marrow biopsy and aspirate are done to determine whether bone marrow disease is present. To diagnose lymphoma, a lymph node biopsy is required to determine pathology. If the pathology reveals a CD 20+ tumor, the client may receive rituximab (Rituxan), a monoclonal antibody specific for CD 20+ cells, as part of the chemotherapy regimen. Option C, a 24-hour urine, is not necessary in the staging of Hodgkin's lymphoma.

11. *Answer:* C
Rationale: Client education regarding side effects of chemotherapy is important. The chemotherapy agents that are part of CHOP chemotherapy include cyclophosphamide, adriamycin, vincristine, and prednisone. These agents may cause myelosuppression and gastrointestinal toxicity, which will result in side effects such as low blood counts, nausea, vomiting, diarrhea or constipation, poor appetite, and mucositis. Side effects of rituximab include fever, chills, rigors, urticaria, fatigue, and headache.

12. *Answer:* A
Rationale: Although other reasons are possible, recurrence of Hodgkin's disease is the most likely cause of itching in this client. A thorough review of systems will assist the nurse in determining the likelihood of other causes of itching like poison ivy, nervousness, and contact dermatitis.

13. *Answer:* C
Rationale: Usually topical treatment of itching in a client with Hodgkin's disease is not effective. Antihistamines may briefly improve symptoms of itching but will not alleviate the symptoms. The most effective treatment for itching in clients with Hodgkin's disease is chemotherapy with or without steroids, because this treats the underlying cause.

14. *Answer:* B
Rationale: Persons with multiple myeloma are at risk for pathologic fractures caused by bone disease. Although other reasons for pain in the forearm could occur, evaluation for fracture must be considered.

15. *Answer:* B
Rationale: Because of bony disease, clients with multiple myeloma are at risk for pathologic fractures. Bisphosphonates such as pamidronate disodium (Aredia) and zoledronic acid (Zometa) have been used monthly for bone strengthening. Other methods such as vitamins and herbal supplements have not been shown to promote bone strengthening. In general, aspirin and aspirin-containing products should be avoided because of risk of bleeding and interference with platelet counts.

BIBLIOGRAPHY

Berenson, J.R., & Casciato, D.A. (1995). Plasma cell disorders. In D.A. Casciato & B.B. Lowitz (Eds.). *Manual of clinical oncology* (3rd ed.). Boston: Little, Brown and Company, pp. 386-401.

Crouch, M.A. (2000). Hematologic cancers. In B.M. Nevidjon & K.W. Sowers (Eds.). *A nurse's guide to cancer care*. Philadelphia: Lippincott, pp. 160-177.

Friedenberg, W.R., Gordon, L.I., & Mazza, J.J. (2002). Malignant lymphomas. In J.J. Mazza (Ed.). *Manual of clinical hematology* (3rd ed.). Philadelphia: Lippincott Williams & Wilkins, pp. 297-354.

Kyle, R.A. (2002). Multiple myeloma and related monoclonal gammopathies. In J.J. Mazza (Ed.). *Manual of clinical hematology* (3rd ed.). Philadelphia: Lippincott Williams & Wilkins, pp. 247-273.

Rosen, P.J. (1995). Hodgkin's disease and malignant lymphoma. In D.A. Casciato & B.B. Lowitz (Eds.). *Manual of clinical oncology* (3rd ed.). Boston: Little Brown and Company, pp. 347-385.

33 Nursing Care of the Client with Bone and Soft Tissue Cancers

ELLEN CARR

Select the best answer for each of the following questions:

1. Cartilaginous tissue sarcoma is called
    A. osteosarcoma.
    B. chondrosarcoma.
    C. fibrosarcoma.
    D. Ewing's Family of Tumors (EFT).

2. The most common type of EFT is
    A. Ewing's Sarcoma of Bone.
    B. Extraosseous Ewing's (EOE).
    C. Primitive neuroectodermal tumor (PNET).
    D. Osteosarcoma (osseous tissue).

3. Leiomyosarcoma is a sarcoma of
    A. involuntary smooth muscle.
    B. adipose tissue.
    C. skeletal muscle.
    D. vascular tissue.

4. A contributing condition toward the development of Kaposi's sarcoma is
    A. human papillomavirus (HPV).
    B. melanoma.
    C. Epstein-Barr virus (EBV).
    D. herpes virus type 8 (HHV-8).

5. If found early, the 5-year survival rate for soft tissue sarcoma is
    A. 25%.
    B. 50%.
    C. 75%.
    D. 90%.

6. A factor **not** considered a risk for bone cancer is
    A. previous high-dose irradiation.
    B. chemicals—vinyl chloride gas, arsenic, dioxin.
    C. trauma to the bone.
    D. familial, genetic connections.

7. Osteosarcoma, when metastasizing, usually goes first to the
    A. brain.
    B. liver.
    C. lung.
    D. skin.

8. Fibrosarcoma commonly affects
    A. babies.
    B. adolescents and young adults.
    C. those over 35 years.
    D. those over 50 years.

9. Successful treatment of EFT is due partly to
    A. new chemotherapy treatment.
    B. late-stage therapy.
    C. early diagnosis.
    D. multimodality therapy.

10. When grading sarcoma, G2 means
    A. looks like normal tissue—fast growing.

B. looks like normal tissue—tends to be slow growing.
C. looks less like normal tissue—fast growing.
D. does not look at all like normal tissue—fastest growing.

11. When amputation is the treatment, one of the postsurgical clinical concerns is
   A. infection and the degree of skeletal immaturity.
   B. calcium levels.
   C. neutropenia.
   D. Wilms' tumor.

12. Soft tissue tumors can be radiosensitive and radioresponsive. The best use of radiation therapy is for tumors that
   A. have metastasized.
   B. are localized.
   C. are only in the brain.
   D. have recurred.

13. A clinical symptom of osteosarcoma is
   A. bleeding.
   B. dysphagia.

C. pain.
D. weight loss.

14. Clinical symptoms of EFT are
   A. specific: weight loss of 10% over 2 months.
   B. vague: pain progressing, lump progressing; sometimes feel heat over lump.
   C. seasonal: cough/wheezing in weather <32° F (0° C).
   D. fleeting: blanching of the skin over the affected area.

15. Clinical symptoms of soft tissue tumors can be
   A. severe (intense pain).
   B. dramatic (plummeting red blood cell counts).
   C. systemic (a rash over the entire body).
   D. minor (an initial report of a painless, swollen mass).

NOTES

ANSWERS

1. *Answer:* B
Rationale: Osteosarcoma originates from osseous tissue, chondrosarcoma originates from cartilaginous tissue, fibrosarcoma originates from fibrous tissue, and the EFT are a form of reticuloendothelial tissue.

2. *Answer:* A
Rationale: The EFT originate from reticuloendothelial tissue. These tumors occur mainly during childhood. Estimates of occurrence in EFT are Ewing's sarcoma of bone (60% to 80%), EOE (8%), and PNET (5%). Osteosarcoma is a form of sarcoma.

3. *Answer:* A
Rationale:. Leiomyosarcoma originates from involuntary smooth muscle. Liposarcoma originates from adipose tissue. Rhabdomyosarcoma originates from skeletal muscle. Angiosarcoma originates from vascular tissue.

4. *Answer:* D
Rationale: Kaposi's sarcoma is a disease of immunosuppression originating from HHV-8.

5. *Answer:* D
Rationale: If found early, the 5-year survival rate for soft tissue sarcoma is 90%. If found after it has metastasized, the 5-year survival rate is 10% to 15%.

6. *Answer:* C
Rationale: Trauma to the bone is not a risk factor for bone cancer. Among risk factors for bone cancer are previous high-dose irradiation, chemicals such as vinyl chloride gas, arsenic, and dioxin, and familial and genetic risk factors.

7. *Answer:* C
Rationale: Osteosarcoma typically first metastasizes to the lung.

8. *Answer:* B
Rationale: Fibrosarcoma is most often seen in adolescents and young adults.

9. *Answer:* D
Rationale: As a result of multimodality therapies and precision in surgery (wide resections), the estimate for disease-free survival for those diagnosed with EFT is 40% to 70%.

10. *Answer:* C
Rationale: Histologic grades for sarcoma: G1: Looks like normal tissue—tends to be slow growing; G2: Looks less like normal tissue – faster growing; G3: Only slightly looks like normal tissue—even faster growing; G4: Does not look at all like normal tissue – fastest growing.

11. *Answer:* A
Rationale: A clinical concern after amputation is infection and the degree of skeletal immaturity. When the lower extremity is not yet fully grown, adding a prosthesis may potentially create a discrepancy in length with the unaffected extremity. Calcium levels are not affected. Neutropenia is a concern after selected chemotherapy administration. Wilms' tumor is a tumor of the kidney.

12. *Answer:* B
Rationale: Usually external beam x-ray therapy is used before or after surgery for soft tissue tumors to debulk or remove a localized tumor. Radiosensitivity means that certain tissues, organs, and cell types are more sensitive to radiation therapy. Radioresponsive means that with radiation therapy the clinical appearance of the tumor is regressing.

13. *Answer:* C
Rationale: Clinical symptoms of osteosarcoma are pain and swelling in the affected area.

14. *Answer:* B
Rationale: Clinical symptoms of EFT can be vague: pain progressing, lump progressing, sometimes feel heat over lump, flu-like symptoms, fever, fatigue, and anemia.

15. *Answer:* D
Rationale: Often clients with soft tissue tumors initially report no symptoms.

Worsening pain is reported in only a third of cases. Late symptoms include peripheral neuralgias, vascular ischemia, paralysis, or bowel obstruction.

BIBLIOGRAPHY

American Cancer Society (ACS). (2004). *Cancer facts and figures—2004*. Atlanta: Author.

American Cancer Society (ACS). (2003). Cancer Reference Information: Sarcoma. Retrieved February 19, 2003 from http://www.cancer.org/downloads/CRI/2002_Sarcoa_Adult_Soft_Tissue. pdf.

American Joint Commission on Cancer (AJCC). (2002). Musculoskeletal sites. *AJCC Cancer Staging handbook* (6th ed.). New York: Springer-Verlag, pp. 211-228.

Antman, K., & Chang, Y. (2000). Kaposi's sarcoma. *New England Journal of Medicine 342,* 1027-1038.

Brennan, M., Alektia, K., & Maki, R. (2001). Sarcomas of soft tissue and bone. In V.T. DeVita, S. Hellman, S.A. Rosenberg (Eds.). *Cancer: Principles and practice of oncology* (6th ed.). Philadelphia: Lippincott Williams & Wilkins, pp. 1841-1891.

Couto, S. (2002). Soft tissue sarcoma: Diagnosing and treating soft tissue sarcomas. Retrieved February 19, 2003 from CancerSource.com. web site http://www.cancersourcern.com/search/getcontent.cfm?DiseaseID=26&Contentid=22684.

Demetri, G. (2002). Management of soft tissue sarcomas. Program and abstracts of the Scripps Cancer Center's Annual Conference. Clinical Hematology and Oncology 2002; February 16-19, 2002; La Jolla, California.

Memorial Sloan-Kettering Cancer Center (MSKCC). (2002). Questions and answers about sarcoma. Retrieved February 19, 2003 from http://www.mskcc.org/mskcc/html/439.cfm.

NANDA. (2001). *Nursing diagnoses: Definitions and classification, 2001-2003*. Philadelphia: Author.

National Cancer Institute (NCI). (2002). Childhood rhabdomyosarcoma. Retrieved February 19, 2003, from CancerNet (PDQ) websites for health professionals: http://www.nci.nih.gov/cancerinfo/pdq/treatment/childrhabdomyosarcoma/healthprofessional/#Section1.

National Cancer Institute (NCI). (2002). Ewing's family of tumors.: Retrieved February 19, 2003, from CancerNet (PDQ) websites for health professionals: http://www.nci.nih.gov/cancerinfo/pdq/treatment/ewings/healthprofessional/#Section1.

National Cancer Institute (NCI). (2002). Soft tissue sarcoma. Retrieved February 19, 2003, from CancerNet (PDQ) websites for health professionals: http://www.cancer.gov/cancer_information/cancer_type/soft_tissue_sarcoma.

Piasecki, P. (2000). Bone and soft tissue sarcoma. In C.H. Yarbro, M.H. Frogge, M. Goodman, S.L. Groenwald (Eds.). *Cancer nursing: Principles and practice* (5th ed.). Sudbury, MA: Jones and Bartlett Publishers, pp. 323-351.

Pisters, P., O'Sullivan, B., & Demetri G. (2000). Sarcomas of nonosseous tissues. In R.C. Bast, D.W. Kufe, R.E. Pollock, et al. (Eds.). *Cancer medicine.* Hamilton, Ontario: BC Decker, pp. 1903-1930.

Yasko, A., Patel, R., Pollack, A., & Pollock R. (2001). Sarcomas of soft tissue and bone. In R.E. Lenhard, R T. Osteen, & T. Gansler (Eds.). *Clinical oncology.* Atlanta: American Cancer Society, pp. 611-632.

34 Nursing Care of the Client with HIV-Related Cancers

JOE BURRAGE, Jr.

Select the best answer for each of the following questions:

1. The most frequently diagnosed human immunodeficiency virus (HIV)–related malignant disease or disorder is
   A. cervical cancer.
   B. Kaposi's sarcoma (KS).
   C. B-cell lymphoma.
   D. cervical dysplasia.

2. HIV-related lymphoma
   A. has a different epidemiologic characteristic than non-HIV-related lymphoma.
   B. usually occurs midway through the trajectory of HIV infection.
   C. is usually characterized by presentation with a B-cell tumor.
   D. is most often systemic in nature.

3. HIV-related KS
   A. progresses slowly.
   B. incidence is increasing.
   C. exhibits skin lesions that blanch with pressure and are flat.
   D. exhibits skin lesions that range from pink to purple to brownish in color.

4. Survival time is shortest with
   A. low-grade HIV-related lymphomas.
   B. HIV-related systemic lymphoma.

   C. HIV-related lymphoma with a central nervous system (CNS) primary lesion.
   D. HIV-related lymphoma in a client with CD4 <100.

5. The prognosis of persons with HIV-related KS is:
   A. not affected when taking HAART.
   B. better in people with gastrointestinal (GI) tract lesions.
   C. not related to nutritional status or lifestyle.
   D. the worst in those with previous major opportunistic infections.

6. A goal of using radiotherapy to treat KS lesions is
   A. curative.
   B. long-term alleviation of lymphedema.
   C. improvement of perceived body image.
   D. achievement of only short-term systemic control.

7. The type of cancer thought to be a complication of advanced HIV disease is generally considered to be
   A. glioblastoma.
   B. multiple myeloma.
   C. squamous cell cancer.
   D. primary central nervous system lymphoma (PCNSL).

8. A proposed etiology of KS is
   A. unknown.
   B. KS herpes virus (KSHV).
   C. herpes simplex virus (HSV) type 1 or 2.
   D. cytomegalovirus (CMV).

9. The Ann Arbor Staging System applied to non–HIV-related lymphoma is also appropriate for
   A. toxoplasmosis.
   B. KS.
   C. HIV-related lymphoma.
   D. Mycobacterium avium-intracellulare.

10. Development of nursing interventions for people with HIV-related cancer(s) should consider
   A. the client's significant other as the primary care provider.
   B. the significant other who is infected with HIV will exhibit signs of guilt.
   C. the client's previous experiences with HIV-related hospitalizations.
   D. the significant other who is not infected with HIV will be less likely to assist with care.

11. A sign or symptom associated with primary CNS acquired immunodeficiency syndrome (AIDS) include which of the following:
   A. Oliguria.
   B. Hemiparesis.
   C. Negative Epstein-Barr virus titer.
   D. CD4 count greater than 500.

12. The nurse knows that in evaluating laboratory data of people with HIV-related cancers:
   A. Chemotherapy will also cause a decrease in the CD4 count.
   B. CD4/T4 lymphocyte count increases in the absence of HAART.
   C. Serum levels of B_2 microglobulin will decrease in progressive infection.
   D. Core antigen p24 serum levels will decrease with progressive infection.

NOTES

ANSWERS

1. *Answer:* C
Rationale: B-cell lymphoma is the most frequently diagnosed disease in HIV+ clients. The incidence of KS has declined dramatically with the use of highly active antiretroviral therapy (HAART). Women with HIV are at increased risk for cervical dysplasia, followed by rapid progression to cervical cancer, but the difference is the aggressiveness of the histology.

2. *Answer:* C
Rationale: The majority of clients who present with HIV-related lymphoma have B-cell tumors of intermediate- or high-grade histologic type and may be either systemic or primary central nervous system lymphomas (PCNSL). HIV-related lymphoma reflects the same epidemiologic characteristics as non–HIV-related lymphoma. It is a late manifestation of HIV disease.

3. *Answer:* D
Rationale: The incidence of KS is decreasing with the usage of HAART. Classic presentation includes skin lesions that range from pink to purple to brownish, are flat or raised, are usually painless, and do not blanch with pressure. HIV-related KS may be very aggressive and progress rapidly compared with non-HIV-related KS. KS can initially present as a skin or any organ system lesion.

4. *Answer:* C
Rationale: The shortest survival time is with CNS primary tumor (median, 1 to 2 months); the longest survival time is with low-grade lymphomas (12 months to 4 years).

5. *Answer:* D
Rationale: Clients with previous or comorbid major opportunistic infection have the worst prognosis, with a median survival time of less than 1 year. Survival depends on multiple factors including HAART, nutritional status, and lifestyle. Survival time is shorter in people with GI tract lesions.

6. *Answer:* C
Rationale: Use of radiotherapy may have effective short- to moderate-term local control, especially for cosmetic effects.

7. *Answer:* D
Rationale: PCNSL is generally a complication of advanced HIV disease. The others are not generally considered to be associated with HIV infection.

8. *Answer:* B
Rationale: Compelling evidence now exists for causative association of KS herpes virus with KS. KS herpes virus is different from herpes simplex type 1 and 2 in that they are not known to cause KS. CMV is associated with vision complications in people with HIV.

9. *Answer:* C
Rationale: Staging for HIV-related lymphoma typically follows the same schema for non–HIV-related lymphoma. The Ann Arbor Staging System is a classification system used to stage lymphomas. The other options are *(A)*, protozoan parasites, *(B)*, nonlymphomas, and *(D)* mycobacteria, and are not staged as lymphomas.

10. *Answer:* C
Rationale: Assessment should include determination of past experiences with HIV disease to develop interventions specific to the client and significant other(s).

11. *Answer:* B
Rationale: Hemiparesis is a neurologic sign. Oliguria is not associated with PCNS. Epstein-Barr titers would be positive, and CD4 cell counts would be less than 100 cells/mm^3.

12. *Answer:* A
Rationale: Chemotherapeulic agents can decrease the CD_4 count. CD4/T4 counts will also decrease in the absence of HAART. B_2 microglobulin (a serum marker for immune

activation) and core antigen p24 (a major structural core protein of the HIV virus that is a highly specific predictor of disease progression) indicate progressive infection so serum levels will increase.

BIBLIOGRAPHY

Calihol, J., Calatroni, M., Roudiere, L., et al. (2003). Increased incidence of lung neoplasms among HIV-infected men and the need for improved prevention. *Journal of Acquired Immune Deficiency Syndrome* 34(2), 247-249.

Cottrill, C., & Bower, M. (2003). The changing role of radiotherapy in AIDS-related malignancies. *Clinical Oncology* 15(1), 2-6.

Engels, E., Biggar, R., Marshall, V., et al. (2003). Detection and quantification of Kaposi's sarcoma-associated herpes virus to predict AIDS-associated Kaposi's sarcoma. *AIDS* 17(12), 1847-1851.

Franceshi, S., Dal Maso, L., Pezzotti, P., et al. (2003). Incidence of AIDS-defining cancers after AIDS diagnosis among people with AIDS in Italy, 1986-1998. *Journal of Acquired Immune Deficiency Syndrome* 34(1), 84-90.

Gerard, L., Galicier L., Boulanger, E., et al. (2003). Improved survival in HIV-related Hodgkin's lymphoma since the introduction of highly active antiretroviral therapy. *AIDS* 17(1), 81-87.

Herida, M., Mary-Krause, M., Kaphan, R., et al. (2003). Incidence of non-AIDS-defining cancers before and during the highly active antiretroviral therapy era in a cohort of human immunodeficiency virus-infected patients. *Journal of Clinical Oncology* 21(18), 3447-3453.

Mbulaiteye, S., Bioggar, R., Goedert, J., & Engels, E. (2003). Immune deficiency and risk for malignancy among persons with AIDS. *Journal of Acquired Immune Deficiency Syndrome* 32(5), 527-53.

Osborne, G., Taylor, C., & Fuller, L. (2003). The management of HIV-related skin disease. Part II: neoplasms and inflammatory disorders. *International Journal of STD/AIDS* 14(4), 235-241.

Powels, T., Nelson, M., & Bower, M. (2003). HIV-related testicular cancer. *International Journal of STD/AIDS* 14(1), 24-27.

Scadden, D. (2003). AIDS-related malignancies. *Annual Review of Medicine* 54, 285-303.

NOTES

35 Nursing Implications of Surgical Treatment

THOMAS J. SZOPA

Select the best answer for each of the following questions:

1. The purpose of an excisional biopsy is to
   A. establish tissue diagnosis and provide definitive treatment.
   B. establish tissue diagnosis and determine surgical stage of disease.
   C. establish tissue diagnosis and perform prophylactic surgery.
   D. establish tissue diagnosis only.

2. A client had a wide excision and groin dissection for synovial cell sarcoma. The client calls the outpatient department complaining of swelling, redness at the incision site, and a low-grade fever. The nurse tells the client:
   A. "These symptoms are postoperative symptoms."
   B. "Take your antidiuretic medication."
   C. "Call me if your fever increases; otherwise do nothing at the present."
   D. "You must come in to be seen."

3. A client has just returned from having a total laryngectomy. The nurse's immediate postoperative care priority would be
   A. pain management.
   B. maintaining an effective airway.
   C. maintaining an effective means of communication.
   D. providing for adequate nutrition.

4. The immediate educational priority for the client who has had a total laryngectomy is
   A. a referral for speech therapy.
   B. a referral to a counselor to help with emotional adaptation.
   C. appropriate nutritional instruction that addresses adequate wound healing and the functional impact on the client's ability to swallow.
   D. appropriate safety measures for life with a stoma.

5. Surgery is often the treatment of choice for those tumors that
   A. are fast-growing and spread via the circulatory system.
   B. have a low growth fraction and therefore are slow growing and confined locally and/or regionally.
   C. adhere to the musculature of a body organ and have not perforated into a space, for example, abdominal cavity.
   D. have a high growth fraction and therefore are fast growing and confined locally and/or regionally.

6. Currently, cancer surgery is performed
   A. as the primary treatment for most cancers.
   B. in a manner to remove the tumor and a very large margin of adjacent tissue to minimize the risk of metastasis.

C. with the goal of tumor removal, regardless of the structural, functional, and/or cosmetic changes that might occur.

D. utilizing surgical strategies that would decrease the local and systemic spread of cancer and minimize the functional and cosmetic impact.

7. The purpose of cytoreductive surgery is

A. to establish a tissue diagnosis.

B. to remove nonvital organs and/or tissues that have a high risk of subsequent cancer.

C. to promote client comfort and quality of life without the goal of cure of disease.

D. to reduce the tumor volume to improve the effect of other cancer treatment modalities.

8. A client receiving preoperative radiation therapy, surgical resection with diverting colostomy, and postoperative chemotherapy for rectal cancer is receiving treatment that is called

A. primary treatment.

B. combination treatment.

C. salvage treatment.

D. palliative treatment.

9. Mrs. S. is undergoing lumpectomy for breast cancer followed by external beam radiation. She asked for clarification of the rationale for the external beam radiation. As her nurse, you explain that

A. this is called adjuvant therapy, or one that is used to eliminate possible microscopic disease, thereby decreasing the risk of local recurrence.

B. this is considered a palliative treatment to improve the quality of her life by decreasing any problematic disease-related symptoms she may experience.

C. this is her primary treatment because the lumpectomy was to establish the type of cancer she has.

D. today's cancer treatment always includes a combination of therapies as primary treatment for the best chance of cure.

10. In assessing the client before surgery, you question the client about what type and when the client may have received other cancer therapies. Your rationale for assessing this is that in experiencing other cancer therapies recently:

A. The client would be sensitized to pain medications and therefore alert you in utilizing a variety of pain relief strategies such as increased medication dosages.

B. The client would have an increased risk of postoperative complications based on the type and how recently these occurred. This would assist you to plan care appropriate for the client.

C. The client has received teaching previously; therefore you will not need to focus on client teaching as part of the care plan.

D. The client has been connected with various support services; therefore you will not need to make such referrals during the postoperative period.

11. Mrs. K. underwent extensive surgery for stage IV ovarian cancer. Within a month of surgery, she began her chemotherapy. She now presents with a partially dehisced incision and wound with continuous yellow-colored drainage. In managing her wound care, your priorities would include

A. use some method of protection for the peri-wound area from the drainage.

B. use dry, sterile dressings to absorb the drainage.

C. consult the social worker to explore the client's concerns with an open wound.

D. discuss the use of total parenteral nutrition with the physician.

12. Your client just returned from having a cystectomy with ileal conduit creation. In conducting your postoperative assessment, you observe the stoma to be pale in color. Based on this finding, you would

A. observe the stoma frequently throughout your shift.

B. change the pouch system, fearing it may be to tight around the stoma.

C. notify the physician. This may be a sign of an impending stomal complication.

D. document your finding and consider it a normal finding for a stoma during the immediate postoperative period.

13. The client's rehabilitation after cancer surgery is most positively affected by
   A. multidisciplinary discharge planning.
   B. referrals to support groups related to the client's specific type of cancer.
   C. appropriate pain management.
   D. specific instruction on any assistive or prosthetic devices used after surgery.

14. A 45-year-old client with a history of moderate ulcerative colitis for over 12 years is scheduled for a total colectomy with ileostomy creation. The surgeon described this surgery as a "prophylactic" cancer surgery, which is defined as
   A. the reconstruction of anatomic defects created by cancer surgery to improve function and cosmetic appearance.

B. surgery performed on an organ that has an extremely high risk of developing cancer.
   C. the insertion of various therapeutic hardware during active treatment periods to facilitate the delivery of treatment and increase client comfort.
   D. the removal of hormonal influence of the cancer.

15. Radiation therapy before cancer surgery can
   A. improve tumor resectability and alter the extent of surgery needed.
   B. alter the extent of surgery needed but increase the functional disabilities after therapy.
   C. provide more appealing options to clients but decrease treatment outcomes.
   D. improve treatment outcomes but increase the functional disabilities after therapy.

NOTES

ANSWERS

1. *Answer:* A
   Rationale: Excisional biopsy removes the entire tumor mass and is therefore definitive therapy. The purpose of all biopsies is to establish tissue diagnosis. Options B, C, and D provide incorrect purposes for performing the procedure.

2. *Answer:* D
   Rationale: Infection is a potential postoperative complication. The incisional site must be assessed to rule out a local infection, abscess or fistula formation, impending wound dehiscence, or the occurrence of lymphedema, a complication of lymph node removal. The client may need antibiotic or other additional therapy to resolve the complication. The other options do not appropriately address the client's problem.

3. *Answer:* B
   Rationale: Options A and C (pain management and providing a means of communication) are very important, but not as important as Option B, which would prevent a life-threatening complication. Option D (providing adequate nutrition) is important over time and becomes more of an issue during the rehabilitation period after surgery.

4. *Answer:* D
   Rationale: Options A, B, and C are very important but not as essential as Option D (appropriate safety measures), which will prevent a life-threatening event from occurring. Protecting the stoma from water, dust, dirt, and small objects and other safety recommendations will help the client avoid harm.

5. *Answer:* B
   Rationale: Option B is correct because cancer that grows slowly remains more local and confined. Thus surgery may have a greater chance in removing most or the entire tumor, providing good control or cure of the disease, and causing the least disruption in normal organ structure and function. Options A and D are incorrect because fast-growing cancers (high growth fraction) metastasize

locally, regionally, and distantly; thus surgery may be used to assist other treatments in being effective in the control or cure of the disease but would not be considered the primary treatment of choice. Surgery is a local type of treatment. In the case of tumor attached to normal organ structure, surgical treatment may be a component of the treatment plan to debulk tumor and free up attached structure, but other treatment would assist in controlling such disease. Thus, Option C is incorrect.

6. *Answer:* D
   Rationale: Historically, surgery was the first and sometimes only treatment. Combination therapy has clarified which tumor types and amount of disease are best suited for surgical intervention. Studies have shown how much tissue and organ structure must be removed. Thus current therapy is based on removing the least amount of tissue and planning the procedure with preservation of structure, function, and cosmetic appearance for successful rehabilitation after surgery. Using surgery in combination with other therapies will allow such surgical therapy to be designed for the client.

7. *Answer:* D
   Rationale: Cytoreductive therapy is defined as the reduction of tumor volume to improve the effect of other cancer treatments. Although cytoreductive surgery may cause the outcome listed in Option C, this option is the definition of palliative therapy and thus is incorrect. Clinical studies have shown that reducing tumor volume increases the impact of other therapies and can reduce the toxicities of all the therapies used. Option A is the definition for biopsy, and option B is the definition of prophylactic surgery; thus both are incorrect.

8. *Answer:* B
   Rationale: Option B, combination therapy, is a treatment plan using several therapies to achieve positive outcomes for the client. Primary therapy is the therapy that has the greatest impact on the disease for control or cure. Salvage therapy is a therapy that would

be used if other, less invasive therapies did not succeed in controlling or curing the disease. Salvage therapies were once considered the primary therapy, but with treatment advances for that specific cancer type, less invasive/extensive therapy has been found to be as effective with less negative impact on the client. Palliative therapy relieves bothersome disease symptoms and improves the quality of life for the client but does not lead to control or cure of the disease.

9. *Answer:* A
   Rationale: The lumpectomy is the removal of the primary tumor in total and is thus considered the primary treatment, so Option C is incorrect. The external beam radiation is additional therapy at the tumor site. This is done to eliminate any local undetectable microscopic disease left behind. Such therapy is called adjuvant, and studies have demonstrated that this increases the disease-free time for clients. Thus Option A is the correct explanation of this treatment plan. This treatment plan is not one for a client with more extensive disease who is in a palliative phase of the disease, so Option B is incorrect. Many cancer treatment plans include a combination of treatments to produce the most positive outcomes, but only one treatment has the greatest impact and thus is considered the primary therapy. Therefore Option D is not an accurate reflection of what primary therapy is and does for the client.

10. *Answer:* B
    Rationale: Other cancer therapies and resultant toxicities have been shown to cause an increased risk in postoperative complications (i.e., wound healing, respiratory status, cardiac complications) due to their previous impact on specific body systems needed for surgical rehabilitation. Option B is correct because you would be able to plan more appropriately for this client's postoperative care and rehabilitation. The client's pain management is a concern and needs assessment but would not have as great an impact as the rationale in Option B; thus Option A is not the best correct option. Although the client may have received teaching and had been connected with supportive services, this is another therapy with its own unique, specific

aspects, and the client may need additional teaching and services based on the procedure performed and the client's response during the postoperative period; therefore Options C and D are incorrect.

11. *Answer:* A
    Rationale: Containing the wound drainage and protecting the peri-wound skin integrity are priorities in caring for this surgical wound. Protecting the skin integrity in the peri-wound area will prevent other skin-related complications and promote client comfort; thus option A is correct. Option B is one option in containing wound drainage but may not be the most appropriate option for this client, who is draining continuously. This intervention would not prevent maceration of the peri-wound tissue, which could break down and increase the wound size; thus Option B is not correct. Options C and D may be issues for this client, but not the most urgent priorities for client comfort, skin protection, and prevention of additional complications.

12. *Answer:* C
    Rationale: The stoma should be very pink, moist, and draining yellow urine for this client. The ileum used to create the stoma has a rich blood supply. A very light colored, dusky, or blackish colored stoma is generally a sign of compromised blood supply and may need urgent surgical intervention to improve the blood supply and viability of the intestinal conduit. The surgeon should be notified immediately for further assessment and care planning.

13. *Answer:* A
    Rationale: Although Options B, C, and D all include strategies to promote positive rehabilitation for specific client populations with specific needs, Option A is critical to addressing the many possible needs of any client who has undergone surgical treatment for cancer. A comprehensive assessment of the client's short- and long-term needs using a multidisciplinary team approach is most helpful in determining what is the best plan of rehabilitation for the specific client involved.

14. *Answer:* B
    Rationale: Surgical removal of a particular body tissue/organ is recommended if that

tissue/organ has a very high risk for the development of cancer within it. A 10+-year history of chronic ulcerative colitis, along with the client's age, increases the client's risk significantly for colorectal cancer. Such surgery is done prophylactically to eliminate or "cure" the client before the occurrence of cancer. Option A describes reconstructive therapy that cosmetically and functionally improves the defect left from the initial cancer surgical procedure. Options C and D describe common rationale for specific surgical procedures, but these are not preventing a cancer occurrence as in prophylactic surgery.

15. *Answer:* A

Rationale: Shrinkage of the tumor will occur whereby its margins will be more discernible by the surgeon and more easily removed. This will reduce the impact on surrounding tissues. Options B, C, and D are incorrect because the goal is optimum cancer treatment outcomes with minimal disability.

BIBLIOGRAPHY

Cady, B. (2001). Fundamentals of contemporary surgical oncology: Biologic principles and the threshold concept govern treatment and outcomes. *Journal of the American College of Surgeons* 192(6), 777-92.

Carrion, R., & Seigne, J. (2002). Surgical management of bladder carcinoma. *Cancer Control* 9(4), 284-292.

Drake, D.B., & Oishi, S.N. (1995). Wound healing considerations in chemotherapy and radiation therapy. *Clinics in Plastic Surgery* 22(1), 31-37.

Frogge, M.H., & Cunnings, S.M. (2000). Surgical therapy. In C.H. Yarbro, M.H. Frogge, M. Goodman, & S.L. Groenwald (Eds.). *Cancer nursing: Principles and practice* (5th ed.). Sudbury, MA: Jones and Bartlett Publishers, pp. 272-285.

Easson, A.M., Asch, M., & Swallow C.J. (2001). Palliative general surgical procedures. *Surgical Oncology Clinics of North America* 10(1), 161-84.

Ignatavicius, D., & Workman, L. (2002) *Medical-surgical nursing: Critical thinking for collaborative care* (4th ed.). Philadelphia: W. B. Saunders.

Lefor, A.T. (1999). Perioperative management of the patient with cancer. *Chest* 115(5 Suppl), 165S-171S.

Marek, J., & Boehnlein, M. (2003). Preoperative nursing. In W. Phipps, F. Monahan, & J. Sands et. al. (Eds.). *Medical Surgical Nursing* (7th ed.). St. Louis: Mosby, pp. 361-390.

Mintzer, D. (1999). The changing role of surgery in the diagnosis and treatment of cancer. *The American Journal of Medicine* 106(1), 81-89.

Pfifer, K. (2001). Surgery. In S. Otto. (Ed.). *Oncology nursing* (4th ed.). St. Louis: Mosby, pp. 585-594.

Rosenberg, S. N. (2001). Principles of cancer management: Surgical oncology. In V.T. DeVita, S. Hellman, & S. Rosenberg (Eds). *Cancer: Principles and practice of oncology.* (6th ed.). Philadelphia, Lippincott Williams & Wilkins, pp. 253-264.

36 Nursing Implications of Radiation Therapy

CINDY CATLIN-HUTH

Select the best answer for each of the following questions:

1. Which of the following statements best describes the purpose of total body irradiation (TBI) as part of the preparatory regimen before allogeneic transplant?
   - A. TBI is used to eliminate from the body any unwanted bacteria before an anticipated period of neutropenia.
   - B. TBI is used to T-cell deplete the transplant recipient, thereby decreasing the chance of graft-versus-host disease (GVHD).
   - C. TBI is used to mobilize increased numbers of progenitor stem cells from the donor's bone marrow into peripheral circulation for collection.
   - D. TBI is used to kill any residual malignant cells and immunosuppress the transplant recipient, thereby giving the donor stem cells a greater chance of engraftment.

2. Mr. B. is scheduled to undergo external beam radiotherapy to his lumbar spine for his metastatic prostate cancer. During the initial nursing assessment his nurse notes that his baseline hemoglobin (Hgb) is 10 g/dl. The treatment plan includes evaluation of his energy level weekly because
   - A. external beam radiation to any field involving bone marrow will decrease by half the baseline Hgb within 1 week.
   - B. Mr. B. will likely be nauseated from his therapy and be unable to maintain an iron-rich diet.
   - C. hematuria commonly results from this type of radiation therapy, resulting in an increase in his anemia.
   - D. standard of care during radiation therapy includes a weekly physical assessment in order to optimally manage all possible side effects of the therapy or underlying disease.

3. For which individual who has received radiation therapy to the pelvis should the nurse question a request to provide instruction on the use of a vaginal dilator?
   - A. A 68-year-old woman who had a hysterectomy 20 years ago and now has intercourse about once a week.
   - B. A 45-year-old woman who is sexually active with her male partner three times a week.
   - C. A 55-year-old woman who completed radiation 10 years ago and now reports vaginal "tightening."
   - D. A married 58-year-old woman who will not discuss her sexual practices but reports that her nurse practitioner uses a pediatric speculum to make her pelvic exams tolerable.

4. Which individual is at greater risk of experiencing radiodermatitis from external beam radiation therapy?
   A. A 50-year-old African American woman receiving treatment after lumpectomy for breast cancer.
   B. A 35-year-old Caucasian woman with fair skin and light blue eyes receiving treatment after lumpectomy for breast cancer.
   C. A 49-year-old Caucasian woman with brown eyes and fair skin receiving treatment after lumpectomy for breast cancer.
   D. A 69-year-old Asian woman receiving pain palliation for metastatic disease to her right femur.

5. Individuals undergoing pelvic radiotherapy for colorectal cancer might experience which of the following secondary side effects?
   A. Hypokalemia.
   B. Hypocalcemia.
   C. Hyperphosphatemia.
   D. Hypermagnesemia.

6. Which of the following individuals is most likely to experience "radiation recall"?
   A. A 14-year-old starting an anthracycline-based chemo regimen who has never received radiation therapy but who was severely sunburned 4 months ago.
   B. A 50-year-old woman receiving her first dose of doxorubicin (Adriamycin) 6 months after completing radiotherapy.
   C. A 55-year-old farmer who quits using sunscreen 4 years after completing radiotherapy.
   D. A 65-year-old woman receiving her first dose of 5-fluorouracil who received an intravenous radioisotope for thyroiditis in her teens.

7. The delivery of radiation therapy is divided into small fractions for what reason?
   A. Delivering the same total dose of radiation at one time can only be done by use of brachytherapy technique.
   B. Fractionation allows for recovery of the surrounding nonmalignant tissues and in some tissues promotes recruitment of the malignant cells into the cell cycle for an improved cell kill.
   C. Daily treatments over several weeks allow for the development of a therapeutic relationship between the health care providers and the individual undergoing treatment.
   D. Fractionation helps to deoxygenate the malignant cells in the radiation field, making them more sensitive to the radiation.

8. While providing client teaching about possible skin changes from radiation therapy, the nurse is correct in the following instruction:
   A. Pruritus is not a side effect of radiation therapy.
   B. Skin changes rarely occur for at least 4 weeks from initiation of therapy.
   C. Hyperpigmentation often occurs after 2 to 3 weeks of standard therapy and may or may not be permanent.
   D. Sunscreen with a minimum of SPF 15 is recommended for 3 months after radiation therapy to prevent radiation recall.

9. Individuals receiving either whole brain or localized radiation therapy to the brain commonly experience which of the following?
   A. Hyperactive hypothalamic-pituitary function.
   B. Secondary neoplasms of the brain several years later.
   C. Permanent hair loss in the radiation field when a cumulative dose of 10 Gy is reached.
   D. Intensification of pre-existing symptoms such as headache, somnolence, irritability, or seizure.

10. Which of the following signs/symptoms of spinal cord compression in an individual with a history of multiple myeloma should alert the nurse that urgent radiation therapy may be needed?
   A. Localized or radicular back pain.
   B. Muscle weakness.
   C. Hyperreflexes.
   D. Loss of bowel or bladder function.

11. Which of the following might the radiation oncologist order to best distinguish

between radiation necrosis and tumor recurrence in an individual who has received radiation to the brain?

    A. Computed tomography (CT) of the brain.

    B. Brain biopsy.

    C. Positron emission tomography (PET) scan of the brain.

    D. Magnetic resonance imaging (MRI) of the brain with gadolinium.

12. Mr. J. calls the radiation oncologist's office with the following complaints: shortness of breath, dry cough, fever, and severe weakness. He is off all medication since he completed his lung cancer radiation 2 months ago. The screening nurse makes this case a priority for discussion with the radiation oncologist because:

    A. He likely has pneumonia requiring antibiotics.

    B. He likely has radiation pneumonitis requiring steroids.

    C. He likely has radiation pneumonitis requiring antibiotics.

    D. He likely has superior vena cava syndrome requiring urgent radiation therapy.

13. Which of the following statements most accurately describes the pathophysiology of late radiation-induced lymphedema?

    A. Radiation therapy causes capillary leak syndrome.

    B. Radiation therapy causes temporary edema in the radiation field, making it difficult for distal extremities to drain.

    C. Radiation therapy causes venous insufficiency, allowing intravascular fluids to escape into the extravascular spaces.

    D. Radiation therapy damages lymph nodes in the radiation field and over time causes interstitial fibrosis of lymphatic tissue, impeding lymph entry into the system.

14. Which of the following medications should the radiation oncology nurse question for an individual undergoing radiation therapy to the head and neck who is experiencing xerostomia?

    A. Nystatin (Mycostatin) swish and swallow qid.

    B. Pilocarpine (Salagen) 5 mg by mouth tid.

    C. Diphenhydramine (Benadryl) 25 mg by mouth qhs.

    D. Over-the-counter (OTC) artificial saliva prn.

15. Which of the following statements is accurate?

    A. Radiation therapy to ovaries during pelvic irradiation always results in infertility.

    B. Male sex partners of females undergoing radiation therapy to the pelvis should use condoms because of teratogenic risk if conception occurs.

    C. Sperm banking should not be offered to all males receiving radiation therapy to the testes because most males have lowered sperm counts for only 1 to 2 years.

    D. Ovarian cryopreservation is inexpensive and has been well proven.

ANSWERS

1. *Answer:* D
   Rationale: TBI is not used for bacterial control. Its purpose is to eliminate remaining cancer cells and to suppress the immune system in an effort to prevent graft rejection. Option C is incorrect because TBI is not undergone by the stem cell donor. Donor stem cells are instead mobilized using once- or twice-daily colony-stimulating factors. T-cell depletion to prevent GVHD is achieved by other methods.

2. *Answer:* D
   Rationale: Option D is correct because standard of care established by the American College of Radiology requires a weekly physical assessment by the physician for evaluation of possible side effects of therapy. The degree of myelosuppression is directly related to the percent of bone marrow in the radiation field. An L-spine field would not be large enough alone to cause a rapid significant anemia. Nausea is an unlikely side effect in this scenario, because the field does not include the stomach or significant small bowel. Hematuria, though possible, would also be unlikely because of present-day treatment planning sparing the bladder.

3. *Answer:* B
   Rationale: Vaginal fibrosis and stenosis can be minimized by use of either a vaginal dilator or sexual intercourse three times a week. The correct answer is therefore Option B. Option A is incorrect, because this individual does not have intercourse frequently enough to prevent this late radiation change. She may not be undergoing Pap smears; however, periodic pelvic exams will still be necessary for postradiation follow-up. Although use of dilators is optimally started about 2 weeks after therapy and maintained for life, the individual in Option C could benefit from the use of increasingly larger dilators over several weeks to arrest and possibly improve her vaginal stenosis. The individual in Option D would benefit from the same therapy to make exams more comfortable.

4. *Answer:* B
   Rationale: Option A is incorrect because individuals with increased pigmentation are at lower risk for radiation skin changes. Individuals with fair complexions and light-colored eyes are at greatest risk, making Option B correct. The individual in Option C has greater pigmentation than the individual in Option B because of her brown eyes. Option D is incorrect because radiation to the bone rarely delivers significant enough energy to the skin to produce a skin reaction.

5. *Answer:* A
   Rationale: Diarrhea is a common side effect of radiation therapy to the pelvis because of inflammation of the mucosal epithelium and loss of villi, thus making it a primary side effect. With decreased gastrointestinal transit time, watery diarrhea occurs and electrolytes can be lost. Any resulting electrolyte imbalances are secondary side effects. Hypokalemia is correct, because stools have a high concentration of potassium. If dehydration occurs, decreased renal blood flow may result in calcium resorption, causing increased serum levels. Calcium and phosphorus have an inverse relationship, making phosphorus levels low whenever calcium levels are high. Hypermagnesemia is incorrect, because magnesium is also excreted in diarrhea stools.

6. *Answer:* B
   Rationale: Radiation recall is a phenomenon in which previously irradiated tissue that exhibited a skin reaction recurs in response to systemic chemotherapy. (Please note that medications other than chemotherapy can also cause this.) Option A is incorrect because this individual has not received x-ray therapy (XRT). Radiation recall is more likely to occur closer in time to the therapy, and anthracyclines are more likely than other chemotherapeutic agents to cause radiation recall; therefore Option B is correct.

7. *Answer:* B
   Rationale: Option B is correct because smaller once- or twice-daily doses allow for

repair and repopulation of surrounding healthy tissues, thus decreasing toxicity. Delivery of the same total dose is possible by methods other than brachytherapy, making Option A incorrect. Time between fractions also allows for recruitment of the malignant cells into the cell cycle, where they are thought to be more radiosensitive. Option D is incorrect because the presence of oxygen enhances the effects of ionizing radiation.

8. *Answer:* C
Rationale: Pruritus is common after receiving a cumulative dose of 20 to 28 Gray (Gy). Hyperpigmentation occurs after 2 to 3 weeks of therapy and usually resolves in 2 to 3 months, but may be permanent. Radiotherapy does damage the skin's ability to protect itself from ultraviolet exposure. Transient erythema may occur within hours of the start of radiation therapy, but it is more common for true erythema to occur after 2 to 3 weeks of therapy. Use of sunscreen is generally advised for everyone for life, but it is especially important in the radiotherapy field for up to 1 to 2 years after treatment to prevent further damage to the tissues. Radiation recall is generally used in reference to a phenomenon in which systemic chemotherapy causes recurrence of a previous radiation-induced skin reaction.

9. *Answer:* D
Rationale: Option D is correct. Often symptoms of increased cerebral vascular edema and tissue irritation from cancer cell destruction occur as soon as the first few hours after start of radiation therapy to the brain. These symptoms are usually successfully treated with corticosteroids starting 2 to 3 days before therapy. Hypoactive hypothalamic-pituitary function, specifically growth hormone deficiency, is the most common endocrine problem after radiotherapy. Early detection and hormone replacement are paramount in children to prevent irreversible damage. At therapeutic doses, secondary brain tumors are rare. Complete hair loss occurs quite predictably when a total cumulative dose of 45 to 55 Gy is reached and may or may not be irreversible.

10. *Answer:* D
Rationale: Back pain is commonly the first sign of spinal cord compression, followed by

the development of muscle weakness. Hyperreflexes are also an early sign of spinal cord compression. Options A, B, and C are incorrect because it is common to first treat early symptoms with steroids while determining whether true spinal cord impingement exists, requiring treatment with radiation therapy or surgery. Option D is the correct answer because loss of bowel or bladder control is a late sign indicating autonomic dysfunction. Radiation therapy may be needed to prevent permanent neurologic damage

11. *Answer:* B
Rationale: Tumor recurrence in the brain is often impossible to distinguish from radiation changes using CT and non-contrast MRI. Addition of contrast with MRI or PET scanning may be helpful but is not always successful. Therefore Option B, or biopsy, remains the best way to make a definitive diagnosis.

12. *Answer:* B
Rationale: Radiation pneumonitis may occur from 1 to 6 months after therapeutic doses of radiation therapy to lung tissue but is most likely to occur at 2 to 3 months after therapy. Option B is correct, because typical presentation includes insidious onset of these symptoms. Because it is treated with steroids, not antibiotics, Option C is incorrect. Pneumonia would be possible but less likely with a nonproductive cough. Option D is incorrect because fever is not associated with superior vena cava syndrome.

13. *Answer:* D
Rationale: The correct Option is D. Radiation therapy can cause interstitial fibrosis of the lymphatic tissue. Radiation therapy does not cause capillary leak syndrome. Option B is incorrect because this is an early, not a late radiation change. Option C is incorrect because venous insufficiency and lymphedema are two distinctly different pathologies. Radiation is not associated with the former.

14. *Answer:* C
Rationale: Option C should be questioned because one of the most common side effects of diphenhydramine is drying of the mouth. This will add to present discomfort and place

the individual at increased risk of mucositis. Nystatin swish/swallow is often used to prevent or treat oral candida infections, which commonly occur during radiation therapy to the oral cavity. Pilocarpine is appropriate because it is used to stimulate saliva production. OTC artificial salivas are intended to moisten and lubricate the oral cavity, which temporarily alleviates xerostomia.

15. *Answer:* B

Rationale: Option B is the correct option because genetic damage may occur to the follicles, resulting in birth defects. Option A is incorrect, because the chance of infertility after XRT to the pelvis is dependent on the total dose received, the degree to which one or both of the ovaries have been blocked from the field, and the viability of the ovary before therapy. Azoospermia is dose-dependent and varies according to the total dose and delivery method. Permanent azoospermia is common but may reverse in 6 to 8 years. Therefore sperm banking should be offered to all males who desire to have children after radiation therapy. Option D is incorrect because success in ovarian cryopreservation has been variable to date.

BIBLIOGRAPHY

ACR Standard for Radiation Oncology (1999). [Online, http://www.acr.org/departments/stand_accred/standards/pdf/Radiati Obtained from the world wide web on 5/30/03. pp 508.

Camp-Sorrell, D., & Hawkins, R. (Eds.). (2000). *Clinical manual for the oncology advanced practice Nurse*. Pittsburgh: Oncology Nursing Society.

Hellman, S. (2001). Principles of cancer management: Radiation therapy. In V. DeVita, S. Hellman, & S. Rosenberg (Eds). *Cancer: Principles and practice of oncology* (6th ed.). Philadelphia: Lippincott Williams & Wilkins, p. 265-288.

Hilderley, L.J. (2000). Principles of radiotherapy. In C.H. Yarbro, M.H. Frogge, M. Goodman, & S.L. Groenwald (Eds.). *Cancer nursing: Principles & practice* (5th ed.). Sudbury, MA: Jones and Bartlett Publishers, pp. 286-299.

Mayer, K.E. (2000). Radiation therapy: Toxicities and management. In C.H. Yarbro, M.H. Frogge, M. Goodman, & S.L. Groenwald. (Eds). *Cancer nursing: Principles and practice* (5th ed.). Sudbury, MA: Jones and Bartlett Publishers, pp. 323-357,

Miyamoto, C. (2000). Radiation therapy principles for high-grade gliomas. *Principles and Practice of Radiation Oncology 3*(1), 2-13.

Tierney, L., McPhee, S., & Papadakis, M. (Eds.). (2000). *Current medical diagnosis & treatment*. New York: Lang Medical Books/McGraw-Hill, p. 338.

37 Nursing Implications of Biotherapy and Molecular Targeted Therapy

PEG ESPER

Select the best answer for each of the following questions:

1. Management of interleukin-2–induced capillary leak syndrome generally includes
   A. aggressive use of diuretics.
   B. administration of vasopressive agents.
   C. administration of dexamethasone.
   D. dietary restriction of sodium.

2. A monoclonal antibody that is made up primarily of mouse protein but has a human protein component is known as what type of monoclonal antibody?
   A. Humanized.
   B. Primatized.
   C. Murine.
   D. Chimeric.

3. When a client receives a monoclonal antibody, the factor that best predicts for an allergic type reaction during administration is
   A. history of reactions to other antineoplastic agents.
   B. extent of tumor burden.
   C. percentage of murine protein in the antibody.
   D. exclusion of steroids in the premedication regimen.

4. A client receiving high-dose interferon therapy for stage 3 melanoma experiences a doubling of transaminases. This is generally associated with
   A. anticipated side effects of treatment.
   B. previous exposure to hepatitis.
   C. improper dosing of interferon.
   D. hepatic metastasis.

5. Granulocyte colony-stimulating factor is administered to promote an increase in
   A. B lymphocytes.
   B. megakaryocytopoiesis.
   C. erythroid progenitor cells.
   D. neutrophil progenitor cells.

6. The dosing of biotherapy agents is aimed at determining the
   A. optimal biologic dose.
   B. minimally toxic dose.
   C. lowest myelosuppressive dose.
   D. maximum tolerated dose.

7. Which comorbid condition will have the greatest effect on the decision to use a cytokine agent such as interleukin-2 in the treatment regimen for a client with cancer?
   A. Type 2 diabetes mellitus.
   B. History of lupus.
   C. History of alcoholism.
   D. Hypertension controlled by beta blockers.

8. Mr. J. completed treatment for a B-cell non-Hodgin's lymphoma (NHL) 3 weeks ago

with ibritumomab tiuxetan (Zevalin). He presents to the clinic today with complaints of increasing fatigue, dyspnea on exertion, and increasing bruising. His current symptoms are likely related to
    A. tumor lysis syndrome.
    B. pulmonary embolism.
    C. disease progression.
    D. myelosuppressive effects of therapy.

9. Inadequate sources of client tumor is an obstacle in clinical trials involving what type of vaccine therapy?
    A. Polypeptide.
    B. Allogeneic.
    C. Autologous.
    D. Dendritic cell.

10. Which of the following statements is true regarding treatment with interleukin-2?
    A. Cardiac arrhythmias are common but do not require cessation of therapy.
    B. Vigorous hydration helps prevent associated hypotension.
    C. Capillary leak syndrome is a rare occurrence.
    D. Weight gain of 5% to 10% of pretreatment weight is anticipated during treatment.

11. The greatest risk for allergic reactions exists when administering which of the following classifications of biotherapy agents?
    A. Monoclonal antibodies.
    B. Interleukins.
    C. Interferons.
    D. Colony-stimulating factors.

12. The two most difficult to manage side effects of interferon therapy are
    A. fatigue and diarrhea.
    B. flulike syndrome and headache.
    C. fatigue and central nervous system (CNS) alterations.
    D. skin reactions and flulike syndrome.

13. The inflammatory response is an example of
    A. adaptive immunity.
    B. innate immunity.
    C. complement activation.
    D. humoral immunity.

14. A client shares with you that he is worried about being part of a biotherapy clinical trial because he has heard about clients dying during this type of treatment. The best response to this would be:
    A. Encourage the client to share his concerns with the physician before signing the informed consent document.
    B. Explain the strict regulatory processes now in place to safeguard clients against harm while on clinical trials.
    C. Review the preclinical trial data with the client and encourage him to ask questions.
    D. Assure the client that deaths are very rare on clinical trials but stress that participation is voluntary.

ANSWERS

1. *Answer:* B
Rationale: Vasopressors are used to maintain urinary output. Dexamethasone and restriction of dietary sodium have no role in the management of capillary leak syndrome. Although diuretics may be used to manage fluid status in clients receiving interleukin-2, they should be used judiciously, not aggressively.

2. *Answer:* D
Rationale: Chimeric monoclonal antibodies are made primarily of mouse protein with a human protein component. Humanized monoclonal antibodies include only a small percentage of the variable component of the antibody from the species used for immunization (such as a mouse), and the rest is human in composition. Murine monoclonal antibodies consist of mouse variable and constant regions, whereas primatized are created from monkey isotypes.

3. *Answer:* C
Rationale: Allergic reactions against murine antibodies may occur in humans, making C the correct option. Monoclonal antibodies are designed to work in conjunction with the host immune system. Previous reaction to chemotherapy would have no bearing on this because chemotherapy agents are not designed to modify immune responses. Tumor burden can increase the risk for sequelae such as tumor lysis syndrome, but not an allergic reaction. Steroids are frequently excluded from the monoclonal antibody regimen with increased risk of anaphylaxis.

4. *Answer:* A
Rationale: Standard high doses of intravenous interferon used in the adjuvant treatment of stage 3 melanomas are known to be associated with increases in alanine aminotransferase (ALT) and aspartate aminotransferase (AST) (elevated AST reported as high as 63% in melanoma induction therapy), making A the correct option. Although a client with previous hepatitis exposure could have an increase in transaminases, this is not the general reason you see this with high-dose interferon. Hepatic metastasis may also cause increases in ALT and AST; however, this would not be the most likely reason to see this in stage 3 clients who do not have evidence of distant metastasis before initiating interferon therapy.

5. *Answer:* D
Rationale: Neutrophil progenitor cells is the only "granulocyte" option. The other cell types listed are from lymphocyte, platelet, and red blood cell origins.

6. *Answer:* A
Rationale: Option A is the desired means of dosing biotherapy agents. The optimal biologic dose (OBD) is the lowest dose in which the biologic activity of an agent is maximally stimulated. Increasing the dose of a biotherapy agent will not necessarily improve its efficacy. In addition, a minimally toxic dose may be insufficient to stimulate the desired immune response.

7. *Answer:* B
Rationale: Interleukin-2 is a cytokine that promotes the activation of a number of immune cells including cytotoxic T cells, natural killer cells, and monocytes. Use of interleukin-2 can lead to exacerbation of symptoms related to autoimmune disorders such as lupus.

8. *Answer:* D
Rationale: One of the side effects seen during administration of the radioimmunoconjugate, Zevalin therapy is a significant delay in myelosuppression. The client's complaints are very consistent with myelosuppression, and therefore blood count evaluation would be the first step in client management with this therapy for NHL.

9. *Answer:* C
Rationale: Autologous vaccine therapy is using a client's own tumor for vaccine preparation. Many clients will not have readily accessible tumor. Vaccine studies with polypeptide or allogeneic antigens do not require that client

tumor cells be available for use. Dendritic cells are readily harvested from donors or from the client by means of leukapheresis.

10. *Answer:* D
    Rationale: Weight gain of greater than 5% above baseline is reported to be seen in 71% of clients receiving high-dose interleukin-2. Interleukin-2 toxicities are believed to result primarily from a capillary leak syndrome. The use of aggressive fluid replacement, especially late in the cycle of treatment, can result in progressive edema and pulmonary congestion and should be avoided. Cardiac arrhythmias are a rare finding in 6% or less of clients receiving therapy.

11. *Answer:* A
    Rationale: Although the possibility of allergic reactions can exist with interferons and colony-stimulating factors, it is a rare occurrence with interleukins but may be seen with much greater frequency in monoclonal antibodies. This is especially true in those monoclonal antibodies that are derived primarily from the mouse or murine isotype.

12. *Answer:* C
    Rationale: Fatigue is by far the most common and most difficult to manage side effect seen with administration of interferon. CNS alterations such as altered memory, decreased attention span, and difficulty concentrating are, along with fatigue, extremely difficult to manage. Diarrhea may occur but is less frequent and generally well managed by administration of antidiarrheals. Flulike syndrome and headache symptoms are commonly seen as part of the interferon tachyphylaxis response. They are generally controlled with acetaminophen or nonsteroidal antiinflammatory drugs in the early phase of treatment.

13. *Answer:* B
    Rationale: Innate immunity does not involve recognizing a specific antigen but is activated by any invasion of the host by a foreign antigen. The inflammatory response does not require immunologic specificity or memory, making A an incorrect option. Complement activation involves serum proteins triggered by the interaction of antibody with specific antigen. Humoral immunity also involves the immune response, which is primarily mediated by antibodies.

14. *Answer:* A
    Rationale: In this question the client is indicating both a fear related to participating in this particular clinical trial and also a lack of understanding related to risks involved. It is the responsibility of the investigator to make certain that clients have the information needed to provide informed consent for clinical trial participation. As the nurse, you must act as advocate on the client's behalf. Options B, C, and D all fail to address the need for the client to have his fears addressed and to completely understand his personal risks associated with the study.

BIBLIOGRAPHY

Brown, K.A., Esper, P., Kelleher, L.O., et al. (Eds.). (2001). *Chemotherapy and biotherapy guidelines and recommendations for practice.* Pittsburgh: Oncology Nursing Society.

Cuaron, L., & Thompson, J. (2001). The interferons. In P.T. Reiger (Ed.). *Biotherapy: A comprehensive overview* (2nd ed.). Sudbury, MA: Jones and Bartlett Publishers, pp. 125-194.

Frogge, M.H., Barhamand, B., & Esper, P. (2002). *Novel therapies deserve novel educational approaches: Teaching peers and patients about monoclonal antibodies.* Monograph. Pittsburgh: Oncology Education Services, Inc.

Mavroukakis, S.A., Muehlbauer, P.M., White, R.L., & Schwartzentruber, D.J. (2001). Clinical pathways for managing patients receiving interleukin 2. *Clinical Journal of Oncology Nursing 5*(5), 207-216.

MICROMEDEX. Healthcare Series (2003). Vol. 116.

Reff, J.E., Hariharan, K., & Braslawsky, G. (2002). Future of monoclonal antibodies in the treatment of hematologic malignancies. *Cancer Control 9*, 152-166.

Rieger, P.T. (1999). *Clinical handbook for biotherapy.* Sudbury, MA: Jones and Bartlett Publishers.

Rieger, P.T. (2001). Optimizing the dose and schedule of biological agents. In P.T. Reiger (Ed.). *Biotherapy: A comprehensive overview* (2nd ed.). Sudbury, MA: Jones and Bartlett Publishers, pp. 85-122.

Schwartzentruber, D.J. (2000). Interleukin-2: Clinical applications. Principles of administration and management of side effects. In S.A. Rosenberg (Ed.). *Principles and practice of the biologic therapy of cancer* (3rd ed.). Philadelphia: Lippincott, pp. 32-50.

Sompayrac, L. (1999). *How the immune system works*, Malden, MA: Blackwell Science, Inc.

Trask, P., Esper, P., Riba, M., & Redman, B. (2000). Psychiatric side effects of interferon therapy: Prevalence, proposed mechanisms, and future directions. *Journal of Clinical Oncology 18*(11), 2316-2326.

Valentine, A., Meyers, C., Kling, M., et al. (1998). Mood and cognitive side effects of interferon-α therapy. *Seminars in Oncology 25*(1 Suppl. 1), 39-47.

Wujcik, D. (2001). Hematopoietic growth factors. In P.T. Reiger (Ed.). *Biotherapy: A comprehensive overview* (2nd ed.). Sudbury, MA: Jones and Bartlett Publishers, pp. 245-282.

NOTES

38 Nursing Implications of Antineoplastic Therapy

SUSAN VOGT TEMPLE AND BARBARA C. PONIATOWSKI[*]

Select the best answer for each of the following questions:

1. Cancer chemotherapy is a systemic form of cancer treatment that is based on concepts of cellular kinetics including the cell life cycle, cell cycle time, growth fraction, and tumor burden. Cell cycle time is
    A. the length of time required for a cell to move from one mitosis to another.
    B. the number of cells that are actively dividing in a tumor.
    C. the process of reproduction that occurs in normal as well as malignant cells.
    D. the number of cells present in a tumor.

2. Cardiac toxicity is most strongly associated with which of the following chemotherapeutic agents?
    A. Vincristine (Oncovin).
    B. Doxorubicin (Adriamycin).
    C. Nitrogen mustard (Mustargen).
    D. Cisplatinum (Cisplatin).

3. The aim of adjuvant chemotherapy is to
    A. offset the existence of resistant cells.
    B. facilitate ease of chemotherapy administration.
    C. eradicate remaining micrometastases after primary treatment.
    D. palliate symptoms of clients in whom cure is not possible.

4. Cell cycle-specific agents
    A. are dose-dependent and must be administered as bolus doses.
    B. are schedule-dependent and most effective if administered in divided doses.
    C. exert their major cytotoxic effects in all phases of the cell cycle.
    D. are most effective when administered as a short infusion.

5. Ms. J. is receiving amifostine (Ethyol) and cisplatin for treatment of her head and neck cancer. Ethyol is
    A. an alkylating chemotherapy agent.
    B. a chemoprotective agent.
    C. adjuvant chemotherapy.
    D. an alternative/complementary therapy.

6. Ms. J. complains of burning and pain at her peripheral intravenous (IV) site during doxorubicin administration. You stop the infusion and aspirate for blood return. There is no blood return. You would
    A. stop the infusion, aspirate for residual, instill dexamethasone, remove the needle, and apply heat.
    B. stop the infusion, instill sodium thiosulfate, remove the needle, and apply cold.
    C. continue the infusion because there is no evidence of swelling or redness.
    D. stop the infusion, aspirate for residual, remove the needle, and apply cold.

* Susan Vogt Temple and Barbara C. Poniatowski are full-time employees of GlaxoSmithKline (GSK). The views and opinions expressed therein are those of the authors/editors and do not necessarily reflect those of GSK.

7. Mr. P. is receiving bleomycin as a systemic therapy. Which of the following toxicities is most commonly associated with bleomycin (Blenoxane)?
   A. Renal toxicity with hemorrhagic cystitis.
   B. Ototoxicity with tinnitus.
   C. Pulmonary toxicity with pneumonitis.
   D. Diarrhea beginning 24 hours after the completion of chemotherapy.

8. Ms. G. is receiving etoposide for small cell lung cancer. You would administer etoposide (VP-16) as a
   A. 5- to 10-minute IV bolus.
   B. 10- to 20-minute rapid infusion.
   C. 30- to 60-minute infusion.
   D. a continuous infusion for 24 hours.

9. Antimetabolites are cell cycle specific for the
   A. S phase.
   B. G_0 phase.
   C. G_2 phase.
   D. M phase.

10. When infusing chemotherapy agents through a central venous line, you should verify a blood return
    A. before the infusion.
    B. before, during, and after the administration.
    C. at the completion of the infusion.
    D. It is not necessary to verify blood return because this is a central line.

11. Ms. S. is receiving intraperitoneal cisplatinum chemotherapy for ovarian cancer. She received her first cycle yesterday via a Tenckhoff catheter. Today she has a temperature of 101° F (38.3° C) and complains of abdominal pain. A potential cause of her symptoms is
    A. peritonitis caused by nonsterile access of Tenckhoff catheter.
    B. tumor responding to the intraperitoneal therapy.
    C. instillation of the chemotherapy too rapidly.
    D. the drug was placed in an incorrect diluent.

12. You have just begun the infusion of the first cycle of paclitaxel (Taxol) for Ms. T. She relates to you that she is feeling very uneasy and is moving around in the chemotherapy chair. You would suspect
    A. an impending hypersensitivity reaction.
    B. the client is overly anxious about getting chemotherapy.
    C. acting out to impress her husband about the seriousness of her illness.
    D. reacting to the prehydration fluids.

13. Ms. S. is receiving ifosfamide. Which of the following drugs would be administered with ifosfamide (Ifex) to prevent hemorrhagic cystitis?
    A. Amifostine (Ethyol).
    B. Dexamethasone (Decadron).
    C. Mesna (Mesnex).
    D. Cimetadine (Tagamet).

14. You are discharging Ms. J. following chemotherapy administration of vincristine. Discharge medication instructions should include
    A. a bowel regimen to prevent constipation.
    B. a muscle relaxant to prevent footdrop.
    C. an anxiolytic to prevent hot flashes.
    D. loperamide (Imodium) to prevent diarrhea.

15. Ms. C. is midway through the infusion of her ninth cycle of carboplatin (Paraplatin) for ovarian cancer. She begins to complain of perioral and palmar itching and slight shortness of breath. Based on her symptoms, you would suspect
    A. paresthesia of her vagus nerve caused by carboplatin.
    B. palmar plantar erythrodysesthesia.
    C. an impending pulmonary embolus caused by abdominal carcinomatosis.
    D. an allergic reaction to the carboplatin.

16. Ms. A. is to begin chemotherapy and is scheduled to receive cyclophosphamide (Cytoxan) and doxorubicin. Which of the following results would necessitate a change in the proposed regimen?
    A. A lactate dehydrogenase (LDH) of 135 international units/L.
    B. A multiple gated acquisition (MUGA) of 30%.

C. A CA 125 of 35.

D. A hematocrit of 34%.

17. Ms. B. is scheduled to receive her first dose of single agent docetaxel (Taxotere) next week. Which of the following premedication schedules is indicated?

A. Dexamethasone 8 mg by mouth bid the day before, the day of, and the day following chemotherapy.

B. Dexamethasone 20 mg IV, cimetidine (Tagamet) 300 mg IV, and diphenhydramine (Benadryl) 50 mg IV 30 minutes before docetaxel.

C. Dexamethasone 20 mg IV and ondansetron (Zofran) 32 mg IV 30 minutes before docetaxel.

D. Dexamethasone 16 mg by mouth for 4 days beginning the day of chemotherapy.

18. Mr. T. is receiving irinotecan (Camptosar). Nursing considerations should include

A. prophylaxis for stomatitis.

B. prophylaxis for constipation.

C. prophylaxis for pneumonitis.

D. prophylaxis for early and late diarrhea.

19. Capecitabine (Xeloda) would exhibit toxicities similar to

A. vinblastine (Velban).

B. tamoxifen (Nolvadex).

C. 5-fluorouracil (5-FU).

D. prednisone.

NOTES

ANSWERS

1. *Answer:* A
Rationale: Cell cycle time is the amount of time required for a cell to move from one mitosis to another mitosis.

2. *Answer:* B
Rationale: Cardiac toxicity is the dose-limiting toxicity of doxorubicin. Peripheral neurotoxicity is the principal toxicity of vincristine, myelosuppression is dose-limiting for nitrogen mustard, and nephrotoxicity is dose-limiting for cisplatin administration.

3. *Answer:* C
Rationale: The theoretical goal of adjuvant chemotherapy is to eradicate remaining micrometastases after primary treatment. To palliate symptoms would relieve or alleviate symptoms. Resistant cells are those tumor cells that no longer respond to a chemotherapeutic agent(s).

4. *Answer:* B
Rationale: Cell cycle specific agents are schedule-dependent and most effective if administered in divided doses or by continuous infusion.

5. *Answer:* B
Rationale: Amifostine is a cytoprotective agent for toxic effects of cisplatin-related renal toxicities.

6. *Answer:* D
Rationale: If extravasation is suspected, discontinue the infusion, leave the needle in place, aspirate for residual medication, instill antidote if there is a known antidote, remove the needle, and apply heat or cold. There is no antidote for Adriamycin. Doxorubicin requires cold following removal of the needle.

7. *Answer:* C
Rationale: The most common toxicity associated with bleomycin is pulmonary toxicity. Risk increases with cumulative doses and high fractional inspirational oxygen (FiO_2) concentrations.

8. *Answer:* C
Rationale: Etoposide should be administered over 30 to 60 minutes. Rapid infusion of etoposide may precipitate hypotension.

9. *Answer:* A
Rationale: Antimetabolites are cell cycle specific for the S phase or synthesis where cellular DNA is duplicated in preparation for DNA division.

10. *Answer:* B
Rationale: Monitoring central or peripheral IV administration requires that you verify presence of blood return before, during, and after administration of therapy.

11. *Answer:* A
Rationale: Infection is a potential complication of intraperitoneal chemotherapy. Peritonitis (infection) may present with temperature elevation and abdominal pain.

12. *Answer:* A
Rationale: Clients receiving paclitaxel are at risk for a hypersensitivity reaction. An early sign of hypersensitivity is generalized uneasiness.

13. *Answer:* C
Rationale: Mesna is administered as a chemoprotective agent for hemorrhagic cystitis. Amifostine is approved by the Food and Drug Administration as a treatment to reduce the nephrotoxicity of cisplatinum and minimize the incidence of xerostomia associated with radiation therapy for clients with head and neck cancer. Cimetadine is a histamine H_2-receptor antagonist, and dexamethasone is a synthetic adrenocortical steroid.

14. *Answer:* A
Rationale: A neuropathic side effect of vincristine is constipation. Stool softeners and laxatives are used to prevent constipation.

15. *Answer:* D
Rationale: Carboplatin reactions generally occur after six cycles of therapy and midway

through the infusion. Prodromal symptoms include perioral and palmar itching.

16. *Answer:* B

Rationale: Evaluation of the client's right ventricular function (cardiac ejection fraction) should be performed before the first cycle of doxorubicin. This is done with a MUGA scan or radionuclide ventriculography (RVG). Ejection fraction results should be communicated to the physician before initiating doxorubicin. Normal values for ejection fractions are above 50%. Normal values for LDH are 105 to 333 international units/L; thus 135 is within normal limits. The CA 125 would not warrant a change in this regimen, and the hematocrit of 34% is slightly less than a normal value of 36.1% to 44.3% in females and would not, by itself, necessitate a change in the regimen.

17. *Answer:* A

Rationale: Dexamethasone 8 mg bid is administered the day before, day of, and day following docetaxel as premedication/prevention of pulmonary edema.

18. *Answer:* D

Rationale: A dose-limiting toxicity of irinotecan is early- and late-onset diarrhea.

19. *Answer:* C

Rationale: Capecitabine an oral antimetabolite, is converted to 5-fluorouracil when metabolized. Thus, it will exhibit toxicities similar to 5-fluorouracil. Vinblastine is a vinca alkaloid,

tamoxifen is a hormone antagonist, and prednisone is synthetic glucocorticoid.

BIBLIOGRAPHY

Brown, K., A. Esper, P., Kelleher, L., D. et al. (Eds.). (2001). *Chemotherapy and biotherapy guidelines and recommendations for practice.* Pittsburgh: Oncology Nursing Society.

Chabner, B., & Longo, D. (Eds.). (2001). *Cancer chemotherapy and biotherapy: Principles and practice* (3rd ed.). Philadelphia: Lippincott Williams & Wilkins.

Chu, E., & DeVita, V.T. (2001). Principles of cancer management: Chemotherapy. In V.T. DeVita, S. Hellman S.A. & Rosenberg (Eds.). *Cancer: Principles and practice of oncology* (6th ed.). Philadelphia: Lippincott Williams & Wilkins, pp. 289-306.

Fischer, D.S., Knobf, M.T., Durivage, H.J., & Beaulieu, N.J. (2003). *The cancer chemotherapy handbook* (6th ed.). Philadelphia: Saunders.

Gullatte, M. (2001). Principles and standards of chemotherapy administration. In M. Gullatte (Ed.). *Clinical guide to antineoplastic therapy: A chemotherapy handbook.* Pittsburgh: Oncology Nursing Society, pp. 31-45.

Kastan, M., & Skapek, S2. (2001). Molecular biology of cancer: The cell cycle. In V. DeVita, S. Hellman, & S.A. Rosenberg (Eds.). *Cancer: Principles and practice of oncology* (6th ed.). Philadelphia: Lippincott Williams & Wilkins, pp. 91-109.

Perry, M. (Ed.) (2001). *The chemotherapy source book* (3rd ed.). Philadelphia: Lippincott Williams & Wilkins.

Yarbro, C.H. Frogge, M.H., Goodman, M., & Groenwald, S.L. (Eds.). (2000). *Cancer nursing: Principles and practice* (5th ed.). Sudbury, MA: Jones and Bartlett Publishers.

39 Principles of Preparation, Administration, and Disposal of Hazardous Drugs

JEAN M. ELLSWORTH-WOLK AND JAN HAWTHORNE MAXSON

Select the best answer for each of the following questions:

1. As a means to possibly minimize reproductive risk, personnel who are pregnant, breastfeeding, or trying to conceive may
   A. wear gloves when administering antineoplastic agents.
   B. refrain from preparing or administering antineoplastic agents.
   C. administer antineoplastic agents only 1 day per week.
   D. administer antineoplastic agents in a well-ventilated area.

2. A potential long-term health risk that may develop as a result of exposure to antineoplastic agents is
   A. renal failure.
   B. hearing loss.
   C. increased risk of cancer.
   D. liver failure.

3. The appropriate apparel to be worn during the administration of antineoplastic agents, according to the OSHA guidelines, is
   A. disposable gown, goggles, nonpowdered surgical thickness latex gloves, and shoe covers.
   B. disposable gown and nonpowdered surgical thickness latex gloves.
   C. nonpowdered surgical thickness latex gloves and goggles.

   D. disposable gown, shoe covers, and nonpowdered surgical thickness latex gloves.

4. Which of the following is a risk factor for cytotoxic exposure for the nurse administering antineoplastic agents?
   A. Flare reactions.
   B. Hypersensitivity reactions.
   C. Inhalation of aerosols.
   D. Extravasation of drugs.

5. A nurse is caring for a client receiving a continuous infusion of 5-fluorouracil (5-FU). The client puts the call light on and announces that the intravenous (IV) line has pulled apart and is leaking. The nurse's first action after stopping the infusion is to
   A. reconnect the IV tubing.
   B. call the safety officer.
   C. locate a spill kit and cordon off the area.
   D. remove the client from the room.

6. What type of biologic safety cabinet should be used when preparing antineoplastic agents?
   A. Class II (type B) or class III biologic safety cabinet.
   B. Any hood that vents to the outside.
   C. Any vertical airflow hood.
   D. Any laminar airflow hood that vents to the outside.

7. Which of the following is an institutional responsibility with respect to antineoplastic agents?
   A. Conduct clinical evaluations of personal protective equipment.
   B. Develop clinical standards for extravasation management.
   C. Encourage personnel to be evaluated by their physician on a regular basis.
   D. Develop a monitoring system to review incident reports involving antineoplastic agents.

8. How long should interventions to minimize the risk of indirect exposure to antineoplastic agents found in the body fluids of clients be maintained after administration?
   A. 2 hours.
   B. 12 hours.
   C. 24 hours.
   D. 48 hours.

9. A potential short-term health risk that may develop as a result of exposure to antineoplastic agents is
   A. dermatitis.
   B. increased risk of cancer.
   C. chromosomal abnormalities.
   D. reproductive risks.

10. Which of the following is an intervention to minimize the risk of exposure during the preparation of antineoplastic agents?
    A. Prepare agents in a cabinet that vents to the outside.
    B. Wear protective clothing during preparation.
    C. Discard excess solution from vials into an absorbent pad underneath the work area.
    D. Clip or recap all needles after reconstitution of agents.

11. Which is an intervention to minimize exposure during the disposal of antineoplastic agents?
    A. Needles should be clipped or recapped after administration.
    B. Unused portions of drug should be discarded down a drain.
    C. Dispose of filled containers and contaminated equipment in a sealable polypropylene bag.
    D. Special labeling is not necessary on waste containers.

12. Which of the following is an intervention to be used when reconstituting antineoplastic agents packaged in vials?
    A. Employ a multiuse dispensing pin.
    B. Add diluent quickly.
    C. Create positive pressure within the vial by adding a volume of air.
    D. Dispel excess solution into the air within the biologic safety cabinet.

13. Which of the following is an intervention to be used when reconstituting antineoplastic agents packaged in ampules?
    A. Clear all contents from the neck of the ampule before opening.
    B. Wipe the ampule with a damp gauze pad before opening.
    C. Break the neck of the ampule between the thumb and forefinger.
    D. Break the neck of the ampule toward the preparer.

14. What would be the nurse's first action after direct contact with an antineoplastic agent?
    A. Complete an incident report.
    B. Remove contaminated personal protective equipment.
    C. Cleanse the area with soap and water.
    D. Seek medical attention.

15. When is aerosolization a problem in the preparation of antineoplastic agents?
    A. When spiking a bag.
    B. When discontinuing an infusion.
    C. When discarding contaminated materials.
    D. When withdrawing needles from vials.

ANSWERS

1. *Answer:* B
   Rationale: American Society of Health System Pharmacists (ASHP) Technical Assistance Bulletin suggests that personnel who are pregnant, breastfeeding, or trying to conceive (or father) a child should be allowed to avoid contact with antineoplastic agents. Policies should be in effect that provide these individuals with alternate tasks or responsibilities if they so desire.

2. *Answer:* C
   Rationale: Occupational Safety and Health Administration (OSHA) guidelines identify that the long-term effects of partial alopecia, chromosomal abnormalities, increased risk of cancer, and reproductive risks can occur within months to years after exposure to antineoplastic agents.

3. *Answer:* B
   Rationale: OSHA guidelines recommend wearing a disposable, long-sleeved gown made of lint-free fabric with knitted cuffs and a closed front and good-quality, nonpowdered, disposable, surgical thickness latex, nitrile, polyurethane, or neoprene gloves with cuffs long enough to tuck over knit cuffs of the gown.

4. *Answer:* C
   Rationale: Potential routes for the nurse to be exposed to antineoplastic agents include absorption through the skin or mucous membranes after direct contact, inhalation of drug aerosols, or ingestion with contaminated food or tobacco products. Extravasation of drugs, flare reactions, and hypersensitivity reactions are a result of client exposure to antineoplastic agents.

5. *Answer:* C
   Rationale: Oncology Nursing Society (ONS) *Chemotherapy and Biotherapy Guidelines and Recommendations for Practice* state that spill kits should be available wherever antineoplastic agents are stored, transported, prepared, or administered. In the event of a spill involving an antineoplastic agent, a spill kit containing personal protective equipment should be obtained and the area cordoned off to prevent others from being exposed.

6. *Answer:* A
   Rationale: OSHA guidelines state that a class II (type B) or class III biologic safety cabinet should be used when preparing antineoplastic agents.

7. *Answer:* D
   Rationale: OSHA guidelines state that institutions are responsible for the development and periodic review of institutional policies and procedures concerning the use of antineoplastic agents. An employee medical surveillance program to provide medical examinations to potentially exposed personnel and a monitoring system to review incident reports involving antineoplastic agents should be in place.

8. *Answer:* D
   Rationale: ONS guidelines, *Safe Handling of Hazardous Drugs,* state that 48 hours is a standard time frame recommended for precautions to be implemented, because most drugs will be excreted within this time frame.

9. *Answer:* A
   Rationale: Contact dermatitis, alopecia, local skin or mucous membrane irritation are potential short-term effects of exposure to hazardous drugs. Short-term effect occur hours or days after exposure. ONS *Chemotherapy and Biotherapy Guidelines and Recommendations for Practice* state that an increased risk of cancer, chromosomal abnormalities, and reproductive risks are potential long-term health risks that may develop as a result of exposure to antineoplastic agents.

10. *Answer:* B
    Rationale: Personal protective equipment should be worn whenever antineoplastic agents are prepared. Needles should never be clipped or recapped. OSHA guidelines describe that the exposure to antineoplastic agents during preparation can be minimized by using a class II (type B) or class III biologic safety cabinet. A disposable, plastic-backed, absorbent pad should be used underneath the work area. It is recommended that any excess

solution be expelled into a closed container within the biologic safety cabinet.

11. *Answer:* C

Rationale: Unused portions of drug should be disposed of intact, and all materials should be discarded in waste containers that have been identified as hazardous waste. OSHA guidelines state that needles should not be clipped or recapped after administration.

12. *Answer:* A

Rationale: OSHA guidelines suggest that extremes of positive or negative pressure in medication vials should be avoided. Venting devices or dispensing pins allow outside air to replace the withdrawn liquid, thus preventing extreme pressure changes. Diluent should be added to vials slowly, and any excess solution should be expelled into a closed container within the biologic safety cabinet.

13. *Answer:* A

Rationale: ASHP Technical Assistance Bulletin suggests that the contents of the ampule should be gently tapped down from the neck of the ampule before it is opened. The outside of the ampule should be wiped with alcohol, and a sterile gauze pad should be wrapped around the neck of the ampule when it is opened. The ampule should be broken away from the preparer.

14. *Answer:* B

Rationale: OSHA guidelines suggest that contaminated personal protective equipment should first be removed after direct contact with an antineoplastic agent. The affected area should then be thoroughly cleansed with soap and water. After these initial interventions, the nurse should then seek medical attention and document the exposure in an incident report or per the institution's policies and procedures.

15. *Answer:* D

Rationale: OSHA guidelines state that splattering, spraying, and aerosolization can occur during the withdrawal of needles from drug vials and during the transfer of drugs using syringes and needles. It can also occur when ampules are opened and when air is expelled from a drug-filled syringe. Spiking a bag, discontinuing an infusion, and discarding contaminated materials are examples of when exposure can occur during the administration of antineoplastic agents.

BIBLIOGRAPHY

American Society of Health System Pharmacists. (1990). ASHP technical assistance bulletin on handling cytotoxic and hazardous drugs. *Am J Hospital Pharmacy 47*(15), 1033-1049.

Brown, K., Esper, Pl, Kelleher, L.O., et al. (Eds.) (2001). *Chemotherapy and biotherapy: Guidelines and recommendations for practice*. Pittsburgh: Oncology Nursing Society.

Occupational Safety and Health Administration. (1995). Controlling occupational exposure to hazardous drugs. (OSHA Instructional CPL 2-2.20B). Washington, D.C.: Occupational Safety and Health Administration.

Polovich, M. (Eds.). (2003). *Safe handling of hazardous drugs*. Pittsburgh: Oncology Nursing Society.

Tennenbaum, L. (1994). *Cancer chemotherapy and biotherapy: A reference guide*. Philadelphia: W.B. Saunders.

Wolk, J.E., & Maxson, J.H. (2005). Principles of preparation, administration, and disposal of hazardous agents. In J.K. Itano & K.N. Taoka (Eds.). *Core curriculum for oncology nursing* (4th ed.). St. Louis: Elsevier, pp. 802-808.

40 Nursing Implications of Hematopoietic Stem Cell Transplantation

PATRICIA C. BUCHSEL

Select the best answer for each of the following questions:

1. The purpose of the conditioning regimen in the hematopoietic stem cell transplantation (HSCT) process is to
   - A. prevent graft-versus-host disease (GVHD).
   - B. eradicate malignant cells and prevent graft rejection.
   - C. reduce the adverse effects of HSCT.
   - D. mobilize HSCT cells from the bone marrow to the peripheral blood.

2. Hematopoietic stem cells can be derived from all sources **except**
   - A. umbilical cord blood and placenta.
   - B. bone marrow.
   - C. peripheral stem cells.
   - D. animal sources.

3. A nonmyeloablative HSCT (mini-HSCT) is performed in clients who are
   - A. young and newly diagnosed.
   - B. scheduled for umbilical stem cell transplant.
   - C. older clients with preexisting comorbid conditions.
   - D. scheduled for autologous stem cell transplants.

4. Mr. O. has just been given the diagnosis of aplastic anemia. His family members are human leukocyte antigen (HLA) typed for a possible match for a transplant. Unfortunately, there is no match. Mr. O. asks his physician if he could be considered for an autologous HSCT. The physician tells the client that an autologous transplantation is not possible because
   - A. autologous transplants for aplastic anemia are performed only on small children.
   - B. aplastic anemia attacks and destroys the hematopoietic system, leaving diseased and insufficient cells to perform an autologous HSCT.
   - C. the national marrow donor registry only recognizes unrelated transplants for clients with aplastic anemia.
   - D. the cure rate for treating aplastic anemia with an autologous transplant is very low.

5. An allogeneic HSCT is one in which donor cells are derived from
   - A. an HLA-matched donor.
   - B. the client's own marrow.
   - C. the client's twin.
   - D. a cadaver.

6. Common acute complications after HSCT are
   - A. chronic GVHD.
   - B. nausea, vomiting, infection.
   - C. herpes varicella zoster.

D. impaired growth and development in children.

7. The target organs of acute GVHD are
   A. skin, liver, gastrointestinal tract.
   B. vagina, heart, spleen.
   C. skin, pancreas, brain.
   D. gastrointestinal tract, eyes, mouth.

8. Veno-occlusive disease (VOD)
   A. occurs 1000 days after HSCT.
   B. occurs only in recipients of allogeneic HSCT.
   C. occurs only in the stomach and heart.
   D. peaks at 7 to 21 days after HSCT.

9. The target organs of chronic GVHD are
   A. mouth, eyes, vagina.
   B. skin, liver, gastrointestinal tract.
   C. brain, skin, lungs.
   D. skin, liver, heart.

10. A newly discharged allogeneic HSCT recipient caregiver calls the home care nurse and states the client is having a shaking chill but has no fever. The nurse knows that
    A. this is not a problem, because a shaking chill without an accompanied fever is not a worrisome situation.
    B. the caregiver can wait to report this symptom to the doctor in the morning.
    C. the client's doctor must be called immediately because a shaking chill without a fever can be the first sign of sepsis.
    D. the caregiver can give the client any antibiotic that the client may have been ordered at discharge.

11. The long-term complications of HSCT classically occur
    A. 20 days after HSCT.
    B. only in recipients of autologous HSCT.
    C. 80 to 100 days after HSCT.
    D. only in recipients who receive steroid treatment for GVHD.

12. Current diseases under investigation for HSCT are
    A. autoimmune diseases such as rheumatoid arthritis and multiple sclerosis.
    B. cardiac and lung disease.

C. diabetes.
D. Alzheimer's disease.

13. Mrs. Y. is currently a client on an HSCT inpatient unit. She received an autologous HSCT 3 days ago. She tells her nurse that her family just arrived in town and asks if there are any restrictions for the visitors. The nurse tells Mrs. Y. that
    A. school-age children are limited because of the risk for childhood infections such as chickenpox or measles.
    B. she can have no visitors because she remains pancytopenic from the immunosuppressive effects of the conditioning regimens.
    C. the family members should bring fresh salads for Mrs. Y. when they visit because salads are very nutritious.
    D. the visitors must wear sterile surgical garments to protect the client from community diseases.

14. Mr. O. had an allogeneic HSCT 16 days ago. On her morning assessment rounds, his nurse notes that Mr. O. has a weight gain of 5 pounds since yesterday. He asks the nurse repeatedly what day it is. He also complains of upper right quadrant pain. The nurse suspects that
    A. Mr. O. may have acute gastrointestinal GVHD.
    B. Mr. O. is manifesting classic symptoms of VOD.
    C. Mr. O. needs aspirin for his pain.
    D. Mr. O. is not a candidate for VOD because he has had an allogeneic HSCT.

15. A transplant center has a teaching program for all clients and their family members to prepare them for discharge. The nurse teaches the clients and family members that the most important method to avoid infections is to
    A. scrub the kitchen and bathrooms vigorously with bleach three times a day.
    B. wash their hands often and meticulously.
    C. stay at home except to come to the clinic.
    D. monitor temperatures every 2 hours.

16. Mrs. A. is scheduled to have a peripheral stem cell transplantation. The nurse explains that her stem cells will be collected through a process called apheresis. She advises her that she may experience uncomfortable chills during the procedure because

    A. the apheresis room temperature is maintained at 65° F (18.3° C) to enhance the stem cell yield.

    B. cooler rather than warmer temperatures reduce infection rates in clients undergoing apheresis.

    C. calcium is lost during the apheresis process, causing the client to chill and tremor.

    D. little can be done to diminish the effects of chilling.

NOTES

ANSWERS

1. *Answer:* B
Rationale: The goals of pretransplant conditioning regimens are to eradicate any malignant cells that may remain in the recipient. The conditioning regimens cannot prevent GVHD. Colony-stimulating factors, granulocytic colony-stimulating factor, granulocytic-macrophage colony-stimulating factor, and sometimes low-dose chemotherapy are used to mobilize marrow stem cells to the peripheral blood. Conditioning regimens cannot minimize comorbid conditions but rather exacerbate them.

2. *Answer:* D
Rationale: Umbilical cord blood and placenta, bone marrow, and peripheral stem cells all are rich stem cell sources. Animal studies have not been done in human HSCT.

3. *Answer:* C
Rationale: Nonmyeloablative HSCTs are currently reserved for older clients (>age 60) or those with comorbidities because the risk of acute toxicities from the conditioning is less. Nonmyeloablative HSCTs are performed only in the allogeneic recipient. One of the goals of a nonmyeloablative HSCT is to create a graft-versus-tumor effect. Young and newly diagnosed clients can usually withstand the toxicities of HSCT.

4. *Answer:* B
Rationale: Aplastic anemia causes pancytopenia, thereby destroying the client's marrow supply. Recipients of an HSCT for aplastic anemia require a matched donor to replace the failing marrow of the client. Although aplastic anemia can be treated in children with HSCT, they must also have a matched donor source. The national marrow donor registry does support untreated allogeneic transplants for treatment of aplastic anemia. The cure rate for treating aplastic anemia is not only low, but HSCT is not performed for the above reasons.

5. *Answer:* A
Rationale: Allogeneic HSCTs are performed with a matched donor; an autologous HSCT is performed using the client's own marrow; donor cells from a syngeneic transplant are donated from a twin. Cadavers are a source of donor cells, although first attempts in the early 1980s were unsuccessful and are no longer done.

6. *Answer:* B
Rationale: Among the early complications resulting from HSCT are nausea, vomiting, and infection. Chronic GVHD and herpes varicella zoster occur around 80 days after HSCT.

7. *Answer:* A
Rationale: The target organs of acute GVHD are the skin, liver, and gut. Chronic GVHD affects the vagina, but not the heart or spleen. The skin is a target organ of acute GVHD but not the pancreas or brain. Acute GVHD targets the gut, and chronic GVHD targets the eyes and mouth.

8. *Answer:* D
Rationale: VOD is an early complication of HSCT and affects both allogeneic and autologous recipients. This complication affects the liver and peaks from 7 to 21 days after HSCT.

9. *Answer:* A
Rationale: The target organs of chronic GVHD are the mouth, eyes, and vagina. The skin, liver, and gut are target organs of acute GVHD. The brain is not affected in chronic GVHD, but the skin is.

10. *Answer:* C
Rationale: The client's doctor must be called immediately, because even in the absence of fever, a shaking chill can herald an impending life-threatening sepsis. If the caregiver waits until the morning to report these systems, the client may not survive. Often HSCT recipients are discharged from the hospital with one or more antimicrobials. The nurse cannot recommend any current antibiotic and must direct the client to a physician for specific treatment of his septicemia.

11. *Answer:* C
Rationale: The short-term complications of HSCT occur approximately 10 days after HSCT and occur in both the allogeneic and autologous recipient. Although steroid treatment for GVHD causes long-term effects such as bone loss, all recipients of HSCT experience long-term side effects approximately 80 to 100 days after HSCT.

12. *Answer:* A
Rationale: Autologous HSCT has recently been found to be effective in some autoimmune diseases such as rheumatoid arthritis and multiple sclerosis. It allows for high doses of immunosuppressive therapy to be given. More definitive research is needed. No studies have been conducted in cardiac disease, liver disease, or Alzheimer's disease.

13. *Answer:* A
Rationale: Most transplant centers limit school-age children from visiting transplant recipients because of the risk of infectious disease. Clients who are pancytopenic are usually allowed visitors, but protective measures such as meticulous handwashing, masks, or gowns may be required. These precautions vary among institutions. Salads are not permitted for transplant recipients because of the risk of microbial infection. Wearing sterile surgical garments is no longer required for visitors in transplant units.

14. *Answer:* B
Rationale: The classic symptoms of VOD are sudden weight gain, mental confusion, and right upper quadrant pain. Clients with acute gastrointestinal GVHD may have some abdominal cramping, but right upper quadrant pain is typical of VOD. Treating Mr. O. with aspirin for his pain is contraindicated because of hematopoietic immunosuppression from the conditioning regimens of HSCT. VOD occurs in both allogeneic and autologous recipients.

15. *Answer:* B
Rationale: Handwashing has been shown to be the most effective way to reduce the spread of infections.

16. *Answer:* C
Rationale: Clients may chill and have substantive rigors from calcium loss during apheresis. Room temperature has no effect on stem cell yield or on infection rates in transplant recipients. Replacement calcium either intravenously or by mouth can reduce hypocalcemia.

BIBLIOGRAPHY

Buchsel, P.C., & Kapustay, P.M. (2000). *Stem cell transplantation: A clinical textbook.* Pittsburgh: Oncology Nursing Society.

Chouinard, M. S. (2004). Nursing management of the nonmyeloblative hematopoietic stem cell transplant recipient. In P.C. Buchsel & P.M. Kapustay (Eds.). *Stem cell transplantation: A clinical textbook.* Pittsburgh: Oncology Nursing Society, pp. 20.1-20.12.

Ezzone, S. (Ed.). (2004). *Hematopoietic stem cell transplantation: A manual for nursing practice.* Pittsburgh: Oncology Nursing Society.

Hacker, E.D. (2003). Quantitative measurement of quality of life in adult patients undergoing bone marrow transplantation: A decade in review. *Oncology Nursing Forum 30,* 613-633.

Hinds, M., & Minor, S. (2004). Nonmyeloablative transplantation: Reducing toxicity utilizing an immunologic approach. In P.C. Buchsel & P.M. Kapustay (Eds.). *Stem cell transplantation: A clinical textbook.* Pittsburgh: Oncology Nursing Society, pp. 19.1-19.28.

Schmit-Pokorny, K., Franco, T., Frappier, B., & Vyhlidal, R.C. (2003). The cooperative care model: An innovative approach to deliver blood and marrow stem cell transplant care. *Clinical Journal of Oncology Nursing 7,* 509-514, 556.

Williams, L. (2003). Informal caregiving dynamics with a case study in blood and marrow transplantation. *Oncology Nursing Forum 30,* 679-689.

41 Complementary and Alternative Medicines

COLLEEN O. LEE

Select the best answer for each of the following questions:

1. Complementary and alternative medicine can best be described in which of the following statements:
   - A. Insertion of a needle into the skin and underlying tissues in special sites for therapeutic or preventive purposes.
   - B. Plant-derived and pancreatic enzymes given orally with the goal of improving the immune and digestive systems.
   - C. Permanent or pulsed magnetic fields applied to parts of the body for relief of symptoms.
   - D. A group of diverse medical and health care systems, practices, and products that are not presently considered to be part of conventional medicine.

2. The strongest study design for obtaining evidence used to make clinical decisions involving complementary and/or alternative medicine is
   - A. double-blinded, randomized, and controlled clinical trial.
   - B. systematic review of preclinical research.
   - C. convenience sample using a small population of adolescents.
   - D. population-based consecutive case series.

3. There are many reasons why people with cancer seek alternative regimens. One reason that you would **not** agree with would be which of the following?
   - A. Possible improvement in quality of life during cancer treatment.
   - B. Mistrust of conventional medicine practice.
   - C. Evidence-based practices that are widely accepted and result in frequent cancer remissions.
   - D. Some alternative regimens can be less expensive than conventional medicine.

4. You are conducting a medication review during an admission assessment. Key aspects to include in your assessment are which of the following:
   - A. Dosage and schedule of prescription medications, herbal medicines, vitamins, dietary supplements, and all over-the-counter medications.
   - B. Dosage and schedule of prescription medications.
   - C. Dosage and schedule of vitamins and herbal medicines.
   - D. Dosage and schedule of over-the-counter medications.

5. Your client is curious about a nontraditional regimen and is asking multiple questions. Which question would cause you to become concerned?

A. "What are the benefits and risks associated with this therapy?"

B. "Will this therapy interfere with my conventional treatment?"

C. "Is this therapy part of a clinical trial? If so, who is sponsoring the trial?"

D. "Because there is so much information about this regimen, it must be effective for my type of cancer, right?"

6. The best approach to adopt when responding to a client seeking shark cartilage for breast cancer treatment is which of the following:

A. Allow the client to verbalize concerns, seek second opinions, validate credentials of practitioners, and obtain valid information in favor of and/or against the intervention.

B. Encourage the client to try any nontraditional technique because the current conventional therapy may not be effective.

C. Encourage the client to try shark cartilage because it is now considered standard therapy for the treatment of hormone-resistant breast cancer.

D. Condone any alternative intervention, especially when the client is receiving a chemotherapeutic agent with known therapeutic potential.

7. Guided imagery can be an effective intervention with clients dealing with cancer symptoms for the following reason:

A. Clients can develop positive images that may produce desirable effects on the mind and body.

B. Randomized controlled clinical trials have revealed a tumor-reducing effect.

C. Most insurance carriers will provide reimbursement for this intervention.

D. An altered state of consciousness allows clients to "escape reality."

8. Oncology nurses can encourage their clients to partner with their oncologists in discussing complementary and alternative interventions. The best approach can be summarized in which statement?

A. Encourage the client to make hostile remarks about conventional medicine in an attempt to convince his or her

oncologist to recognize an alternative regimen.

B. Give full attention to the client as he or she expresses concerns and support the client's right to choose his or her own therapy.

C. Avoid talking to the client about any intervention other than the traditional or conventional intervention he or she is currently receiving.

D. Support the client in his or her pattern of not disclosing the use of complementary or alternative intervention to the oncologist and health care team.

9. Oncology nurses can assist clients in identifying reliable information on the Internet. Which suggestion would you **not** include in your client education?

A. Read and accept the client testimonials and anecdotal data as accurate depictions without further investigation.

B. Conduct an online literature search through Medline to determine what is known about the effectiveness of the nontraditional therapy in treating cancer or alleviating cancer-related symptoms.

C. Browse reputable Internet sites such as the American Cancer Society, the National Cancer Institute, and the National Center for Complementary and Alternative Medicine to locate reliable information and links to other trustworthy sites.

D. Determine the following about each website: purpose of the site, source of information, author of the information, source of funding, frequency of updates, ability to contact the site manager, and links to other sites before making a final decision for or against an alternative therapy.

10. Your primary client is considering megavitamin therapy along with her chemotherapy and radiation treatment schedule. Your suggestions include which of the following:

A. Vitamins A, B complex, C, D, E, and K with doses twice the recommended dietary allowance because these doses are still considered to be safe.

B. Water-soluble and fat-soluble vitamins with doses twice the recommended dietary allowance because these doses are still considered to be safe.

C. Vitamins C, beta-carotene, and E in doses four times the recommended dietary allowance because recent research has shown their efficacy without toxicity.

D. A nutritional consultation to review current dietary intake and discuss the value of supplemental vitamins and the risks associated with megadosing.

11. The sale of herbal medicine is one of the fastest growing industries in the United States. The most reliable sources of information for the efficacy of herbal medicine are available at which locations:

A. Advertisements in lay complementary and alternative medicine journals.

B. Sale associates in health food and general nutrition stores.

C. Databases available through hospital pharmacies and medical libraries, written documents available through professional organizations, manuscripts published in peer-reviewed journals.

D. Internet sites selling products without offering a sample or money-back guarantee.

12. During a telephone triage interview with a client, you discover that he or she has been taking cyclosporine, acyclovir (Zovirax), docusate sodium (Colace), trimethoprim-sulfamethoxazole (Bactrim), furosemide (Lasix), and St. John's wort while at home for the past several weeks. Which medication combination would you question?

A. Acyclovir and trimethoprim-sulfamethoxazole.

B. Colace and furosemide.

C. Colace and St. John's wort.

D. Cyclosporine and St. John's wort.

13. Acupuncture has been used to alleviate cancer-related symptoms such as pain. The best description of one of the mechanisms of action of acupuncture is summarized in which of the following statements:

A. The placebo effect of acupuncture allows clients to believe they never had pain.

B. The introduction of pain at the point of needle contact on the skin allows the client to refocus his or her perception of the original site of pain.

C. The stimulation of the nerve fibers entering the dorsal horn of the spinal cord mediates the impulses at other parts of the body and allows the client to experience less pain at the original site.

D. The pressure applied by exerting a finger and thumb on specific points on the surface of the skin acts as an entrance and exit for an internal healing force, thereby eliminating the overall sensation of pain.

14. Homeopathy can be best described as

A. a system of healing that uses diluted substances to alleviate disease or symptoms of disease.

B. a system of healing using extracts of crude products to alleviate a variety of diseases.

C. a system of healing using large doses of herbal products given over a period of weeks for symptom relief.

D. a system of healing using small amounts of a raw herb in a cup of water steeped or soaked for several minutes into a tea for daily consumption.

15. Laetrile, a purified form of the chemical amygdalin, was a popular alternative cancer therapy in previous decades. The Food and Drug Administration (FDA) does not approve Laetrile at this time because

A. Laetrile was found to be ineffective in treating cancer or relieving cancer-related symptoms in randomized clinical trials.

B. The FDA approves only those nontraditional avenues that are used by a small portion of cancer clients.

C. it is a traditional medicine approach that does not fall under FDA regulation.

D. the FDA approves only those medications that are administered in intravenous or oral routes, and Laetrile can be administered in more than two routes.

16. A macrobiotic diet consists of
    A. approximately 50% whole grain cereals, 25% vegetables, 10% beans, 5% fish, fruits, nuts, and 5% soup.
    B. approximately 75% fresh and dried fruits, 25% nuts, honey, and olive oil.
    C. approximately 75% saturated fats and 25% polyunsaturated fats.
    D. approximately 75% low antioxidant-containing fruits and vegetables, 25% saturated fats

17. Your client is interested in massage therapy for her right arm lymphedema. Your best response would be:
    A. "Go ahead. I'm sure it will help right away."
    B. "Oh no, I wouldn't do that. It will probably make it worse."
    C. "Would it be all right with you if we discussed this with your oncologist? There are specialists in rehabilitation medicine that use massage therapy for lymphedema, and this intervention may be covered under your insurance."
    D. "Don't trust anyone outside of this clinic. I heard terrible stories of patients who were told that massage therapy could cure their conditions."

NOTES

ANSWERS

1. *Answer:* D
   Rationale: Complementary and alternative medicine is a complex clinical field composed of numerous and diverse nontraditional approaches in comparison with Western medicine, which is the more widely accepted medical practice system in the United States. Complementary approaches are used together with traditional or conventional medical approaches. Alternative approaches are used instead of traditional or conventional medical approaches. The term "integrated medicine" is the use of various complementary approaches along with traditional or conventional approaches. Option A is not correct because it is a definition of acupuncture. Option B is not correct because it is the definition of enzyme therapy. Option C is not correct because it is the definition of magnetic field therapy.

2. *Answer:* A
   Rationale: Randomized controlled clinical trials are studies in which participants are assigned by chance to separate comparison groups. Clients choose to be involved in the randomized trials, but neither the client nor researcher can choose the placement group. Using chance to choose the group in which a client is placed helps to secure similar groups and an objective review of the comparison group. A double-blinded trial conceals the comparison treatment from both the client and the researcher, which supports the highest level of objectivity. Option B is not correct because a systematic review of preclinical data provides in vitro or small animal in vivo data with data that cannot be generalized to a larger population. Option C is not correct because clinical trials should be open to individuals of all ages unless precluded by a specific tumor type. Also, convenience samples are the weakest form of sampling because the risk of bias is greater. Option D is not correct because results from population-based consecutive cases are obtained from a series of clients who received the same treatment but with the absence of a control group. Studies of this type are termed consecutive because the data are obtained from individuals in the order identified by the researcher.

3. *Answer:* C
   Rationale: The field of complementary and alternative medicine does not have a foundation of evidence-based practice as does the field of traditional or conventional medicine, although the practices are widely accepted in some geographic areas. Claims of cancer remission associated with certain complementary or alternative medicine are frequent and not based on reliable clinical data. Options A, B, and D are actual reasons cited by clients for seeking alternative regimens.

4. *Answer:* A
   Rationale: All prescription, nonprescription, dietary supplements (i.e., minerals, elements), herbal medications, and vitamins should be listed in a medication review. Medications are defined as any drug or remedy. Options B, C, and D are not correct because they would only contain a partial listing of all the medications consumed by the client.

5. *Answer:* D
   Rationale: The mere volume of information available on any approach, whether it is nontraditional or traditional, should not be interpreted as evidence of clinical effectiveness. Clients should be informed that the popularity of an approach or therapy does not equate with its efficacy. Oncology nurses can assist clients in accessing credible information by asking a series of questions about the therapy itself and about the practitioner who will be administering the therapy. Essential questions are listed in options A, B, and C. Essential defining attributes of a practitioner, whether traditional or nontraditional, are (1) graduation from an accredited program, (2) possession of a state license, (3) certification by a national board in the specific approach, and (4) membership in the professional association that supports the specific approach.

6. *Answer:* A
   Rationale: Oncology nurses need to provide an open atmosphere in which the client can express his or her feelings and concerns about treatment regimens and to offer concrete advice

as to how to screen potentially harmful interventions from potentially helpful interventions. Option B is incorrect because it undermines the current treatment regimen as prescribed by the client's oncologist and may be harmful. Option C is incorrect because shark cartilage remains in clinical trials, and published data on its effectiveness are forthcoming. Option D is not correct because oncology nurses need to listen to all client concerns regarding standard therapy and to assist clients in selecting the optimal treatment from the available options.

7. *Answer:* A
Rationale: Imagery is a form of behavior rehearsal with the goal of relaxation. Guides can often be helpful in leading clients through the progressive relaxation necessary for the mind and body to focus. Option B is not correct because guided imagery has not demonstrated a tumor-reducing effect. Option C is not correct because insurance carriers have not characteristically reimbursed this intervention. Option D is not correct because "escaping reality" is not a recommended intervention for clients with cancer, because it focuses on what is not real versus what is real.

8. *Answer:* B
Rationale: As stated in the Oncology Nursing Society (ONS) Position Statement on the *Use of Complementary and Alternative Therapies in Cancer Care*, oncology nurses must assess clients for the use of these therapies, and when asked, provide credible information regarding these therapies and facilitate referrals to qualified practitioners. Options A, C, and D do not provide an atmosphere of open communication and collaboration between the client and the health care team.

9. *Answer:* A
Rationale: Clients should be informed that testimonials and anecdotal data related to a certain intervention may be fictitious and may not equate with reliable clinical evidence. Options B, C, and D are excellent suggestions in guiding clients to obtain reliable information on the Internet.

10. *Answer:* D
Rationale: A nutritional consultation will provide an assessment of current dietary intake and suggest dietary alterations to maintain a balanced intake of protein, carbohydrates, fats, fiber, and fluids. After a consultation, the nutritionist may discuss possible vitamin supplements with safe dosing with the client's oncologist. Options A, B, and C are not correct because the recommended dietary allowances are maintained at safe levels for adults and children, and exceeding the recommended dietary allowances may cause harm. Several vitamins, minerals, and elements are in preclinical and clinical trials at this time under controlled conditions.

11. *Answer:* C
Rationale: Several reliable herbal products and medication databases are accessible for health care providers and consumers in addition to client education materials through professional organizations. Peer-review journals generally have higher standards when reviewing manuscripts so that the most current, accurate, and nonbiased information is published. Options A, B, and D are not correct because the advertisement industry and health products industry are profit-based and may be inclined only to discuss favorable results.

12. *Answer:* D
Rationale: St. John's wort has been clinically shown to decrease the plasma concentration of cyclosporine and should not be taken in combination with cyclosporine. St. John's wort is an inducer of the metabolic pathway cytochrome P450 and thereby decreases plasma concentrations of protease inhibitors and may also affect nonnucleoside reverse transcriptase inhibitors. Consequently, concomitant use of St. John's wort and human immunodeficiency virus (HIV) drugs such as indinavir (Crixivan) and chemotherapy agents such as irinotecan hydrochloride (Camptosar) is not recommended. Options A, B, and C are not correct because there are no known contraindications for these combinations of medications.

13. *Answer:* C
Rationale: Acupuncture needles in one part of the body can affect the pain sensation in another part of the body through the mediation process that occurs when impulses stimulate the nerve fibers in the dorsal horn of the spinal

cord. Option A is not correct because although a placebo effect may be present for some clients, the mechanism of action in acupuncture is not to convince the clients that they never had pain. Options B and D are not correct because these are not mechanisms of action in acupuncture. Pressure applied to the skin surface with the finger and thumb describes the process in acupressure. Acupressure is similar to acupuncture without needles.

14. *Answer:* A

Rationale: Homeopathy is a system of healing founded by Samuel Hahnemann using substances in hyperdiluted concentrations for symptom management or disease resolution. Option B is not correct because extracts are an example of herbal remedies. Option C is not correct because large doses of herbals have not been proven safe for human consumption. Option D is not correct because this is a description of a tea. Options B, C, and D are not systems of healing.

15. *Answer:* A

Rationale: Laetrile has not been shown to be effective in treating cancer in randomized controlled clinical trials in the United States. Option B is not correct because any FDA-approved medication undergoes years of in vitro and in vivo testing before it is an approved medication for market. Option C is not correct because Laetrile is a compound that is a concentrated form of amygdalin or B_{17}, a naturally occurring substance in fruits and several plant products. Option D is not correct because the FDA approves multiple routes of administration for medications, although laetrile can be given in intravenous, intra-arterial, oral, and colonic methods.

16. *Answer:* A

Rationale: Macrobiotics is a way of eating and living that stems from an intuitive understanding of the orderliness of nature. Diets emphasize whole grains such as wheat, barley, buckwheat with fresh vegetables and greens, nuts, beans, and fruits. Option B is not correct because it constitutes a fruitarian diet. Option C is not correct because high saturated fats in the daily diet are associated with certain cancers, heart disease, and obesity. Option D is not correct because antioxidant advocates would encourage an increased dietary intake versus a decreased dietary intake.

17. *Answer:* C

Rationale: Oncology nurses should promote partnering between clients and health care providers when discussing nontraditional methods of symptom management. Also, insurance carriers may not reimburse clients if their care is provided at a facility or clinic outside of their primary care unless the specialist is on their approved list. Option A is not correct because espousing an intervention without first discussing it with the client and oncologist may not ensure the best case possible for the client. Options B and D are not correct because oncology nurses should promote an open atmosphere for discussion.

BIBLIOGRAPHY

Beckner, W.M., & Berman, B.M. (2003). *Complementary therapies on the Internet.* St. Louis: Churchill Livingstone.

Decker, G.M. (Ed.). (1999). *An introduction to complementary and alternative therapies.* Pittsburgh: Oncology Nursing Society.

Edwards, D. (Ed.). (2002). *Voice massage: Scripts for guided imagery.* Pittsburgh: Oncology Nursing Society.

Ernst, E. (Ed.). (2001). *The desktop guide to complementary and alternative medicine.* Edinburgh: Mosby.

Fetrow, C.W., & Avila, J.R. (2001). *Professional's handbook of complementary and alternative medicines.* Springhouse, PA: Springhouse Publishers.

Freeman, L.W., & Lawlis, G.F. (2001). *Mosby's complementary and alternative medicine: A research-based approach.* St. Louis: Mosby.

Skidmore-Roth, L. (2001). *Mosby's handbook of herbs & natural supplements.* St. Louis: Mosby.

Spencer, J.W., & Jacobs, J.J. (2003). *Complementary and alternative medicine: An evidence-based approach* (2nd ed.). St. Louis: Mosby.

PART SEVEN

HEALTH PROMOTION

42 Epidemiology and Prevention of Cancer

SUZANNE M. MAHON

1. Colon cancer prevention strategies include which one of the following?
   A. Reduction of red meat in the diet.
   B. Modification of dietary fat intake.
   C. Pursuit of a diet rich in vegetables.
   D. Pursuit of a diet rich in fiber and vegetables.

2. From a client's history, the nurse discerns that the client does not practice breast self-examination regularly, is a heavy coffee drinker, is infected with condyloma acuminatum (HPV), and follows a diet that is high in fat and low in fiber, fruits, and vegetables. Of these risk factors, which has been specifically linked with a type of cancer?
   A. Lack of practice of monthly breast self-examination.
   B. Caffeine consumption.
   C. Infection with HPV.
   D. A diet high in fat and low in fiber, fruits, and vegetables.

3. Of all the classes of chemotherapy, which class has the strongest potential for carcinogenic activity?
   A. Alkylating agents.
   B. Antibiotics.
   C. Antimetabolites.
   D. Plant alkaloids.

4. The director of your state's environmental health program has asked you to consult on the development of a new public health services grant proposal. The purpose of this grant is to significantly reduce the number of cancer deaths related to a select environmental cause. A focus on which of the following would potentially have the greatest public health impact?
   A. Electromagnetic field exposure (EFE) and childhood cancer.
   B. Cellular telephone use and cancer of the brain and nervous system.
   C. Ultraviolet exposure and skin cancer.
   D. Hazardous waste dump exposure and leukemia.

5. Chemoprevention trials with calcium supplements have been associated with a reduction in risk for which of the following cancers?
   A. Breast cancer.
   B. Colon cancer.
   C. Melanoma.
   D. Osteosarcoma.

6. The three leading sites for cancer deaths worldwide are
   A. lung, stomach, and liver.
   B. lung, breast, and prostate.
   C. lung, colorectal, and pancreatic.
   D. lung, skin, and colorectal.

7. Risk factors associated with pancreatic cancer include

A. cigarette smoking, consumption of smoked or processed meat, *Helicobacter pylori*, and history of diabetes mellitus.

B. age, diet high in fat and calories and low in fiber, and a history of ulcerative colitis.

C. increasing age and history of radiation exposure.

D. cigarette smoking and history of radon exposure.

8. According to a recent report by the Institute of Medicine, the United States could decrease cancer deaths and new cancer cases if the following things were done:

A. Ban the use of alcohol.

B. People stopped eating red meat.

C. People changed their behaviors and a system was in place to allow people to take advantage of cancer detection procedures.

D. Prophylactic surgery was performed on patients at risk for developing cancer.

9. A nurse is preparing to give a program to the public on breast cancer. She wants the participants to understand how many women will be affected by a diagnosis of breast cancer. She might begin this by expressing breast cancer statistics for

A. risk.

B. incidence.

C. mortality.

D. case-fatality.

10. A nurse recommends that a family at high risk for developing colorectal cancer begin colonoscopy at age 40. This is an example of

A. primary prevention.

B. secondary prevention.

C. tertiary prevention.

11. A nurse completes a risk assessment on an individual. The biggest benefit to the individual in undergoing this assessment is to

A. select appropriate cancer prevention tools.

B. help establish a pattern of inheritance.

C. contribute to the biologic understanding of cancer.

D. identify individuals at risk for developing cancer.

12. A nurse completes a cancer risk assessment on a 28-year-old woman with multiple female relatives with breast cancer. The nurse best communicates this woman's risk using

A. absolute risk.

B. attributable risk.

C. cumulative risk.

D. relative risk.

NOTES

ANSWERS

1. *Answer:* D
Rationale: A diet high in fiber and vegetables promotes regular evacuation of stool.

2. *Answer:* C
Rationale: HPV is a virus that has been directly linked with but not proven as a single cause of carcinoma of the cervix. Breast self-examination is not associated with a cancer; it is a screening tool. A diet high in fat and low in fiber, fruits, and vegetables is associated with several cancers including colorectal, breast, prostate, and endometrial cancer.

3. *Answer:* A
Rationale: Alkylating agents are known chemical carcinogens and have the greatest potential for producing a second malignancy. Recognition of this iatrogenic risk factor has nursing implications for long-term follow-up and regular screening.

4. *Answer:* C
Rationale: Sunlight exposure contributes to approximately 90% of skin cancers including melanoma. A statewide campaign to reduce sun exposure could significantly affect the number of skin cancer deaths. Overall, environmental risk factors contribute to only 2% of all cancer deaths. Further, the link between ultraviolet light exposure and skin cancer is better understood than the risks associated with EFE, cellular telephones, and hazardous waste exposure.

5. *Answer:* B
Rationale: Calcium supplements have been found to reduce hyperproliferation of the colonic mucosa cells, thereby providing a potential protective effect against colon cancer.

6. *Answer:* A
Rationale: Lung, stomach, and liver are the most common cancers worldwide. Lung, breast, and prostate are the most common cancers in the United States. Lung is the leading cause of death in both men and women in the United States, colorectal is the second leading cause of cancer death irrespective of gender in the United States, and pancreatic is the fourth most common cause of cancer death in the United States. Skin cancer is a common cancer but not a leading cause of cancer death.

7. *Answer:* A
Rationale: Cigarette smoking, consumption of smoked or processed meat, *Helicobacter pylori,* and history of diabetes mellitus increase risk. In addition, a history of chronic pancreatitis is also considered a risk factor. Option B is incorrect because age, a diet high in fat and calories and low in fiber, and a history of ulcerative colitis are risk factors for colorectal cancer (CRC). Other risk factors for CRC include polyps, familial polyposis, women with a history of cancer of the ovary, uterus, or breast, personal history of CRC, and family history of CRC. Option C is incorrect because increasing age, family history of breast cancer, and history of radiation exposure are risk factors related to breast cancer. In addition, early menarche; late menopause; nulliparity; older age at first live birth; personal history of proliferative benign breast disease; and BRCA1, BRCA2, p53, or PTEN (phosphatase and tensin homolog deleted on chromosome 10) mutations have been considered risk factors. Option D, cigarette smoking, and history of radon exposure, are risk factors associated with lung cancer. Other risk factors for lung cancer are exposure to asbestos, recurring inflammation of the lung, and marijuana use.

8. *Answer:* C
Rationale: If people changed their behaviors and a system were in place to allow people to take advantage of cancer detection procedures, overall a healthier lifestyle would be achieved. Instituting these behaviors and providing access to early detection of cancer could result in the prevention of 60,000 cancer deaths and 100,000 new cancer cases annually by 2015. Options A and B are ways to reduce the number of cancer cases, but they are not realistic to implement. Option D is a drastic measure. Surgical removal of organs to prevent disease has been suggested to prevent the development of some cancers in people at high

risk, especially those with a known mutation for cancer predisposition. Some of these include prophylactic oophorectomy in women at risk for inherited ovarian cancer, mastectomy for women at risk for breast cancer, and removal of adenomatous polyps to reduce the risk of colorectal cancer. These measures are usually not used with the general population.

9. *Answer:* B

Rationale: Incidence is the number of new cancers of a specific type that occur in a defined population during a 1-year period. The American Cancer Society publishes incidence rates annually. Incidence rates will help the audience to understand how many individuals a cancer affects each year. Option A, risk, describes those factors that are associated with an increased susceptibility for developing the disease. They do not define why a particular cancer might be a significant health problem. Option C, mortality, is the number of deaths attributed to cancer in a defined population during a 1-year period. Mortality is helpful in understanding the significance of a public health problem, but it must be interpreted with the incidence to provide useful information. Some cancers have a high incidence (i.e., skin cancer) but a low mortality rate. Other cancers have a relatively low incidence but a high mortality rate. Option D, case-fatality, refers to the number of persons among all those with the same diagnosis of cancer who die of it during a specified period of time. It provides a measure of the aggressiveness of cancer or the degree of success of treatment for a specific cancer.

10. *Answer:* B

Rationale: The term *secondary prevention* is often used interchangeably with cancer screening, cancer detection, or cancer surveillance. Secondary prevention includes efforts to detect the disease in persons without symptoms when treatment should be most effective. Option A, primary prevention, refers to efforts to prevent disease or delay the development of disease. Examples of primary prevention include chemoprevention, eating a healthy diet, exercising, ensuring a diet with adequate vitamins, or preventing exposure to carcinogens such as ultraviolet light. Option C, tertiary prevention, refers to monitoring long-term

survivors of cancer for second primary cancers or other long-term complications associated with treatment.

11. *Answer:* A

Rationale: The selection of appropriate cancer prevention tools is the primary benefit to the individual undergoing cancer risk assessment. Once an individual's risk for developing cancer is better understood, the individual can decide which tools for primary and secondary cancer prevention would be appropriate for this individual. Option B, helps establish a pattern of inheritance, may be an outcome from completing a cancer risk assessment. Approximately 10% of all individuals diagnosed with cancer have a hereditary predisposition for developing the disease and once identified, these families may benefit from further evaluation including genetic testing. Option C, contributes to the biologic understanding of cancer, is a benefit to completing a cancer risk assessment. The benefit is more to the population at large than the individual, because epidemiologic evidence provides a better understanding of cancer risk. Option D, identify individuals at risk for developing cancer, is an outcome of completing a cancer risk assessment. An assessment is only beneficial, however, if the individuals understand the risk and it assists them in making appropriate choices about cancer prevention.

12. *Answer:* D

Rationale: Relative risk is the best means to communicate risk to the woman. Relative risk is an estimate of one's increased probability of developing a certain cancer based on exposure to a risk factor compared with those without the risk factor. In this case, the woman with multiple female relatives with breast cancer risk is compared with those women who do not have a significant family history. The higher the relative risk, the higher the chance of developing that cancer. Sometimes relative risk is known as risk ratio, hazard ratio, or odds ratio. Option A, absolute risk, is a measure of cancer in terms of cancer incidence or mortality. In individuals with multiple risk factors, it will greatly underestimate risk because it is based on averages of all women in a population. Option B, attributable risk, is the amount of disease in a population that could be avoided by reducing or eliminating risk factors. It is useful for those creating public health policy. In this case it is not particularly helpful, because the woman cannot change her family history. Option C refers to cumulative risk, which is the total amount of risk of developing a disease over time.

BIBLIOGRAPHY

Clark, R.A., & Reintgen, D.S. (1996). Principles of cancer screening. In D.S. Reintgen & R.A. Clark (Eds.). *Cancer screening.* St. Louis: Mosby, pp. 1-20.

Foltz, A.T., & Mahon, S.M. (2000). Application of carcinogenesis theory to primary prevention. *Oncology Nursing Forum 27* (Suppl - October), 5-11.

Jemal, A., Tiwari, R., Murray T., et al. (2004). Cancer statistics, 2004. *CA: A Cancer Journal for Clinicians 54,* 8-29.

Jennings-Dozier, K., & Mahon, S.M. (2000). Introduction: Cancer prevention and early detection from thought to revolution. *Oncology Nursing Forum 27* (Suppl — October), 3-4.

Jennings-Dozier, K., & Mahon, S.M. (Eds.). (2003). *Cancer prevention, detection and control: A nursing perspective.* Pittsburgh: Oncology Nursing Society.

Mahon, S.M. (2000). The role of the nurse in developing cancer screening programs. *Oncology Nursing Forum 27* (Suppl — October), 19-27.

Mahon, S.M. (2001). Cancer prevention and early detection. *Clinical Journal of Oncology Nursing 5,* 105-117.

Mahon, S.M. (2003a). Patient education regarding cancer screening guidelines. *Clinical Journal of Oncology Nursing 7*(5), 581-584.

Mahon, S.M. (2003b). Skin cancer prevention: Education and public health issues. *Seminars in Oncology Nursing 19*(1), 52-61.

NOTES

43 Early Detection of Cancer

ROBIN L. COYNE

Select the best answer for each of the following questions:

1. Annual mammographic screening for breast cancer is an example of what type of screening technique?
   A. Mass screening.
   B. Single screening.
   C. Multiphasic screening.
   D. Selective or prescriptive screening.

2. Which tumor marker, when elevated in an adult, may suggest a primary liver or germ cell cancer?
   A. CA 15-3.
   B. Neuron-specific enolase (NSE).
   C. Alpha-fetoprotein (α-FP).
   D. CA 125.

3. The use of CA 27-29 to monitor for recurrence of stages II and III breast cancer is an example of
   A. surveillance.
   B. secondary prevention.
   C. diagnosis.
   D. treatment.

4. The relative risk of developing a disease or cancer is defined as
   A. the amount of preventable disease when considering the incidence of the disease that is likely to occur in the absence of risk factors.
   B. the risk for cancer development associated with a hereditary predisposition.
   C. an estimation of the increased probability of developing a certain cancer based on exposure to associated risk factors.
   D. the number of persons among all those who have a certain type of cancer who die of it during a specified period of time.

5. According to the U.S. Preventive Services Task Force, which of the following cancers lack proven screening interventions?
   A. Cervical cancer.
   B. Breast cancer.
   C. Skin cancer.
   D. Colorectal cancer.

6. Which of the following statements regarding colorectal screening is true?
   A. Screening for men should begin at the age of 40.
   B. Screening for women should begin at the age of 40.
   C. Screening for both genders should begin at the age of 60.
   D. Screening for both genders should begin at the age of 50.

7. Which of the following mnemonic is helpful in teaching clients the "Seven Warning Signals of Cancer?"

A. WARNING.
B. CAUTION.
C. CANSTOP.
D. STOPCAN.

8. Which statement is true regarding the prostate-specific antigen (PSA)?
A. PSA is 100% specific and sensitive for prostate cancer.
B. PSA may be elevated in men with benign prostate conditions.
C. Men age 40 and older should obtain an annual PSA to screen for prostate cancer.
D. This tumor marker meets the criteria set forth by the U.S. Preventive Services Task Force as an effective screening test.

9. Which of the following statements regarding socioeconomic status is true?
A. Increased tobacco use is commonly seen among wealthier populations.
B. Low socioeconomic groups use screening services less often.
C. Urbanization is associated with lower incidences of disease.
D. More advanced disease presentations are evident in urban and metropolitan areas.

10. Which statement regarding cancer-directed physical examination is true?
A. A physical examination is not necessary in asymptomatic individuals.
B. Cancer checkups should be conducted annually in asymptomatic individuals 39 years of age or younger.
C. Cancer checkups are not necessary for asymptomatic individuals over the age of 65.
D. Cancer checkups should be conducted annually in asymptomatic individuals age 40 and older.

11. Ms. W., a 20-year-old, presents to the clinic for her first well-woman examination. Which of the following statements regarding cervix cancer screening recommendations best reflects the information the nurse would need to review with Ms. W.?
A. Cervical cancer screening is recommended annually until there is a mini-mum of three consecutive normal Papanicolaou (Pap) smears.
B. Asymptomatic women need not be screened for cervical cancer.
C. Cervical cancer screening is recommended every 3 years for women under the age of 40.
D. There is no evidence that tobacco is a risk factor for cervical cancer.

12. The incidence of a disease is defined as
A. the number of cancer cases, both existing and new, during a specified time period in a defined population.
B. the number of deaths attributed to a cancer during a specified time period in a defined population.
C. the study of distribution and determinants of disease in a defined population.
D. the number of new cases of cancer during a specified time period in a defined population.

13. Appropriate education and follow-up care for the client with positive screening test results should include
A. explaining to the client that he/she has cancer.
B. scheduling annual follow-up for cancer screening.
C. identifying resources for cancer information and referral for further evaluation.
D. explaining to the client that the condition is terminal and he/she should get his/her affairs in order.

14. Which statement best describes selection bias?
A. Appearance of improved survival in screen-detected cases that results by merely lengthening the interval from diagnosis to death rather than lengthening life.
B. Bias that occurs if those individuals undergoing screening have better health habits than the general population, lowering mortality because of increased resistance to the disease or being more compliant with therapy.
C. Bias associated with a greater proportion of individuals who have less

aggressive disease, appearing to lengthen survival.

D. Bias created by the exclusion of individuals from screening with a history of excessive alcohol and tobacco use, which are known cancer risk factors.

15. Which of the following, if identified during the male genitalia examination, is considered suspicious for cancer?
    A. Testicular mass.
    B. Inguinal hernia.
    C. Undescended testes.
    D. Varicosities of the scrotal skin.

16. At what age does the American Cancer Society recommend that women at average risk for breast cancer begin annual mammography?
    A. 20.
    B. 30.
    C. 40.
    D. 50.

17. Carcinoembryonic antigen (CEA) is a tumor marker used to monitor what type of cancer?
    A. Colon.
    B. Leukemia.
    C. Sarcoma.
    D. Endometrial.

18. Which of the following tumor markers may be elevated in most types of cancer, is not routinely used as a diagnostic tool, but may be a helpful monitoring test?
    A. Lactate dehydrogenase (LDH).
    B. PSA.
    C. NSE.
    D. CEA.

19. A key component of the client history to be obtained during the cancer-directed screening examination is
    A. number of siblings.
    B. marital status.
    C. place of birth.
    D. medical and cancer history of relatives.

20. A cancer-directed physical examination should include the following:
    A. Assessment of cranial nerves.
    B. Assessment of the oral cavity.
    C. Assessment of muscle strength.
    D. Assessment of vision.

21. When conducting a clinical breast examination, which of the following findings would be considered suspicious for breast cancer?
    A. A firm, fixed mass.
    B. One breast that is smaller than the other.
    C. Breast tenderness upon palpation of the breasts.
    D. Chronic bilateral nipple inversion.

22. Which of the following is a useful technique to lower barriers to early cancer detection?
    A. Offer free cancer screening examinations each Saturday at your church.
    B. Use scare tactics to motivate individuals to undergo screening.
    C. Personalize recommendations based on individual history and risk profiles.
    D. Begin cancer prevention and early detection education in elementary school.

23. Which test for colorectal cancer screening is recommended every 5 years?
    A. Laparoscopy.
    B. Colonoscopy.
    C. Fecal occult blood test.
    D. Flexible sigmoidoscopy.

24. The efficacy of tumor markers for cancer diagnosis is often limited because
    A. the risks of testing do not outweigh the benefits.
    B. the tests are often cost-prohibitive.
    C. clients are often reluctant to undergo venipuncture.
    D. the result may not be elevated in every person with the cancer.

25. The percentage of persons with a negative screening test result who clearly do not have the disease being tested describes the
    A. specificity.
    B. sensitivity.
    C. negative predictive value.
    D. positive predictive value.

26. A comprehensive assessment of a client's symptoms describes the

A. social history.
B. review of systems.
C. medical history.
D. history of present illness.

27. The digital rectal examination (DRE) is performed annually for men over the age of 50 to screen for which of the following cancers?
A. Colon cancer.
B. Rectal cancer.
C. Testicular cancer.
D. Prostate cancer.

28. Which of the following statements regarding prostatic acid phosphatase (PAP) is true?
A. Elevation in PAP is always associated with prostate cancer.
B. PAP is used less frequently than PSA to diagnose prostate cancer.
C. PAP is a tumor marker used in conjunction with DRE to screen for prostate cancer.
D. PAP is a tumor marker used in conjunction with PSA to screen for prostate cancer.

29. Elevation of CA 19-9 is common for what cancer?
A. Pancreatic.
B. Breast.
C. Cervical.
D. Ovarian.

30. Marijuana use may result in elevated levels of which of the following tumor markers?
A. α-FP.
B. LDH.
C. CEA.
D. Human chorionic gonodotropin (HCG).

31. Which of the following tests is recommended every 10 years for the purpose of screening for colorectal cancer?
A. Colonoscopy.
B. Flexible sigmoidoscopy.
C. Fecal occult blood test.
D. Double-contrast barium enema.

32. What is the recommended interval for clinical breast examination in asymptomatic women between the ages of 20 and 39?
A. Annually.

B. Every 2 years.
C. Every 3 years.
D. Every 5 years.

33. The American Cancer Society recommends annual screening for cervical cancer begin no later than _____ years after a women initiates vaginal intercourse?
A. 1.
B. 2.
C. 3.
D. 4.

34. The American Cancer Society supports the discontinuation of cervical cancer screening in women with three or more normal Pap tests and no abnormal Pap tests within the past 10 years for women over the age of
A. 60.
B. 70.
C. 75.
D. 80.

35. When evaluating outcomes of cancer screening, both short-term and long-term measures are considered. Which of the following is an example of long-term measures for cancer screening?
A. Impact of early detection on quality of life.
B. Sensitivity and specificity of the screening test.
C. Cost of the screening test per cancer detected.
D. The number of individuals in a target population offered screening.

36. The best and most effective treatment for cancer is
A. surgery.
B. chemotherapy.
C. radiation therapy.
D. prevention or early detection.

37. The rationale for the development of risk profiles and screening guidelines is to
A. enhance screening efficacy and decrease costs.
B. promote uniform staging.
C. provide an estimate of the burden of the disease in a defined population.
D. improve the sensitivity and specificity of screening tests.

ANSWERS

1. *Answer:* B

Rationale: The purpose of annual mammography is to screen for one single condition: breast cancer. Mass screening refers to the process of screening an entire population or group. Selective or prescriptive screening looks for specific problems within a high-risk population, and multiphasic screening refers to an evaluation that occurs over an extended period of time.

2. *Answer:* C

Rationale: α-FP is produced by a developing fetus. When α-FP is elevated in adults, there may be an associated primary liver or germ cell cancer. CA 125 is a tumor marker for ovarian cancer. An elevation of CA 15-3 may occur with advanced breast cancer. NSE is most commonly used in clients with neuroblastoma or small-cell lung cancer.

3. *Answer:* A

Rationale: The use of tumor marker CA 27-29 to monitor for breast cancer recurrence is considered a process of surveillance for further disease. Secondary prevention is the act of screening individuals in an asymptomatic phase with the goal of diagnosing a condition at a stage when cure is possible. Diagnosis is the process of identifying the disease, and treatment would be planned if there were evidence of a recurrence based on surveillance tests.

4. *Answer:* C

Rationale: The relative risk is an estimate of the increased probability of cancer development based on the amount of exposure to the associated risk factors. The amount of preventable disease in the absence of all identified risk factors is the attributable risk. The risk of a cancer development associated with a hereditary predisposition is based on the assessment of an individual's family history of cancer. Case fatality is the number of persons with a certain type of cancer who die of the disease during a specified period of time.

5. *Answer:* C

Rationale: Routine screening for skin cancer has not been proven to effectively reduce morbidity or mortality of the disease. Data on cervical, breast, and colorectal cancer screening have revealed a reduction in mortality when implemented as recommended by current guidelines.

6. *Answer:* D

Rationale: All individuals at average risk of developing colorectal cancer should begin screening at the age of 50. Screening after the age of 60 is not as effective and may result in delayed cancer diagnosis. Colorectal cancer screening at age 40 may be considered for individuals with an increased risk for the disease. Individuals with a family history of colorectal cancer or adenomas in one or more first-degree relatives are at moderate risk for developing the disease. A history of inflammatory conditions of the colon, such as Crohn's disease, also increases the risk for colorectal cancer. Women with a history of breast, ovarian, or endometrial cancer are at some increased risk. Colorectal cancer screening is likely to be initiated early and performed more frequently for those individuals at increased risk. Personalized guidelines would be initiated and be dependent on risk assessment.

7. *Answer:* B

Rationale: The CAUTION mnemonic reminds clients and health care providers of common symptoms that may be related to cancer. They include **C**hange in bowel or bladder habits, **A** sore that does not heal, **U**nusual bleeding or discharge, **T**hickening or lump in breast or elsewhere, **I**ndigestion or difficulty swallowing, **O**bvious change in wart or mole, **N**agging cough or hoarseness.

8. *Answer:* B

Rationale: The PSA may be elevated in men with benign prostate conditions, resulting in false-positive results. Men of average risk for prostate cancer should begin PSA and digital rectal examinations at the age of 50.

According to the U.S. Preventive Services Task Force, there is not sufficient evidence to recommend the use of PSA to screen for prostate cancer.

9. *Answer:* B
Rationale: Individuals of lower socioeconomic status often lack the resources that allow them to obtain cancer screening. Increased tobacco use is often seen in poorer populations. Advanced disease presentation is more common in rural or lower socioeconomic groups. Urbanization is associated with increased incidences of disease.

10. *Answer:* D
Rationale: Annual physical examinations directed at screening for cancer should begin at the age of 40 for asymptomatic individuals. Individuals between the ages of 20 and 39 should be encouraged to have a cancer screening examination every 3 years. There is currently no upper age limit for conducting cancer-directed physical examinations. Asymptomatic individuals should be actively screened for cancer with the goal of diagnosing the condition early. Individuals with symptoms that could be related to cancer should be evaluated based on the presenting complaint.

11. *Answer:* A
Rationale: Women should be screened annually for cervical cancer. If the client meets certain criteria, less frequent cervical cancer screening may be considered. Symptoms of cervical cancer do not typically occur until late stages of the disease, so women should be educated on the benefits of screening. There is significant evidence that tobacco use is associated with an increased risk for cervical cancer.

12. *Answer:* D
Rationale: Incidence is defined as the number of new cases of cancer in a given population within a specified time period. Prevalence is defined as both existing and new cancer cases during a specified time period in a defined population. The study of distribution and determinants of disease is the definition of epidemiology, and the number of deaths attributed to a cancer during a specified time period in a defined population is considered the mortality rate.

13. *Answer:* C
Rationale: The client should be assisted to identify resources for cancer information, and a referral for further evaluation and diagnosis should be initiated. Follow-up in 1 year may result in a missed cancer diagnosis. The significance of a positive test result should be reviewed. The client should understand that a positive test result does not always lead to a cancer diagnosis. The nurse may speak with the client regarding the accuracy of the screening test and other conditions that may result in a positive test and give him/her information about the diagnosis process.

14. *Answer:* B
Rationale: Selection bias may occur when individuals participate in screening programs because they generally have better health habits than the general population. Better health may contribute to improved outcomes after a cancer diagnosis. When a bias is associated with the appearance of improved survival resulting from a longer interval between diagnosis and death, this is considered a lead-time bias. Length bias is when a greater proportion of individuals undergoing screening have less aggressive disease. Exclusion of individuals from screening because of excessive alcohol and tobacco use is not a common practice, although these individuals may be less likely to actively participate in cancer screening.

15. *Answer:* A
Rationale: A palpable testicular mass may be indicative of testicular cancer, and further evaluation is warranted promptly. History of an undescended testis may increase the risk of testicular cancer, but it is not a symptom of testicular cancer. An inguinal hernia is a significant finding to communicate to the client but is not a symptom of cancer. Varicosities of the scrotal skin are a benign and common finding.

16. *Answer:* C
Rationale: The American Cancer Society recommends that women ages 20 to 39 have a clinical breast examination performed every 3 years. Beginning at age 40, women should

have a clinical breast examination accompanied by a mammogram to screen for breast cancer.

17. *Answer:* A
Rationale: CEA is a tumor marker commonly used to monitor colorectal cancer, especially when there is metastasis. CEA is not effective for monitoring the progression of leukemia, sarcoma, or endometrial cancer.

18. *Answer:* A
Rationale: LDH is not routinely used to assist in the diagnosis of a specific type of cancer but may be helpful in surveillance after treatment. PSA is a tumor marker widely used in men over 50 years of age to screen for prostate cancer. NSE is a tumor marker used in neuroblastoma and small-cell lung cancer. CEA is a tumor marker for colon cancer.

19. *Answer:* D
Rationale: Assessment of family history is an important part of the risk assessment and screening process. The number of siblings, the client's marital status, and place of birth represent important information about the client's social history but are of less importance.

20. *Answer:* B
Rationale: A thorough evaluation of the oral cavity is an essential component of the cancer-directed physical examination. The mucous membranes and tongue should be inspected for color and integrity and presence of lesions and plaques. The tongue should be palpated for masses and tenderness. Although assessment of cranial nerves, vision, and muscle strength is an important component of a comprehensive physical examination, it is not a key component of a cancer-directed physical.

21. *Answer:* A
Rationale: A firm, fixed mass identified in the breast tissue is considered suspicious for a breast cancer until proven otherwise. It is not uncommon for women to have breasts that are different sizes. Breast tenderness in conjunction with an otherwise normal breast examination is not considered suspicious for breast cancer. New-onset, asymmetric nipple inversion may be associated with a breast cancer,

but chronic bilateral nipple inversion is not considered suspicious.

22. *Answer:* C
Rationale: Providing clients with an individualized risk assessment based on their personal and family history helps to lower perceived barriers to cancer screening. Scare tactics are unlikely to be an effective motivator for cancer screening and may result in increased anxiety about a potential cancer diagnosis. Introducing children to healthy lifestyle practices and cancer prevention recommendations (i.e., use of sunscreen to prevent skin cancer) can be beneficial. Formal cancer screening is not necessary until young adulthood. Free cancer screening serves as an opportunity to reach out to a population to facilitate cancer screening but may not result in ongoing screening over an individual's lifetime.

23. *Answer:* D
Rationale: Flexible sigmoidoscopy is recommended every 5 years to screen for colorectal cancer. Fecal occult blood testing is recommended annually. It may be used alone or in combination with endoscopy examination. Colonoscopy is recommended every 10 years, and laparoscopy is not a screening test for colorectal cancer.

24. *Answer:* D
Rationale: Not all individuals with a particular cancer will have an associated elevation of the tumor marker. The sensitivity of tumor marker testing varies. The cost of tumor marker testing varies. Although the cost may prohibit individuals of lower socioeconomic status from screening, the cost of the tumor marker does not decrease efficacy. The risk associated with venipuncture required for tumor marker testing is minimal, and clients typically tolerate it well.

25. *Answer:* C
Rationale: The percentage of persons with a negative screening test result without disease describes negative predictive value. Specificity is a measure of the probability that a test result will be positive if the disease is present. Sensitivity is a measure of the probability that a test result will be negative if the disease is not present. Positive predictive value is the

percentage of persons with a positive screening test who have the disease.

26. *Answer:* B
Rationale: The review of systems consists of a comprehensive review of the organ systems to assess for symptoms that may be associated with cancer. The social history is the assessment of a client's personal history, marital status, occupation, and tobacco, drug, and alcohol use. The medical history serves to document any previous or chronic medical problems. History of present illness is a description of the client's current problem and reason for visit.

27. *Answer:* D
Rationale: DRE and PSA are used in combination to screen men 50 years of age and older for prostate cancer. Although the DRE is often performed during a general cancer screening examination, it offers a very limited assessment of colon. Endoscopic evaluation is the preferred method of screening for colorectal cancer. DRE is not an exam that is used to screen for testicular cancer.

28. *Answer:* B
Rationale: PAP is a tumor marker that is less frequently used than PSA to screen for or diagnose prostate cancer. PAP elevations may be associated with other types of cancer and benign conditions. The PSA is used in conjunction with DRE to screen for prostate cancer. The PSA and PAP are not commonly used together for screening purposes.

29. *Answer:* A
Rationale: Elevated levels of CA 19-9 have been identified in individuals with pancreatic cancer and other gastrointestinal malignancies. Breast, cervical, and ovarian cancer does not result in elevations of CA 19-9.

30. *Answer:* D
Rationale: Marijuana use may elevate levels of HCG. This phenomenon is not reported with α-FP, LDH, or CEA.

31. *Answer:* A
Rationale: Colonoscopy is recommended every 10 years to screen for colon cancer. Modalities such as flexible sigmoidoscopy and double-contrast barium enema are recommended every 5 years. Fecal occult blood testing is recommended annually and may be used alone or in combination with flexible sigmoidoscopy, colonoscopy, and double-contrast barium enema.

32. *Answer:* C
Rationale: The American Cancer Society recommends clinical breast examination every 3 years for asymptomatic women between the ages of 20 and 39.

33. *Answer:* C
Rationale: The American Cancer Society recommends that cervical cancer screening begin within 3 years of initiation of vaginal intercourse but no later than 21 years of age.

34. *Answer:* B
Rationale: The American Cancer Society supports the discontinuation of Pap tests in women over the age of 70 who meet the appropriate criteria. The decision to stop screening for cervical cancer is made at the discretion of the health care provider and client.

35. *Answer:* A
Rationale: The impact of early detection through cancer screening on quality of life is a long-term measure of effectiveness. Determining the sensitivity and specificity of the screening test, cost per cancer detected, and the number of individuals offered screening are all short-term measures.

36. *Answer:* D
Rationale: Prevention and early detection are the best and most effective treatments for cancer.

37. *Answer:* A
Rationale: The other options are not rationales for developing risk profiles and screening guidelines. Staging and test sensitivity and specificity are irrelevant. Option C describes an aspect of prevalence.

BIBLIOGRAPHY

American Cancer Society. (2004). *Cancer facts & figures – 2004*. Atlanta: Author.

Daly, M. (1999). NCCN Practice Guidelines: Genetics/familiar high-risk cancer screening. *Oncology 13*, 161-183.

Jennings-Dozier, K., & Mahon, S.M. (Eds.). (2002). *Cancer prevention, detection, and control: A nursing perspective*. Pittsburgh: Oncology Nursing Society.

Mahon, S.M. (1998). Cancer risk assessment: Conceptual considerations for clinical practice. *Oncology Nursing Forum 25*, 1535-1547.

Mahon, S.M. (2000). Principles of cancer prevention and early detection. *Clinical Journal of Oncology Nursing 4*, 169-176.

National Cancer Institute Web site. Available at: http:/ *www.cancernet.nci.nih.gov.* Accessed June 2003.

National Comprehensive Cancer Network (NCCN). (2003). Breast cancer screening and diagnosis: clinical practice guidelines in oncology. *Journal of the National Comprehensive Network 1*, 242-263.

U.S. Preventive Health Task Force Prevention Guidelines. Available at: http:/*www.ahrq.gov/clinic/prevnew.htm.* Accessed July 2003.

NOTES

PART EIGHT

PROFESSIONAL PERFORMANCE

44 Application of the *Statement on the Scope and Standards of Oncology Nursing Practice* and Evidence-Based Practice

LINDA U. KREBS

1. The Standards of Care from the Oncology Nursing Society (ONS) *Statement on the Scope and Standards of Oncology Nursing Practice* can be used to
   - A. identify performance roles for advanced practice nurses.
   - B. test quality assurance protocols.
   - C. assist in the development of performance appraisal tools.
   - D. meet Joint Commission on Accreditation of Healthcare Organizations (JCAHO) standards.

2. The 14 high-incidence problem areas in oncology nursing cited in the *Statement on the Scope and Standards of Oncology Nursing Practice* are
   - A. key areas in which oncology nurses assess, plan, and intervene.
   - B. the problems with the highest incidence rates in cancer care.
   - C. problems that most often affect the client in the acute care setting.
   - D. clinical indicators that are measurable dimensions of the quality of client care.

3. Professional Performance Standard II, Practice Evaluation, states that the oncology nurse evaluates his or her own nursing practice in relation to professional practice standards and relevant statutes and regulations. Which of the following statements reflects a measurement criterion that indicates this standard has been met?

The oncology nurse
   - A. shares knowledge and skills with colleagues and others during practice.
   - B. seeks regular, constructive feedback regarding own practice and role performance from peers, professional colleagues, clients, and others.
   - C. collaborates with other health care providers in educational programs and consultation, management, and research endeavors as opportunities arise.
   - D. evaluates factors related to safety, effectiveness, and cost when two or more practice options would result in the same expected client outcome.

4. Standard of Care III, Outcome Identification, states that the oncology nurse identifies expected outcomes individualized to the client. Which of the following measurement criteria supports this standard? The oncology nurse
   - A. communicates the client's responses with the health care team.
   - B. ensures that expected outcomes provide direction for continuity of care.
   - C. incorporates preventive, therapeutic, rehabilitative, palliative, and comforting nursing actions into the plan of care.
   - D. reviews and revises the nursing diagnoses, expected outcomes, and plan of

care based on the findings of the evaluation.

5. Using evidence to influence clinical practice is a multistep process. After clarifying the problem of interest, the next step in the process is
    A. conducting a literature review of relevant research.
    B. getting "buy in" from colleagues and administration.
    C. identifying the information needed to solve the problem.
    D. developing a clinical protocol to address the problem

6. In critiquing a research report, before making a decision about the scientific validity and clinical usefulness of the report, the oncology nurse's evaluation should focus on
    A. the problem statement and methodology.
    B. the data collection and analysis plans.
    C. the methodology and conclusions.
    D. every component of the research report.

7. The oncology nurse generalist's most common role in oncology nursing research is
    A. as the principal investigator overseeing the research protocol.
    B. helping to implement the protocol through client accrual and data collection.
    C. evaluating the outcomes of the protocol.
    D. interpreting the outcomes for use in clinical practice.

8. Evidence-based practice (EBP) can be best explained as practice that
    A. incorporates both research-based and nonresearch-based evidence.
    B. is based solely on findings from multiple, randomized, controlled clinical trials.
    C. takes the outcome of a single research study and uses it in practice with a specific client.
    D. uses previous clinical experiences and client outcomes to inform current practice.

9. The components of an oncology standard of care include
    A. statement, rationale, measurement criteria.
    B. statement, explanation, evaluation measures.
    C. standard, rationale, evaluation measures.
    D. standard, explanation, measurement criteria.

10. The research priority ranked highest in the ONS Year 2000 Research Priorities Survey is
    A. neutropenia/immunosuppression.
    B. pain.
    C. fatigue.
    D. prevention/risk reduction.

11. For the oncology client, the ONS standards ensure that
    A. nursing care will be the same from nurse to nurse.
    B. the client will be able to participate in aspects of care.
    C. the nurse has an adequate education.
    D. the client will receive state-of-the-art care.

12. The primary goal of EBP is to
    A. guide nursing interventions to enhance quality and outcomes.
    B. ensure new findings are incorporated into nursing care.
    C. develop protocols of care for use in multiple settings.
    D. use best evidence to develop clinical algorithms.

13. A Phase IV treatment clinical trial is designed to evaluate
    A. drug toxicities.
    B. what tumor will be responsive to a drug.
    C. new areas of use after Food and Drug Administration (FDA) approval.
    D. activity of a new combination in relation to the standard of treatment.

14. A Phase I treatment clinical trial is designed to evaluate
    A. drug toxicities.
    B. what tumor will be responsive to a drug.

C. new areas of use after FDA approval.

D. activity of a new combination in relation to the standard of treatment.

15. The overall title for the research methodology that explores phenomena is

A. quantitative.

B. qualitative.

C. historical.

D. ethnographic.

NOTES

ANSWERS

1. *Answer:* C
   Rationale: The standards can be used to develop performance appraisal tools for the oncology nurse generalist. They are not designed for the advanced practice nurse (see the ONS *Statement on the Scope and Standards of Advanced Practice Nursing in Oncology)*, nor are they designed to test quality assurance protocols or meet JCAHO standards.

2. *Answer:* A
   Rationale: The 14 high-incidence priority areas refer to clinical problems that oncology clients most often experience, regardless of setting. They are integrated throughout the standards and are the focus of assessment, intervention, and evaluation.

3. *Answer:* B
   Rationale: Although all four options are measurement criteria for the Standards of Professional Performance, Option B is the only one that pertains to practice evaluation.

4. *Answer:* B
   Rationale: According to the Standards, Option B supports the outcome standard, Option A supports implementation, Option C supports planning, and Option D supports evaluation.

5. *Answer:* C
   Rationale: After the problem of interest has been clearly identified, the next step is to identify the information needed to solve the problem. Once the information has been identified, then the literature review is conducted. Getting "buy in" from colleagues and the administration is essential but is not part of the process to use evidence to inform clinical practice.

6. *Answer:* D
   Rationale: All components of the research report are important and need to be evaluated. Focusing on only one or a few components of the report may lead to an inaccurate or inadequate evaluation of the evidence.

7. *Answer:* B
   Rationale: The most likely role for the oncology generalist nurse is in helping to implement the research protocol through such roles as data collection and client accrual. The other roles are more common for the advanced practice nurse or a nurse with advanced educational preparation in nursing research.

8. *Answer:* A
   Rationale: Identifying the best evidence for practice requires evaluation of evidence that comes from both research studies and from evidence based on other aspects of disease and clinical care. A single study or merely the incorporation of previous experience or practice outcomes is not sufficient evidence upon which to base practice changes.

9. *Answer:* A
   Rationale: The components of the standard include the statement, the rationale, and the measurement criteria.

10. *Answer:* B
    Rationale: All of the items are among the top 10 research priorities from the ONS Year 2000 Research Priorities Survey; however, pain was identified as the top priority.

11. *Answer:* B
    Rationale: One of the most important aspects of the standards is the mandate for client participation in health promotion, restoration , and maintenance.

12. *Answer:* A
    Rationale: While the outcome of EBP should lead to incorporation of new findings into practice and the development of standardized protocols, practices, and algorithms, the primary goal is to guide nursing interventions to enhance quality and outcomes.

13. *Answer:* C
    Rationale: The primary goal of a Phase IV treatment clinical trial is to evaluate new uses (different tumor types or settings such as outpatient use, etc.) after a drug has received FDA

approval. Phase I trials evaluate toxicities, Phase II trials identify tumor types in which the drug is most likely to be effective, and Phase III trials compare the current standard of care with a new drug or combination that is hoped to be better or have fewer side effects.

14. *Answer:* A

Rationale: The primary goal of a Phase I treatment clinical trial is to evaluate the new drug/compound's toxicities. Phase II trials identify tumor types in which the drug is most likely to be effective, Phase III trials compare the current standard of care with a new drug or combination that is hoped to be better or have fewer side effects, and Phase IV trials evaluate new uses after FDA approval.

15. *Answer:* B

Rationale: Qualitative methodology is the global title given to research investigations that look at phenomena or try to gain understanding of the area of interest. Quantitative research is a formal, objective, systematic process used to describe and test relationships and to examine the cause-and-effect relationships among variables. Historical research studies the recent or remote past. By studying the past, researchers often gain insight into present and future issues and trends. Ethnographic research studies issues related to culture.

BIBLIOGRAPHY

Brant, J.M., & Wickham, R.S. (Eds.). (2004). *Statement on the scope and standards of oncology nursing practice.* Pittsburgh: Oncology Nursing Society.

Burns, N., & Grove, S.K. (2003). *Understanding nursing research* (3rd ed.). Philadelphia: W.B. Saunders.

Cooke, L., & Grant, M. (2002). Support for evidence-based practice. *Seminars in Oncology Nursing 18,* 71-78.

Cope, D. (2003). Evidence-based practice: Making it happen in your clinical setting. *Clinical Journal of Oncology Nursing 7,* 97-98.

Goode, C. J. (2003). Evidence-based practice. In K.S. Oman, M.E. Krugman, & R.M. Fink (Eds.). *Nursing research secrets.* Philadelphia: Hanley & Belfus, pp. 7-14.

Krebs, L.U. (2005). Application of the *Statement on the Scope and Standards of Oncology Nursing Practice and Evidence-Based Practice.* In J.K. Itano & K.N. Taoka (Eds.). *Core curriculum for oncology nursing* (4th ed.). St. Louis, Elsevier, p. 875-892.

Mast, M. (2000). Evidence-based practice: What it is, what it isn't. *ONS News 15*(6), 1, 4, 5.

Mooney, K. (2001). Advocating for quality cancer care: Making evidence-based practice a reality. *Oncology Nursing Forum 28*(2 Supp.), 17-21.

Oman, K.S. (2003). Reading, understanding, and critiquing research reports. In K.S. Oman, M.E. Krugman, & R.M. Fink (Eds.). *Nursing research secrets.* Philadelphia: Hanley & Belfus, pp. 37-45.

45 The Education Process

CAROL S. BLECHER

Select the best answer for each of the following questions:

1. A 48-year-old woman is discharged after a lumpectomy for a newly diagnosed malignant breast tumor. What would her priority learning needs include?
   - A. Education regarding postmastectomy wound care.
   - B. Education regarding breast self-examination.
   - C. Education regarding breast cancer and its treatment.
   - D. Education regarding follow-up mammography.

2. The purpose of the educational component of nursing practice is to help people acquire the knowledge they need in order to
   - A. comply with the physician's orders.
   - B. learn what health professionals believe they need to know.
   - C. understand the particular diagnosis.
   - D. participate in their treatment decisions and self-care.

3. A nurse prepares an educational plan for a client who is about to receive chemotherapy. The client verbalizes a desire to continue working during the treatment. Which of the following statements represents an important learning principle in addressing the client's needs?

   A. Learning should be subject-centered, not client-centered.
   B. Learner's needs should receive priority.
   C. Learning is often negated by life experiences.
   D. Learning occurs when the teaching plan is completed.

4. A nurse is responsible for developing an educational program for clients starting their first regimen of chemotherapy. Outcomes must be identified to evaluate the program. Which of the following statements represents an appropriate outcome? Upon completion of this program the client will be able to
   - A. describe strategies for managing common side effects of chemotherapy.
   - B. understand the role of chemotherapy in cancer treatment.
   - C. learn about community resources available for cancer care.
   - D. know the names of the chemotherapy drugs he/she will be receiving.

5. Participation in cancer-related public education is an important nursing activity because
   - A. these programs have potential impact on cancer prevention, incidence, morbidity, and mortality.

B. these programs enhance the professional image of cancer nursing.

C. the participants' fear of cancer will be modified.

D. the competence of the nurse as a cancer-client educator will improve.

6. Mr. A. had a hemicolectomy with colostomy 2 days ago. In assessing his readiness for attending a 15-minute teaching session on ostomy care, you would be most interested in

A. his education level.

B. his pain level.

C. his ability to walk.

D. his socioeconomic status.

7. Which of the following emotional states increases a client's receptivity to learning?

A. Mild anxiety.

B. Anger.

C. Grief.

D. Fear.

8. A busy, private practice nurse is educating a client regarding self-administration of interferon. In choosing a place to conduct the session, the nurse takes into consideration that

A. the client has excellent family support.

B. the insurance is paying for the medication.

C. the area chosen is conducive to learning.

D. the client is a college professor.

9. Mrs. J. is hospitalized for shortness of breath. A mass is seen on chest x-ray, and a biopsy reveals non–small cell lung cancer (NSCLC). She smokes two packs of cigarettes per day and has for the last 20 years. Her mother died of lung cancer when Mrs. J. was 15. How would you begin the educational process with this client?

A. Teach Mrs. J. about the pathophysiology of lung cancer.

B. Educate Mrs. J. regarding the causes of lung cancer.

C. Enroll Mrs. J. in a smoking cessation program.

D. Ask Mrs. J. what she knows about lung cancer and about her past experiences with cancer.

10. You are meeting with a client for the second time for ostomy teaching after colon surgery. During the last session you reviewed basic information with the client, and he seemed eager to learn how to manage his ostomy. You gave him printed material, which he said he would read later when it was quiet. Today you ask the client if he has read the material, and the reply is, "My eyes were blurry, so I gave it to my wife to read." You might suspect that

A. this client is not interested in learning about ostomy care.

B. this client may have literacy problems.

C. the client has a low IQ.

D. the client is learning impaired.

11. The nurse is responsible for developing a public education program regarding prostate cancer. Information that she might need to assist her in the development of this program would include

A. target audience.

B. date and time of the program.

C. names of the individuals who will be attending.

D. knowledge of the JCAHO standards.

12. In developing staff education programs in the ambulatory setting, the nurse educator would do which of the following first?

A. Determine a meeting time and place.

B. Perform a needs assessment to identify the staff's educational needs.

C. Comply with the JCAHO standard requiring that ambulatory care meet the same quality standards as inpatient care.

D. Certify chemotherapy competency as needed.

13. Printed materials should be written at what reading level:

A. 5th to 6th grade.

B. 7th to 9th grade.

C. 10th to 12th grade.

D. College level.

14. When planning public education programs, the nurse should take into consideration the following factors:

A. Problems identified by the nurse, behaviors related to the health problem, development and implementation of a program, and evaluation of the program.

B. Problems of concern to the community, specific behaviors related to the health problem, development and implementation of a program, and evaluation of the program.

C. Problems of concern to the community, general behaviors that might address the health problem, and presentation of a program.

D. Problems identified by the nurse, general behaviors that might address the health problem, presentation of a program, and evaluation of the program.

15. Some of the barriers to public education include the fact that
   A. people react favorably to fear.
   B. people believe that science is truth.
   C. people are future-oriented.
   D. health risk is an intangible concept.

16. One of the initial steps involved in planning a health education program is:
   A. promotion and distribution of materials.
   B. evaluation of the results of the program.
   C. writing goals and objectives.
   D. development of materials.

17. A method for producing reading materials that are easy to read includes
   A. using primarily graphics.
   B. using lengthy paragraphs.
   C. using abbreviations and lots of medical terminology.
   D. using short words and sentences.

18. Some resources for cancer client education materials include
   A. Chemotherapy and You, Radiation and You, Eating Hints.
   B. Y-ME, I Can Cope, Reach for Recovery.
   C. The National Cancer Institute, The American Cancer Society, and The National Coalition for Cancer Survivorship.
   D. *Oncology Nursing Forum, CA:A Cancer Journal for Clinicians, Cancer Nursing: An International Journal for Cancer Care.*

19. One of the mistakes that is often made when initiating client education includes
   A. assessing the person's current level of knowledge.
   B. teaching people what the nurse thinks the client should know.
   C. individualizing teaching to accommodate the individual's background, attitudes, and motivation.
   D. coordinating teaching efforts across the continuum of care.

20. When educating the older client, the following should be taken into consideration:
   A. The need for others to take control and guide them.
   B. Decreased intellectual ability.
   C. Differences in culture, language, and physical impairments.
   D. No fear of being tested on the information presented.

ANSWERS

1. *Answer:* C

   Rationale: People need information that addresses their immediate concerns. This woman has a new diagnosis of breast cancer, and her immediate need would be to learn about breast cancer and its treatment. She does not need education regarding mastectomy, because her surgery was lumpectomy. It is too early to begin teaching about continued breast self-examination and follow-up mammography, because this would not be a priority for the client at this time.

2. *Answer:* D

   Rationale: The overall purpose of client education is to enable full participation, acceptance of responsibility, and shared decision making. Compliance often implies instructions that the client is expected to obey. Client education focuses on empowering the individual for self-care.

3. *Answer:* B

   Rationale: Learning occurs when a person perceives a need to learn something; therefore learner-identified needs should receive priority. Learning should be problem-centered, is influenced by accumulated life experiences, and may not be accomplished even with instruction.

4. *Answer:* A

   Rationale: A well-stated expected outcome identifies a behavior or an action that the learner will begin to do. Understanding, learning, and knowing are not actions and are difficult to measure.

5. *Answer:* A

   Rationale: Participation in public cancer-related programs is believed to positively affect cancer prevention and detection activities and ultimately cancer morbidity and mortality.

6. *Answer:* B

   Rationale: Physical responses such as pain can decrease motivation and receptiveness to learning.

7. *Answer:* A

   Rationale: Research indicates that mild or moderate anxiety may be helpful to learning. Emotional responses including anger, fear, and grief may decrease motivation, ability to concentrate, and receptiveness to learning.

8. *Answer:* C

   Rationale: One of the criteria for client education resources is that an environment conducive to learning is maintained. It is a strength that the client is well educated and has good family support and good insurance. All of these factors affect the learning process, but in a busy practice there must be a private quiet area with good lighting for client education.

9. *Answer:* D

   Rationale: Theories of adult learning indicate that people have had life experiences that are resources on which to base new learning. These experiences must be acknowledged and dealt with before new learning can take place. Adult learners rarely want an anatomy lesson when what they need are the basics. The nurse would not want to cause/increase guilt with the implication that Mrs. J. is responsible for causing her cancer, and her consent would be necessary to enroll her in a smoking cessation program.

10. *Answer:* B

    Rationale: About one adult in five is functionally illiterate — with poor reading skills. Clients need to be assessed for literacy. The client appeared eager to learn the first time, so the problem would not be interest. Individuals with low literacy are not necessarily learning impaired, nor do they necessarily have low IQ. Low literacy is due more to poverty, unemployment, minority/immigrant status, and advanced age. People with low literacy skills can function well by compensating in other ways for their lack of reading skills.

11. *Answer:* A

    Rationale: Knowledge regarding the target audience will enable the nurse to present appropriate data regarding risk factors and community resources. The nurse will develop material that is respectful of the religious, cultural, and ethnic beliefs and practices of the target audience. Knowing the date and time of the program and the JCAHO standards is important, but it will not help in developing a program for a specific audience. Participant names are not helpful in program development.

12. *Answer:* B
Rationale: The educator would perform a needs assessment before the development of staff education programs. The educator would need to determine a time and meeting place, but that activity would not affect program development. In developing programs the educator is striving to comply with JCAHO standards, but JCAHO does not dictate the content of programs. Certifying chemotherapy competence is certainly one of the programs that is developed, but ongoing education is the major focus.

13. *Answer:* A
Rationale: One in five Americans reads at the 5th grade reading level or below, so materials need to be written at this level. Much of our printed material is written on an 8th to 9th grade level, and some of it is on the 9th to 11th grade or 12th grade level, which means that the material is overwhelming for much of the population.

14. *Answer:* B
Rationale: An organizational framework that provides a framework for health education includes the identification of problems that are of concern to people within a community, specific behaviors that are health-related and will address the identified problem, and, as with all educational activities, the program must be individualized for the target community and evaluated after presentation to ensure that it meets the needs of the community. Problems identified by the nurse may not be pertinent to the community. Behaviors must be specifically identified; generalizations cannot be measured and will not demonstrate the effectiveness of the program. Programs must be developed specifically for the population targeted, just as all educational efforts are specifically targeted to the person or group being addressed.

15. *Answer:* D
Rationale: The National Cancer Institute has identified the fact that health risk is an intangible concept. Most people underestimate their risk of developing cancer; they believe that it "will not happen to them." People do not react favorably to fear. When placed in a fearful situation, people will deny. People doubt science and do not believe in the predictive ability of science. People lack a future orientation, especially the lower socioeconomic population. Individuals have problems changing their behaviors, especially if they feel that cancer will not happen to them.

16. *Answer:* C
Rationale: In Stage 1 of program planning the nurse would develop written goals and objectives. These will identify the purpose of the program. Development and testing of materials will follow once there are goals and objectives. Promotion and distribution of materials occur during the implementation phase, and the evaluation occurs after the program has been implemented.

17. *Answer:* D
Rationale: Materials given to clients should have short words (two syllables or less) and short sentences for simplicity. Paragraphs should be short and limited to one idea. Abbreviations should not be used at all, and medical terminology should be explained in layman's terms. The text should be broken up with the use of graphics, and it is useful to repeat the same information in print, pictorial, and graphic formats.

18. *Answer:* C
Rationale: Option C is a listing of some of the resources for client education materials. Option A consists of the names of some printed material that can be obtained for the client from the National Cancer Institute. Option B is a listing of some support services available to clients. Option D lists some professional cancer journals.

19. *Answer:* B
Rationale: Client education should always be individualized to meet the needs of the client, not the nurse. The nurse should always assess clients to determine what they

are ready and willing to learn, as opposed to teaching what the nurse thinks they should know. The nurse should always assess current level of knowledge as well as client background, attitudes, and motivation to learn. Teaching efforts must be coordinated across the continuum of care from inpatient to outpatient and home care or hospice

20. *Answer:* C

Rationale: As with all clients, the nurse should consider the cultural and language differences when educating the older adult. Language differences should be addressed with attempts to provide materials in the person's primary language. Older individuals may have hearing or visual losses caused by aging, which must be considered when planning educational activities. Older adults do not have a decrease in intellectual ability, although they may learn more slowly than younger people, and they may have concerns and be uncomfortable in testing situations.

Older adults are used to being in control of their lives, and they have no need or desire for this control to be taken away from them.

BIBLIOGRAPHY

Agre, P. (2004). The education process. In J.K. Itano and K.N. Taoka (Eds.). *Core curriculum for oncology nursing* St. Louis Elsevier, pp. 893-898.

Blecher, C.S. (Ed.). (2004). *Standards of oncology education: Patient/significant other and public.* Pittsburgh: Oncology Nursing Society.

Doak, C., Doak, L., & Root, J. (1996). *Teaching patients with low literacy skills* (2nd ed.). Philadelphia: J.B. Lippincott.

Jacobs, L.A. (2003). *Standards of oncology nursing education: Generalist and advanced practice levels* (3rd ed.). Pittsburgh: Oncology Nursing Society.

Rankin, S.H., & Stallings, K.D. (2001). *Patient education: Principles and practice* (4th ed.) Philadelphia: J.B. Lippincott.

Yarbro, C.H., Frogge, M.H., Goodman, M., & Groenwald, S.L. (2000). *Cancer nursing: Principles and practice* (5th ed.). Sudbury, MA: Jones and Bartlett Publishers.

NOTES

46 Legal Issues Influencing Cancer Care

KIM K. KUEBLER

1. What primary source of law serves as the basis for most malpractice litigation?
   - A. Statutes.
   - B. Legislation.
   - C. Common law.
   - D. Administrative law.

2. State-specific definitions of nursing practice are found through
   - A. licensure.
   - B. credentialing.
   - C. nurse practice acts.
   - D. required continuing education.

3. A nurse applies evidence-based practice and participates in the symptom management of a client dying from metastatic lung cancer. The client's family blames the nurse, who administered opiates, believing it contributed to client weakness, and threaten legal action. The nurse feels secure with her clinical decision making because she
   - A. practices under protocol.
   - B. is familiar with the current literature.
   - C. is a member of her state nursing organization.
   - D. follows the nurse practice acts and professional standards of care.

4. A cognitively impaired client who is unable to participate in his/her medical decision making can rely on appropriate medical care by having a(n)

   - A. legal will.
   - B. insurance policy.
   - C. durable power of attorney and advance directive.
   - D. organ and tissue donation.

5. A registered nurse who calls in a new prescription for her client without a physician order is an example of
   - A. duty.
   - B. malpractice.
   - C. negligence.
   - D. breach of duty.

6. Litigation can result from the nurse's actions as described in question 5 and will most likely involve placing the nurse in what legal situation or action?
   - A. Trial by jury.
   - B. Institutional sanctions.
   - C. Out-of-court settlement.
   - D. Professional sanctions by state board of nursing.

7. Professional documents used in legal decision making to establish minimal standards of care include state-specific nurse practice acts and
   - A. statutes.
   - B. licensure requirements.
   - C. professional standards of care.
   - D. state-determined competencies required for practice.

8. Many health care agencies act to reduce liability stemming from the hiring of independent contractors by
    A. providing a wide range of benefits.
    B. employing fair labor practices.
    C. identifying the professional as a contract employee.
    D. equitable hiring and promotion practice.

9. A client, dying from advanced disease, follows all of the instructions given to him by the nurse, who is an independent contractor for a home health care agency, though that is never revealed to the client. After death, the client's family files a lawsuit against the home health care agency, believing the care was inappropriate. The family is acting on its belief that
    A. the nurse has violated protocol.
    B. the home health care agency is incompetent.
    C. the nurse did not adequately evaluate the client's symptoms.
    D. the nurse had apparent authority to act on behalf of the home health care agency.

10. A "no solicitation" rule enforced in a health care institution suggests?
    A. Fair labor standards.
    B. Fair and competitive wages.
    C. No discrimination of sex, race, and religion.
    D. A way to inhibit union solicitation within the health care agency.

11. The nurse manager often calls the night staff while intoxicated. She comes to work late and is often reluctant to follow through on important tasks. You are hesitant to address her behaviors of addiction but understand the importance of protecting clients and the health care agency from harm and liability. To confront her you should also
    A. record her telephone calls with staff.
    B. perform frequent urinalysis evaluations.
    C. ask her to attend an Alcoholics Anonymous meeting.
    D. offer support through peer or employee assistance programs.

12. Nurses who have an addiction problem are frequently undetected because
    A. colleagues fail to report suspicious behaviors.
    B. nurses often undergo routine drug screening.
    C. nurses are not considered addicts but rather caregivers.
    D. 10% of the general population has a substance abuse problem.

13. An Advance Directive is
    A. a living will.
    B. a do not resuscitate order.
    C. appointing an agent whom the client trusts to make medical decisions.
    D. a document that informs health care providers of medical management requests.

14. The Patient Self-Determination Act requires that clients
    A. designate a durable power of attorney.
    B. understand state-specific legislation related to health care.
    C. retain an attorney to legally enforce their medical requests.
    D. be informed of their rights to accept or refuse medical treatments should they become incapacitated.

15. Informed consent documents delineate certain
    A. client rights.
    B. professional standards of care.
    C. agency or institutional policies and decisions.
    D. client wishes in the event of respiratory or cardiac failure.

16. To provide a "union free" workplace, it is suggested that health care organizations
    A. orient and train staff properly.
    B. establish a board of nursing.
    C. provide free parking.
    D. establish equitable hiring and promotion practices.

ANSWERS

1. *Answer:* C
   Rationale: Common law is the body of law that is interpretative by the courts and not legislative in nature. Option A: A statute is an act of the legislature declaring, commanding, or prohibiting something: a particular law enacted and established by the legislative department of government. Option B: Legislation is the act of giving or enacting laws: the making of laws through the legislation, in contrast to court-made laws. Option D: Administrative law is a body of law created by administrative agencies in the form of rules, regulations, orders, and decisions.

2. *Answer:* C
   Rationale: State law is the most powerful source of authority for nursing practice and is found in the state-specific nurse practice acts. Option A: Licensure is the permission by state authority to practice the act of nursing. Option B: Credentialing is the documented evidence of the nurse's authority. Option D: Continuing education is a state-specific requirement for nursing education.

3. *Answer:* D
   Rationale: Nurse practice acts and professional standards of care are sources used in legal decision making relevant to oncology nursing practice. Protocol is an agreement about how specific care is provided. Familiarity with the literature supports evidence-based practice. A member of the state nursing organization provides the nurse with professional resources.

4. *Answer:* C
   Rationale: Durable power of attorney is the designated client advocate to participate in medical decisions should the client be incapacitated. An advance directive is a written document from the client that is used to inform health care providers of medical management requests in the event they are incapacitated. Option A: A legal will is an instrument by a person to dispose of his/her property upon death. Option B: An insurance policy does not address a client's medical care. Option D:

Organ and tissue donation is an election by the client in the event of death.

5. *Answer:* B
   Rationale: Malpractice is professional misconduct or unreasonable lack of skill. Duty is a legal or moral obligation: obligatory conduct or service. Negligence is the failure to provide care as a reasonably prudent and careful nurse would use under similar circumstances. Breach of duty is the failure to perform any legal or moral duty.

6. *Answer:* A
   Rationale: Trial by jury is a judicial examination and determination of issues by a selected panel within the community. Institutional sanctions reflect the enforcement of a penalty resulting from a violation of law. Out-of-court settlement is a determination by agreement of the parties outside a court of law. Sanctions by the state board of nursing enforce penalties to the nurse violating rules or regulations.

7. *Answer:* C
   Rationale: State nurse practice acts and professional standards of care (i.e., American Nurses Association, Oncology Nursing Society) provide sources that can be used in legal decision making. A statute is an act of the legislature declaring, commanding, or prohibiting something: a particular law enacted and established by the legislative department of government. Licensure is the permission by state authority to practice the act of nursing. State-determined competencies vary from state to state and are not used to discern professional standards of care.

8. *Answer:* C
   Rationale: Acts of independent contractors will not pose liability on a health care agency as long as it takes prudent measures to limit its exposure, one of which is to identify the staff as an independent contractor. Providing a wide range of benefits may attract the contract employee to become an employee of the health care agency. Employing fair labor

practices is a federal mandate for all employers. Equitable hiring and promotion practice is an incentive for employers to retain and recruit employees.

9. *Answer:* D
Rationale: Ostensible agency or apparent authority may render an institution liable unless steps are taken to reduce its liability, one of which is to identify a contract employee as such. The lawsuit is against the health care agency and not on specific practice; this would be evidence in the case. Incompetence would need to be determined through the legal process. Inadequate assessment by the nurse would also require further investigation to determine cause.

10. *Answer:* D
Rationale: A "no solicitation" rule is often in effect to inhibit union solicitation within the health care agency. Fair labor standards are a federal act that sets a minimum standard wage and a maximum work week (40 hours). The act created the Wage and Hour Division in the Department of Labor. Discrimination is constitutional law that prohibits unfair treatment or denial of normal privileges to persons because of their race, age, nationality, or religion.

11. *Answer:* D
Rationale: Seven percent of nurses have problems associated with substance use. Supportive measures should be encouraged first with appropriate documentation of action. Recording a telephone call, performing routine urinalysis, and requesting attendance to Alcoholics Anonymous meetings all violate the nurse manager's protected privacy. The Federal Privacy Act prevents against a breach of privacy without the consent of the person accused.

12. *Answer:* A
Rationale: It is reported that peers and colleagues are often reluctant to report suspicious behaviors. Drug screening is not a routine practice in health care. The perception that nurses are caregivers without addictive propensity is false. It is a fact that 10% of the American population is identified with an addiction problem, but this is not the reason for the nurse addiction to go undetected.

13. *Answer:* D
Rationale: An Advance Directive is a written document that informs health care providers of their medical management requests in the event that they are unable to do so themselves. A living will provides specific instructions about the kinds of health care that should be provided or prevented in certain situations; it is not recognized in all states. A do not resuscitate order is used in inpatient settings that support an advance directive. A durable power of attorney is an appointed health care advocate or surrogate.

14. *Answer:* D
Rationale: The Patient Self-Determination Act is a federal law enacted in 1991 that requires that clients are informed of their rights to accept or refuse medical treatment and to specify, in advance, the care they would like to receive should they become incapacitated. Durable power of attorney is the appointed health care advocate to make decisions on behalf of the client should he/ she become incapacitated. The Patient Self-Determination Act is a federal law that supersedes state legislation. An attorney can help to develop an advance directive.

15. *Answer:* A
Rationale: Client rights are identified by:
• American Hospital Association (AHA)— Patient's Bill of Rights
• Joint Commission on Accreditation of Healthcare Organizations (JCAHO)— standards of care related to client rights
• Right of self-determination
• Informed consent documents
Professional standards relate to health care providers and not client consent for care or services. Agency and institutional policies reflect client rights through accreditation bodies. Advance directives delineate client wishes for care.

16. *Answer:* D
Rationale: Among the recommendations for maintaining a "union free" workplace, health care organizations should establish equitable hiring and promotion practices. Orienting and training reduces the incidence of liability. Establishing a board of nursing is a

sanction by the state. Free parking is not a benefit that can be linked to retaining employees.

BIBLIOGRAPHY

Buppert, C. (1999). *Nurse practitioner's business practice and legal guide*. Gaithersburg, MD: Aspen Publication.

Garner, B. (Ed.). (2001). *Black's law dictionary* (2nd pocket ed.). St. Paul, MN: West Group.

Kuebler, K., & Berry, P. (2002). Clinical practice guidelines for advanced practice nursing. In K. Kuebler, P. Berry., & D. Heidrich (Eds). *End-of-life care: Clinical practice guidelines*. Philadelphia: W.B. Saunders, pp. 15-22.

Taylor, C. (2002). Advance directives. In K. Kuebler & P. Esper (Eds.). *Palliative practices from A-Z for the bedside clinician*. Pittsburgh: Oncology Nursing Society, pp. 1-4.

NOTES

47 Selected Ethical Issues in Cancer Care

GABRIELA KAPLAN

1. Randomization is an example of
   A. autonomy.
   B. beneficence.
   C. justice.
   D. nonmaleficence.

2. The following would **not** be an intent of informed consent:
   A. Assurance of success.
   B. Protection from harm.
   C. Autonomous choice.
   D. Avoidance of exploitation.

3. Phase I trials generally
   A. study the efficacy of a specific drug against a specific cancer.
   B. compare standard therapy with new therapy.
   C. determine long-term safety of a treatment.
   D. determine safe drug levels of the new drug.

4. Phase IV trials
   A. determine long-term safety and efficacy of a new drug or treatment.
   B. determine safe drug levels and/or schedules of a new drug.
   C. focus on a particular form of cancer.
   D. compare standard therapy with the new therapy.

5. A risk of clinical trial participation is
   A. participant may benefit from the new drug.
   B. results of the clinical trial may be helpful to clients in the future.
   C. insurance may not cover all of the costs associated with the trial.
   D. access to a new drug that is available only in the clinical trial.

6. A benefit of clinical trial participation is
   A. side effects that are worse than the standard treatment.
   B. increased health care attention than that received with standard care.
   C. insurance may not cover all of the associated costs.
   D. new drug may not be superior to standard care.

7. The role of the Data and Safety Monitoring Board (DSMB) is to maintain client safety in
   A. phase I clinical trials.
   B. phase II clinical trials.
   C. phase III clinical trials.
   D. phase IV clinical trials.

8. The role of the nurse in a clinical trial is
   A. advocate for all issues related to the trial and participation.
   B. obtain informed consent.

C. maintain minutes of institutional review board (IRB) meetings.

D. write the protocol.

9. The role of the nurse in clinical research is
   A. attend the DSMB meetings.
   B. collaborate with the sponsoring agency.
   C. ensure access to all medical records.
   D. manage symptoms related to treatment or intervention.

10. Ms. J. has agreed to participate in a clinical trial. She approaches the nurse and says, "I'm so worried my insurance company won't pay." The nurse's **best** response would be:
   A. "Don't worry. Research isn't all that important."
   B. "I will call and speak with your case manager."
   C. "Can you afford to put out the initial costs?"
   D. "You need an appointment with the financial counselor."

11. Mr. R. signed the informed consent to participate in a phase I trial. After two treatment cycles, he calls the nurse and says, "I don't want to do this anymore. This is just too hard." The nurse's **best** response would be:
   A. "Can you tell me what the issues are?"
   B. "OK. I'll let your doctor know."
   C. "Thank you for your past participation."
   D. "If you quit now, you'll jeopardize the study."

12. Ms. S. has been approached to participate in a prevention trial. She questions the purpose of randomization, stating, "I will only participate if I get into the 'real' prevention arm." The nurse's **best** response is:
   A. "We can make sure you get the 'real' medication."
   B. "The study coordinator will be notified of your request."
   C. "Randomization ensures equal access and opportunity."
   D. "You can't participate, if you won't take a chance."

13. Dr. T. is speaking to his client about clinical trial participation. He is overheard to say,

"Don't worry. We can make sure you end up in the real treatment arm." The nurse's best **first** response would be to:
   A. Notify hospital administration of Dr. T.'s remarks.
   B. Notify the IRB of Dr. T.'s remarks.
   C. Tell the client he is ineligible to participate in the study.
   D. Speak with Dr. T. privately about his overheard remarks.

14. The following statement best serves to illustrate the role of the IRB:
   A. The IRB reports toxicities to trial participants.
   B. The IRB ensures compliance with Health Insurance Portability and Accountability Act (HIPAA) regulations.
   C. The IRB protects the rights of research participants.
   D. The IRB can waive exclusion criteria.

15. Mr. L. is being evaluated for participation in a clinical trial. During the course of the physical exam, he says, "I'm not sure I want to be a guinea pig." The nurse's best response is:
   A. "We have a lot of patients participating in this trial."
   B. "Can you share your concerns?"
   C. "Why not?"
   D. "There are many safeguards in place."

16. Informed consent is an example of
   A. justice.
   B. randomization.
   C. eligibility criteria.
   D. autonomy.

17. Mr. Q. gave consent to receive chemotherapy. His daughter, a hospice nurse, strongly objects to her father's receiving this treatment. Mr. Q.'s consent is an example of
   A. autonomy.
   B. beneficence.
   C. justice.
   D. coercion.

18. The following would **not** be an element of an informed consent:
   A. Protection from harm.
   B. Coercion.

C. autonomy.

D. exploitation avoidance.

19. A client with an advance directive requesting "no heroics" is brought to the emergency room after a car accident. The emergency room physician determines that the client's condition is a reversible event and institutes treatment. This is an example of

A. justice.

B. autonomy.

C. beneficence.

D. nonmaleficence.

20. Beauchamp and Childress are the proponents of

A. virtue-based ethics.

B. case-based ethics.

C. narrative-based ethics.

D. principle-based ethics.

21. Social Security, Medicare, and Medicaid exemplify the principle of

A. justice.

B. beneficence.

C. autonomy.

D. nonmaleficence.

22. Paternalism is an expression of

A. autonomy.

B. beneficence.

C. nonmaleficence.

D. justice.

23. The first step in an ethical workup is

A. making a decision.

B. determining a course of action.

C. ascertaining the facts.

D. determining the values.

24. A client with breast cancer does not appear for her outpatient follow-up. This happens twice. Social work becomes involved, leading to further information being shared by a friend and her daughter. The resulting decision to continue treatment is an example of

A. virtue-theory.

B. casuistry.

C. justice.

D. hermeneutics.

25. Mrs. S. tells the nurse, "I want to live, I need to be cured." The nurse's **best** response is:

A. "I'm sure the doctor will do her best."

B. "What did the doctor tell you today?"

C. "Sometimes cure is not possible."

D. "Your condition is very serious."

26. Mr. J. is considering entering a phase II study for treatment of refractory prostate cancer. The physician and research nurse are eager to enroll Mr. J. An ethical principle that the research nurse and physician must be careful to protect is

A. veracity.

B. autonomy.

C. beneficence.

D. justice.

27. Mrs. R. is having difficulty choosing among several treatment options for her metastatic breast cancer. She asks the nurse, "If you were me, what would you do?" The nurse's **best** response would be:

A. "I would choose the treatment with the best response rate."

B. "The decision is totally up to you."

C. "I can see that making this decision is very difficult. What would you like to know about the different treatment options?"

D. "I have seen patients do well on all of the proposed therapy options."

28. Mrs. W. informs the nurse that she does not intend to read the informed consent document for her participation in a phase III chemotherapy trial. She states she finds the diagnosis and its associated treatment too upsetting. The nurse's best response would be:

A. "You need to read and sign the document before therapy is started."

B. "Let's go over it together. We can discuss anything you find confusing or upsetting."

C. "I will get the doctor so we can decide what to do next."

D. "There are risks associated with therapy and being a part of a trial. That is why you must sign the document before we start therapy."

29. Mr. T.'s family would like to remove his tube feeding and other extraordinary means of life support. Which of the following groups should the nurse consult?

A. IRB.
B. Hospital ethics committee.
C. Hospital lawyer.
D. Hospital cancer committee.

30. Informed consent is both an ethical and legal consideration. One element of informed consent includes
    A. offering the client your personal feelings about the treatment.
    B. encouraging the client to think about his/her decision because once the consent form is signed, no changes can be made.
    C. assessing the mental status of a client with depression, other mental illness, dementia, or retardation.
    D. strongly encouraging the client to participate because the doctor wants him/her to.

31. A written document that allows a person to name another individual to make health care decisions for a client if he/she is unable to make them is called
    A. Advance directive.
    B. Power of attorney.
    C. Medical power of attorney.
    D. Living will.

NOTES

ANSWERS

1. *Answer:* C
Rationale: The principle of justice addresses the concept of equal access. Each clinical trial participant should have the same chance to participate in each arm. Participants should not be prequalified to a certain arm based on physical or emotional characteristics. Each person coming to the trial should have equal opportunity to be chosen. Randomization ensures this opportunity. Autonomy means to honor client confidences and practice shared decision making. Beneficence means to act in the best interests of others. Nonmaleficence ensures that anticipated treatment benefits outweigh any anticipated harms. Thus clients should be offered only potentially therapeutic interventions.

2. *Answer:* A
Rationale: The purposes of an informed consent is to ensure autonomous choice (the participant makes up his/her own mind), protection from harm (the participant will be protected from adverse effects as best as possible), and the participant will not be coerced, or forced, into participation or a decision they are not comfortable with. An informed consent cannot ensure the success of the trial as stated in Option A.

3. *Answer:* D
Rationale: Phase I studies are set up to determine the Maximum Tolerated Dose (MTD) of a specific agent. Phase II trials are to determine the efficacy of the new drug against a specific cancer. Phase III trials are to compare the new treatment against the approved/standard treatment. Phase IV trials study long-term effects of treatment and quality of life issues.

4. *Answer:* A
Rationale: Phase IV trials study long-term effects of treatment and quality of life issues. Phase I studies are set up to determine the MTD of a specific agent. Phase II trials are to determine the efficacy of the new drug against a specific cancer. Phase III trials are to compare the new treatment against the approved/standard treatment.

5. *Answer:* C
Rationale: Insurance companies generally are not eager to cover the costs of clinical trial participation. Generally, clients who participate in clinical trials need more frequent monitoring of their status, leading to increased use of resources, leading to increased costs. Options A, B, and D are potential benefits from participating in a clinical trial.

6. *Answer:* B
Rationale: Because the participant in a clinical trial requires more frequent monitoring, he has greater access to the health care team, allowing for more vigilance of the disease/health state, allowing for greater educational opportunities. Options A, C, and D are all potential risks of participating in a clinical trial.

7. *Answer:* C
Rationale: The role of the DSMB is to review the progress of the clinical trial. Typically, the board asks two questions: Are there any expected or severely toxic effects, and what is the treatment outcome so far? Because phase III trials are designed to assess the treatment in large groups of clients, these questions become more relevant.

8. *Answer:* A
Rationale: While the role of the nurse is to ensure that an informed consent has been obtained, the nurse's primary responsibility is to advocate for the client. The nurse needs to assess the participant's level of understanding, clear up confusion, and help the participant get the answers that are needed. Options C and D are not necessarily a role of the nurse.

9. *Answer:* D
Rationale: The role of the nurse in clinical research is to manage any and all symptoms related to the treatment or intervention. It is through this activity that potential and actual side effects and adverse reactions are identified, treated, and reported to the DSMB and the IRB.

10. *Answer:* B

Rationale: As the client advocate, it is the nurse's role to call and coordinate care with the client's insurance carrier. Often, the carrier would be willing to pay for services if the parameters were explained ahead of time, not after the fact. An appointment with a financial counselor is a good strategy; it does not speak to the client's immediate concern about clinical trial participation.

11. *Answer:* A

Rationale: It is certainly the client's right to withdraw from a study whenever he wants. However, the nurse would be doing a terrible injustice to the client if she did not determine the reason for the client's change of heart. Notifying the physician and thanking the client for his participation are correct actions, but they do not address the client's immediate concerns. Perhaps the client is having symptoms or logistical (transportation) issues that can be addressed so that the participation can continue. Telling the client that if he quits he will jeopardize the study will cause the client to distrust the health care system, as well as being extremely unethical.

12. *Answer:* C

Rationale: Option C is correct because it emphasizes the purpose of randomization and opens the communication for the nurse to re-explain the purpose of a prevention trial. Option A is incorrect because in a randomized study, the participant is randomized (assigned) to a particular arm based on statistical formulations. There is no way to ensure one arm over another. Option B is incorrect because notifying the study coordinator may help, as he/she will be able to re-explain the purpose of randomization. However, the coordinator cannot guarantee anything. Option D is incorrect because it is not helpful to be rude, and it does not educate the participant about the true nature of a randomized prevention trial.

13. *Answer:* D

Rationale: Although Options A and B are correct, it would be inappropriate to take either of those actions without approaching Dr. T. first. The nurse should ask Dr. T. the "why" of his remark (in a nonjudgmental,

nonaccusatory manner). This would open the door to education about randomization and its importance in clinical trials. Option C is not relevant to Dr. T.'s remarks. The client eventually needs to be informed that a specific treatment arm cannot be guaranteed in a randomized trial.

14. *Answer:* C

Rationale: Option C is the most encompassing option. The primary purpose of the IRB is to protect the rights and welfare of participants in research. This is done by ensuring that risks are minimized and reasonable in relation to anticipated benefits. The IRB ensures that the selection of participants is equitable, informed consent is obtained and documented, and provisions exist for the privacy of participants and confidentiality of data. The IRB does not report toxicities directly to trial participants and does not waive exclusion criteria. All clients are subject to HIPAA guidelines, not just those participating in clinical trials.

15. *Answer:* B

Rationale: The public has many fears about clinical trial participation. These fears are not allayed by stories in the media about deaths, unethical researchers, etc. The nurse's role is to ascertain the client's state of mind, provide education and clarification, and answer the client's questions. Nurses need to be effective listeners and effective purveyors of information. Options A, C, and D do not respect the client's concerns.

16. *Answer:* D

Rationale: Autonomy is the principle of self-determination. According to the Patient Self-Determination Act, clients have the right to decide for themselves on the course of action they wish to pursue. While the informed consent document (and process) covers the concepts of randomization and eligibility criteria, autonomy is the overriding principle involved.

17. *Answer:* A

Rationale: Autonomy means to honor client confidences and practice shared decision making. The client has the right to choose for himself. Beneficence means to act in the best interests of others. Justice or fairness means to allocate scarce resources fairly and abide by institutional and/or insurance allocation policies. Coercion violates the principle of autonomy.

18. *Answer:* B

Rationale: The informed consent process exists to provide education and clarification and to enhance participation in clinical trials. In no way should coercion be implemented, or hinted at, when soliciting participants.

19. *Answer:* C

Rationale: Beneficence is the principle of "doing good." In this case, the emergency room physician determined that the client's condition was reversible, that the client could be returned to his/her previous state of health, and that the action of "doing good" outweighed the "no-heroics" advance directive. Justice or fairness means to allocate scarce resources fairly and abide by institutional and/or insurance allocation policies. Autonomy is the principle of self-determination. Nonmaleficence ensures that anticipated treatment benefits outweigh any anticipated harms.

20. *Answer:* D

Rationale: Beauchamp and Childress identify four core ethical principles. They are autonomy, nonmaleficence, beneficence, and justice.

21. *Answer:* A

Rationale: Justice is the principle concerned with equal access and equal opportunity. Social Security, Medicare, and Medicaid seek to level the field in terms of health care access for less advantaged citizens. Beneficence means to act in the best interests of others. Autonomy is the principle of self-determination. Nonmaleficence ensures that anticipated treatment benefits outweigh any anticipated harms.

22. *Answer:* B

Rationale: Paternalism is best symbolized by the concept of "father knows best," or, in medicine's case, by "the doctor knows best." Beneficence, the concept of "doing good," lends itself easily to the "doctor knows best" scenario. Autonomy is the principle of

self-determination. Nonmaleficence ensures that anticipated treatment benefits outweigh any anticipated harms. Justice or fairness means to allocate scarce resources fairly and abide by institutional and/or insurance allocation policies.

23. *Answer:* C

Rationale: The first step in any process is gathering facts. Although it may be tempting to apply values as a beginning, values may only cloud the issues. The values the client/family/health care provider determine to be important are the values that will factor into the decision-making process after all relevant facts have been gathered.

24. *Answer:* D

Rationale: Hermeneutics mean interpreting the case in its whole context: the individual's life plans and values, the family's values, social and cultural factors, etc. In this case, the noncompliant client does not come for her appointments. Information is sought and gathered from family and friends. The resulting contributions add to the decision making, resulting in a broader understanding of the client's situation, values, fears, and desires.

25. *Answer:* B

Rationale: The first step in any conversation is to ascertain facts. It is always a good idea to find out what the client knows versus what the client suspects. It is not the nurse's role to provide information that was not sought. It is the nurse's role to determine what the client is asking. By exploring the information the client was given (or the client's interpretation of the information), the nurse is in an excellent position to provide education, comfort, and support.

26. *Answer:* A

Rationale: The purpose of informed consent is to assist the client to make an appropriate informed decision regarding proposed therapy. Individuals must make treatment decisions based on information that is factual, unbiased, and noncoercive. Veracity is the obligation to tell the truth. The physician and nurse have a need to disclose to Mr. J. that they are very eager to enroll clients in this study.

Autonomy means to honor client confidences and practice shared decision making. Beneficence means to act in the best interests of others. Justice refers to the fair allocation of scarce resource and abiding by institutional and/or insurance allocation policies.

27. *Answer:* C
Rationale: Informed consent enables an autonomous choice. By providing additional education on the different treatment options, the nurse is providing the client with informed consent. Options A and D are the nurse's personal opinion. Option B is not a supportive response.

28. *Answer:* B
Rationale: Individuals undergoing therapy in a trial need to be aware of what to expect regarding risks, benefits and alternatives. When the risks have been discussed, the client can make an informed choice about treatment and participation in the trial. Options A and D are coercive. Further, without knowledge of risks and side effects, the client will not know what to expect or how to manage complications if they should occur. Option C does not respect the autonomy of the client.

29. *Answer:* B
Rationale: An objective third party often can be of great assistance in helping the family to better understand and weigh the moral issues and arguments of a proposed intervention and assist the family in coming to a thoughtful resolution. This is a common function of hospital ethics teams. Option A is incorrect because the purpose of the IRB is to protect the human subjects involved in research. Option C is incorrect because the lawyer will probably only consider the hospital's liability. Option D is incorrect because the hospital cancer committee functions to oversee cancer-related activities in the institution and set hospital policies.

30. *Answer:* C
Rationale: Informed consent is an ethical and legal concept that requires health care professionals to provide sufficient information about the client's condition and the recommended treatments to enable the client to make a reasonable decision. For the client to make an informed decision, the nurse must consider the several elements. The client must be capable of making a decision. Option C is correct: Clients who have a mental illness, dementia, retardation, and other types of disabilities may still possess decision-making capacity; however, assessment is required. Other essential elements of informed consent include disclosure (reasonable person standard is disclosing what an ordinary person in the client's position considers significant, and subjective standard is what this client needs or wants to know); comprehension (providing information in a way the client can understand); voluntarism (no coercion or undue pressure influence is acceptable); and authorization (the client must make a clear choice as evidenced by an oral or written agreement). Options A and D oppose voluntarism. This client would not be making his/her own decision but doing what the doctor or nurse suggested. Option B is incorrect because no decision is absolute or permanent.

31. *Answer:* C
Rationale: Medical power of attorney is the written document that allows another individual to make health care decisions for a client if he/she is unable to make them. Some states include special provisions about the types of decisions that can be made and under what circumstances. Option A: Since the passage of the federal Patient Self-Determination Act (PSDA), all health care institutions receiving federal funds are required to give clients written information about their right to participate in their own health care decisions and complete advance directives or specifications about their health care wishes. The legal document must be signed by a competent person to provide guidance for medical and health care decisions in the event the person becomes incompetent to make such decisions. A living will and medical power of attorney are two examples of advance directives. Option B is a legal instrument granting power for someone to act as an agent. Option D: A living will is a written document that directs a person's physician to withhold or withdraw life-prolonging interventions if the person is unable to make the decision. The nurse's role in any PSDA directives includes educating the client and family about the use of the document, referring the client to

the appropriate resource for initiating the document, and ensuring the health care team is aware of the document.

BIBLIOGRAPHY

Ahronheim, J.C., Moreno, J.D., & Zuckerhman, C. (2001). *Ethics in clinical practice* (2nd ed). Gaithersburg, MD: Aspen Publishers, Inc., pp. 368-381.

ANA Code www.nursingworld.org.

Arras, J.D., & Steinboch, B. (1995). *Ethical issues in modern medicine.* Mountainview, CA: Mayfield Publishing Co., pp. 1-39.

Beauchamp, T.L., & Childress, J.F. (2001). *Principles of biomedical ethics* (5th ed). New York: Oxford University Press.

Beltran, J.E., & Coluzzi, P.H. (1997). Medical ethics: A model for comprehensive palliative care. *The Talbert Journal of Health Care.* Spring/Summer, 47-57.

Buckman, R. (1992). *How to break bad news: A guide for health care professionals.* Baltimore, MD: The Johns Hopkins University Press.

Clinical trials: Questions and Answers. Cancer Facts 2.11 http://cis.nci.nih.gov/fact/2 11.htm.

Health Insurance Portability and Accountability Act (HIPAA). (1996). Pub.L.No. 104-191.

Moss, A.H. (2003). *Course book for health care ethics.* West Virginia University Center for Health Ethics and Law. Morgantown, West Virginia University, www.wvethics.org.

Nelson-Marten, P., & Braaten, J.S. (2001). Common ethical dilemmas. In R.A. Gates & R.M. Fink (Eds.). *Oncology nursing secrets* (2nd ed). Philadelphia: Hanley & Belfus, Inc., pp. 565-573.

Oncology clinical trials. www.nci.nih.gov/clinical-trials.

The Patient Self-Determination Act (PSDA). (1994). (Pub.L.No. 101-508, '4206, 4751 (hereinafter OBRA) 104 Stat. 1388-115 to 117, 1388-204 to 206 (codified at 42 U.S.C.A.'1395cc(f)(l) & id. '1396a(a) (West Supp. 1994).

Quill, T. (2001). *Caring for patients at the end of life: Facing an uncertain future together.* New York: Oxford University Press.

Rosse, P.A. & Garcia, M.T. (2001). Clinical trials. In R.A. Gates & R.M. Fink (Eds.). *Oncology nursing secrets* (2nd ed.) Philadelphia: Hanley & Belfus, Inc., pp. 97-102.

Scanlon, C., & Glover, J.J. (1995). A professional code of ethics: Providing a moral compass in turbulent times. *Oncology Nursing Forum 22*(10), 1515-1521.

Works, C. (2000). Principles of treatment planning and clinical research. In C.H. Yarbro, M.H. Frogge, M. Goodman, & S.L. Groenwald (Eds.). *Cancer nursing: Principles and practice* (5th ed.). Sudbury, MA: Jones and Bartlett Publishers, pp. 259-271.

48 Cancer Economics and Health Care Reform

MOLLY LONEY

Select the best answer for each of the following questions:

1. The current national health care crisis means that there are
    A. fewer clients than nurses.
    B. more clients than nurses.
    C. sicker clients with fewer nurses.
    D. more clients than health care reimbursement funds.

2. The reorganization of hospitals over the past decade has resulted in
    A. improved access to quality health care services.
    B. decreased number of oncology-specialized nurses.
    C. increased frequency of acute care hospitalizations.
    D. reduced costs of prescription drug benefit programs.

3. A major factor influencing the U.S. health care crisis is
    A. rising cancer incidence.
    B. rising cancer mortality.
    C. rising cancer prevention.
    D. rising cancer clinical trials.

4. Cancer occurs in individuals over the age of 65 with which of the following incidence?
    A. 38%.
    B. 45%.
    C. 57%.
    D. 70%.

5. Cancer is a major health care problem in the United States largely because of which of the following?
    A. More elderly are participating in cancer screening programs.
    B. More women than men are being diagnosed with cancer.
    C. More people are living longer with cancer.
    D. More people die of cancer than are diagnosed each year.

6. Characteristics of managed care include which of the following?
    A. Episodic, financially focused care.
    B. Choice among physician groups.
    C. Reimbursement based on standard practice guidelines.
    D. Unlimited use of referrals to ancillary support services.

7. One of the most challenging cancer care costs that is difficult to measure is the
    A. direct medical costs.
    B. quality of life costs.
    C. indirect mortality costs.
    D. indirect morbidity costs.

8. What intervention is needed to decrease the rising health care costs at the end of life?
    A. Aggressive treatment of disease.
    B. More research into causes of cancer.
    C. Early decision making about advance directives.
    D. Early recognition of symptoms needing emergency treatment.

9. Enrollment in preferred provider organizations (PPOs) has been growing as consumers are searching for
    A. greater choice of physicians outside the health maintenance organization (HMO).
    B. greater access to a wide range of health care services.
    C. a clear understanding about how managed care works.
    D. lower copay rates with a universal health care reimbursement plan.

10. Medicare reimbursement can best be described as
    A. a private health insurance program for families.
    B. a state-regulated health insurance program for teachers.
    C. an HMO program for adults.
    D. a government-regulated health insurance program for people over 65.

11. Major disparities in cancer demographics include which of the following?
    A. Higher mortality rate in Asians.
    B. Higher morbidity rate in Hispanics.
    C. Higher incidence in American Indians.
    D. Higher incidence in African Americans.

12. How many individuals in the United States are estimated to be uninsured? More than
    A. 25 million.
    B. 41 million.
    C. 50 million.
    D. 71 million.

13. A key factor that will affect the nursing shortage in the future is
    A. hospitals have reduced RN positions.
    B. the average age of RNs in practice is 45 years.

C. the average age of RN entering practice is 22 years.
    D. 16% of RNs recently surveyed report they belong to a union.

14. Surveyed nurses report dissatisfaction in their work environments in which of the following areas:
    A. Lack of flexible scheduling.
    B. Working with too many agency staff.
    C. Lack of a collaborative professional environment.
    D. Working with demanding clients and their families.

15. A recent landmark study by Needham and others demonstrated that more time with care provided by an RN gives hospitalized clients which of the following?
    A. Higher client satisfaction.
    B. Better recovery after a stroke.
    C. Lower incidence of procedural and surgical complications.
    D. Lower frequency of urinary tract infection and pneumonia.

16. The lifetime probability of developing cancer has increased to which of the following?
    A. 38.5% in men and 43.5% in women.
    B. 38.5% in women and 43.5% in men.
    C. 50% in men and 60% in women.
    D. 75% in both men and women.

17. The 5-year relative survival rates from cancer include only clients
    A. living 5 years after diagnosis.
    B. receiving current cancer treatment.
    C. in cancer remission for 3 years.
    D. cured for 5 years or more.

18. An increased risk for cancer incidence and mortality has been linked to which of the following environmental or lifestyle factors?
    A. Drinking city water.
    B. General physical inactivity.
    C. Consuming a high-fiber diet.
    D. Anorexia with loss of 10% of total body weight.

19. Many consumers have described which of the following as a significant barrier to seeking medical care?

A. Cost of medical care.
B. Fear about cancer diagnosis.
C. Lack of information about health.
D. Lack of nurses when hospitalized.

20. An ethical issue often identified with the managed care system involves which of the following?
    A. Provides specialized care only for clients who can pay for a referral.
    B. Provides an incentive to undertreat clients needing diagnostic workup.
    C. Provides an incentive to treat clients through specialty service referrals.
    D. Provides care by using affiliating physicians in a preselected HMO network.

21. A community's stability can be negatively affected by a
    A. rising number of cancer diagnoses.
    B. rising number of uninsured residents.
    C. rising number of resident cancer survivors.
    D. rising number of managed care organizations.

22. By 2020, an increase in clients with cancer is projected to reach which of the following percentages in the United States?
    A. 20%.
    B. 35%.
    C. 50%.
    D. 75%.

23. Academic issues affecting the growing nursing shortage include
    A. not enough nursing school applicants.
    B. not enough nursing school faculty.
    C. not enough schools of nursing.
    D. not enough experienced PhD nursing faculty.

24. The nursing shortage has significantly affected quality cancer care in which of the following ways?
    A. Increased paperwork.
    B. Increased client acuity.
    C. Care is often given by unlicensed staff.
    D. Chemotherapy is often given by non-oncology nurses.

25. Competing economic demands that have reduced governmental funds available to address cancer care and the nursing shortage include which of the following?
    A. Uninsured.
    B. Ethnic disparities.
    C. Aging of Americans.
    D. Managed care organizations.

26. The ONS Health Policy Agenda focuses on which of the following as its #1 priority?
    A. Nursing shortage.
    B. Medicare reform.
    C. Cancer prevention and detection.
    D. Cancer in underserved population.

27. Besides its Health Policy Agenda, ONS is involved in which of the following advocacy activities?
    A. Workforce Study.
    B. Job Shadowing Kit.
    C. Public image promotion campaign.
    D. Generating grassroots support for major health policy legislation.

28. Hospital initiatives to address the health care crisis in the United States include
    A. nursing unions.
    B. physician-directed administration.
    C. mandatory overtime of nursing staff.
    D. partnerships between nurses and physicians.

29. Individual ONS members can make a difference by taking action in which of the following ways?
    A. Vote in all elections.
    B. Trust legislators to act in their best interest.
    C. Picket legislators who do not support health policy reform.
    D. Encourage legislators to keep the current Medicare system intact.

30. Nurses can constructively change their work environments by
    A. asking for a raise.
    B. going back to nursing school.
    C. looking for the evidence behind practice.
    D. sharing "war" stories about how hard it is to be a nurse.

ANSWERS

1. *Answer:* C
Rationale: The United States is facing a critical shortage of health care resources to meet complex and changing health care needs. Health care resources include nurses. As the aging population increases, clients are sicker with more complex health care problems. Although health care reimbursement funds also make up health care resources, and the reimbursement system needs reform, the funds have not been totally depleted yet.

2. *Answer:* B
Rationale: As hospitals have reorganized with the elimination of many positions and services, access has actually been decreased. With hospitals focusing on the nurse as a generalist and closing oncology units, the number of oncology-specialized nurses employed in the hospital setting has decreased. Care has shifted to outpatient and home care over acute care with hospitalizations. The cost of prescription drugs and benefit programs has increased.

3. *Answer:* A
Rationale: A major factor influencing the U.S. health care crisis is the expected rise in cancer incidence with an aging population. Cancer incidence is rising with a 50% increase in the number of clients with cancer projected by 2020. Cancer mortality has actually decreased. Although increased consumer awareness has increased cancer prevention, it has not affected the health care crisis. Enrollment in clinical trials remains a challenge, with only 3% of clients with cancer participating in such trials.

4. *Answer:* C
Rationale: More than 57% of all cancers occur in individuals over the age of 65.

5. *Answer:* C
Rationale: Cancer is a major health care problem in the United States because it is a chronic, multifaceted disease. Clients are living longer with the need to monitor and manage long-term side effects. Mortality rates for cancer have dropped in the past few years. The estimated number of new cancer cases was 1,368,030 for 2004, while estimated cancer deaths equal 563,700. Participation in cancer screening actually decreases with age. More men than women are being diagnosed with cancer.

6. *Answer:* C
Rationale: Managed care uses standard practice guidelines, care maps, and clinical pathways to help determine health care reimbursement. It focuses on prevention and continuity of care, not episodic care. Managed care does focus on financial efficiency, a limited number of physicians/groups from which to choose, and a primary care that controls referrals.

7. *Answer:* B
Rationale: Intangible and challenging costs to quality of life from unrelieved and distressing symptoms from cancer and its treatment cannot be measured in dollars and cents. Indirect morbidity and mortality costs can be estimated from lost productivity at work related to illness or death.

8. *Answer:* C
Rationale: End-of-life costs may be reduced with coordinated, expert, end-of-life care that promotes early decision making about advance directives and prevents emergency room visits and hospitalizations. Aggressive treatment is appropriate in the acute phase of care, not at the end of life. More research into what causes cancer is important but will not directly affect costs at the end of life. Early recognition of symptoms is also important to promote quality of life, but symptoms should be managed proactively, not with emergency treatment.

9. *Answer:* B
Rationale: The enrollment in PPOs has been growing as consumers search for more choice in physicians within the PPO network and access to the full range of health care services to meet their needs. No universal plan currently exists for health care reimbursement.

10. *Answer:* D
Rationale: Medicare is defined as a government-regulated program that provides health insurance for all individuals age 65 and older, regardless of socioeconomic status or income.

11. *Answer:* D
Rationale: African Americans have a higher cancer incidence, morbidity, and mortality than other ethnic groups:
- 10% higher incidence than whites; 50% to 60% higher incidence than Asians and Hispanics, and twice as high incidence as American Indians.
- 30% higher mortality than whites and more than twice the mortality in Hispanics, Asians, and American Indians.

12. *Answer:* B
Rationale: According to the Institute of Medicine (IOM), more than 41 million people are uninsured in the United States.

13. *Answer:* B
Rationale: Although hospital cost cutting has reduced the number of RNs working in hospitals now, the average age of an RN working in practice is 45 years old. Fifty percent of RNs working in 2003 will reach retirement age in 15 years. At the same time, fewer people are going into nursing. The average age of a new graduate RN is 31. Sixteen percent of RNs surveyed did report belonging to a union, but this will not directly affect the nursing shortage in the future.

14. *Answer:* C
Rationale: In Aiken's survey, reported sources of dissatisfaction included lack of a collaborative professional work environment, high nurse/client ratios, lack of adequate support services, lack of administrative support, increased non-nursing work, mandatory overtime, lack of tools to do the job, inadequate compensation, and poor standards of care.

15. *Answer:* D
Rationale: In the study by Needham and colleagues, more RN-provided care was associated with better care for hospitalized clients, including shorter length of stay, lower rates of urinary tract infection (UTI), pneumonia, gastrointestinal bleeding, thrombosis, sepsis, shock, and cardiac arrest, and lower rates of "failure to rescue."

16. *Answer:* B
Rationale: The lifetime probability of developing cancer has increased to 38.5% in women and 43.5% in men.

17. *Answer:* A
Rationale: The 5-year relative survival rates for cancer include people living 5 years after diagnosis, whether undergoing treatment, symptom management, in remission, cured, or with advanced disease.

18. *Answer:* B
Rationale: An increased risk for cancer incidence and mortality has been linked to general physical inactivity, consuming a high-fat diet, obesity, smoking, infectious disease, and exposure to chemicals and/or radiation.

19. *Answer:* A
Rationale: The cost of health care has been described by many consumers as a barrier to seeking medical care. Fear about a cancer diagnosis and lack of information about health may affect whether a person seeks care, but they have not been identified by consumers as a barrier. Lack of nurses has been described as a factor affecting client satisfaction rather than a barrier to seeking care in the first place.

20. *Answer:* B
Rationale: An ethical issue with managed care involves financial incentives given to primary care physicians to keep costs to a minimum, with the potential to undertreat clients who need a laboratory and diagnostic workup for symptoms. By its nature, managed care is a system that provides care by using affiliating physicians in a preselected HMO network, based on contract agreements.

21. *Answer:* B
Rationale: Although an increase in the number of residents with a cancer diagnosis may indirectly affect the workforce of a community, a rising number of uninsured residents can threaten a community's stability, with reduced services available, poorer general community health, and a less prosperous

local economy. An increase in managed care organizations may actually bring more money and stability to a community.

22. *Answer:* C
Rationale: A 50% increase in clients with cancer is projected by 2020 by the American Cancer Society and National Cancer Institute.

23. *Answer:* B
Rationale: Although enrollment in schools of nursing has decreased, schools are turning away nursing applicants because of a shortage of nursing faculty in general. Experienced and older PhD faculty are more prevalent, with the average age of 53.5 in 2000 for PhD faculty. Younger PhD faculty need to be recruited.

24. *Answer:* D
Rationale: Nononcology nurses giving chemotherapy has had a direct and significant impact on quality cancer care. Although a reality, increased paperwork and client acuity are reported sources of nurse dissatisfaction that affect workload demands. Care given by unlicensed staff has affected quality care in general but is not specific to cancer care.

25. *Answer:* C
Rationale: Factors like the aging population in the United States, urbanization, competition for energy sources, terrorism, and war have reduced available governmental funds to address cancer care and the nursing shortage. Issues involving health care access of the uninsured and ethnic groups have not been addressed with funding programs. The government does not regulate or fund managed care organizations.

26. *Answer:* A
Rationale: The nursing shortage is the #1 priority in ONS's Health Policy Agenda. Medicare reform, cancer prevention and detection, and cancer in underserved populations are also highlighted as needing action.

27. *Answer:* D
Rationale: Generating grassroots support for major health policy legislation is a strong advocacy activity for ONS. The ONS Workforce Study from 2002 is an example of professional activities. The Job Shadowing Kit and public image promotion campaign are examples of community outreach activities.

28. *Answer:* D
Rationale: Hospital initiatives to address the health care crisis include a major focus on recruitment and retention of nurses and efforts to change the work environment through shared governance and nurse/physician partnerships. Hospitals do not seek nursing unions as a solution to the health care crisis. Mandatory overtime is often used by hospitals as a temporary solution to the nursing shortage but has been identified by nurses as a source of dissatisfaction. Physician-directed administration perpetuates a work environment that has been identified as noncollaborative by nurses.

29. *Answer:* A
Rationale: Individual ONS members can make a big difference by voting in all —local, national, and ONS elections. Nurses need to share their stories and let legislators know what they think about upcoming legislation. They also need to partner with legislators from their areas, not picket them. Members need to advocate for Medicare system reform to provide access to quality cancer care.

30. *Answer:* C
Rationale: Nurses can constructively change their work environments by finding the evidence behind nursing practice and using it to make practice improvements. Asking for a raise and going back to school do not directly affect the environment. Sharing negative stories only reinforces nurses' dissatisfaction. Success stories can offer powerful examples of how nurses can and do make a difference.

BIBLIOGRAPHY

Aiken, L., Clarke, S., Sloan, D. et. al. (2002). Hospital nurse staffing and patient mortality, nurse burnout and job dissatisfaction. *Journal of the American Medical Association* 288(16), 1987-1993.

American Cancer Society. (2004). *Cancer facts and figures 2004*. Atlanta: Author.

Boyle, D.M., Engelking, C., Blesch, K., et al. (1992). *Oncology nursing society position paper on cancer and aging: The mandate for oncology nursing*. Pittsburgh: Oncology Nursing Society.

Heinrich, J., & Thompson, T. (2002). Organization and delivery of health care in the United States: A patchwork system. In D. Mason, J. Leavitt, M. Chafee, (Eds.). *Policy and politics in nursing and health care.* Philadelphia: W.B. Saunders, pp. 201-213.

Institute of Medicine. (2003a). *A shared destiny: Community effects on uninsurance.* Washington, DC: National Academies Press.

Institute of Medicine. (2003b). *Improving palliative care: We can take better care of people with cancer.* Washington, DC: National Cancer Advisory Board Publication, National Academies Press.

Jemal, A., Tiwari, R.C., Murray, T., et al. (2004). Cancer statistics, 2004. *CA: A Cancer Journal for Clinicians 54*(1), 8-29.

Lamkin, L. (2003). *The nursing shortage and what ONS is doing about it.* Ohio Health presentation on March 28, Columbus.

Mee, C., & Robinson, E. (2003). What's different about this nursing shortage? *Nursing 2003*(1), 51–55.

Needham, J., Buerhaus, P., Mattke, S. et al. (2002). Nurse staffing and quality of care in hospitals in the United States. *Policy, Politics & Nursing Practice* 3(4):306-308.

Oncology Nursing Society (2002a). *The impact of the national nursing shortage on quality cancer care.* Pittsburgh: Author.

Oncology Nursing Society (2002b). *Patient's bill of rights for quality cancer care.* Pittsburgh: Author.

Oncology Nursing Society (2002c). *Quality cancer care.* Pittsburgh: Author.

Oncology Nursing Society. (2003a). *Average wholesale price (AWP) and oncology nursing practice expenses issue brief.* Pittsburgh: Author.

Oncology Nursing Society (2003b). *Cancer research and cancer clinical trials.* Pittsburgh: Author.

Oncology Nursing Society (2003c). *Ensuring high-quality cancer care in the Medicare program.* Pittsburgh: Author.

Ruetter, L., & Duncan, S. (2002). Preparing nurses to promote health-enhancing public policies. *Policy, Politics, & Nursing Practice* 3(4), 294-305.

NOTES

49 Professional Issues in Cancer Care

CONSTANCE B. ELLIS

1. A newly developed position for a certified oncology nurse is created at an acute care facility, and the nurse in this position is attempting to engage the nurses on the medical surgical oncology unit in the care of clients with cancer. Which intervention is likely to be the most useful in obtaining the cooperation of staff nurses with these clients' care?
   A. Conduct an education program about the importance of symptom management of clients receiving chemotherapy.
   B. Require staff nurses to complete an evaluation form on the care provided to their oncology clients.
   C. Collaborate with the nursing staff to develop critical pathways and reach individual discharge goals.
   D. Provide a 24-hour pager number so that the staff can reach the certified nurse when clinical decisions are needed.

2. Nurses on the oncology unit notice during an audit of the nursing admission assessment forms that nurses are consistently leaving blank or putting N/A (not applicable) on the sexuality portion of the tool. They further evaluate that the nurses are reluctant to ask clients questions to assess for sexuality concerns. The auditing nurses would best correct this deficiency by
   A. suggesting deletion of the sexuality category from the admission form.
   B. designing a sexuality continuing education program to enhance the nurses' knowledge.
   C. developing a poster of the admission form highlighting the sexuality portion.
   D. recommending the use of Annon's PLISSIT (P=Permission; LI=Limited Information, SS=Specific Suggestions, IT=Intensive Therapy) model for sexuality assessment.

3. What is the main purpose of certification for an oncology nurse?
   A. Protecting the public by helping to ensure the safe practice of nurses who provide oncology nursing care.
   B. Upgrading the nursing services provided by the institution in which the certified nurse practices.
   C. Increasing revenue to the institution and to the practicing nurses.
   D. Improving the nurse's knowledge about oncology nursing care.

4. To become a leader in oncology care, it is important for the nurse to be an active member in which organization:
   A. American Nurses Association (ANA).
   B. Home Health Nurses Association. (HHNA)
   C. Sigma Theta Tau International.
   D. Oncology Nursing Society (ONS).

5. Registered nurses who work on the oncology unit are planning to attend a specialized course on oncology nursing. What is the primary advantage to the nurses who attend this course?
   A. Become familiar with current techniques and resources based on the care of oncology clients.
   B. Meet with vendors who supply medications used in the care of clients with cancer.
   C. Discuss the etiology and prognosis of cases that should be referred to an extended care facility.
   D. Identify methods to reduce costs to health maintenance organizations (HMOs) for the care of clients with cancer.

6. A 48-year-old male client was diagnosed with bladder cancer. He has had chemotherapy and radiation and received an ileal conduit. Now several months after surgery he presents to the nurse, fearful of resuming sexual activities. The nurse, who is uncomfortable in the situation, can best advocate for this client by
   A. acknowledging the client's feelings.
   B. explaining to the client that his fears are unfounded.
   C. referring the client to a social worker.
   D. suggesting he seek gratification through other activities.

7. The primary purpose of states having nurse practice acts is to
   A. collect licensing fees to be used for continuing education projects.
   B. protect the public by describing the scope of professional nursing and requirements for licensure.
   C. set accreditation requirements for schools of nursing.
   D. promote continuing education for relicensure.

8. Collaboration between industry and clinical sites fosters research and improves client care. The key to successful collaboration is that
   A. all products are provided free to the clinical site.

B. the negotiated agreement spells out responsibilities.
   C. the industry provides the specific protocol to be followed.
   D. clinical sites complete all data collection and analysis.

9. A nurse who conveys a client's needs and concerns to the client's physician is practicing which type of advocacy?
   A. Consumer advocacy.
   B. Paternalistic advocacy.
   C. Simplistic advocacy.
   D. Consumer-centric advocacy.

10. After a nurse clarifies a procedure for a client, the client decides he does not want to have it. The nurse supports the client by informing the physician of the client's decision. Indicate the type of advocacy.
   A. Simplistic advocacy.
   B. Consumer-centric advocacy.
   C. Paternalistic advocacy.
   D. Consumer advocacy.

11. One intended outcome of the *Standards of Oncology Education: Patient/Significant Other and Public* is to
   A. provide a generic curriculum to students and educators.
   B. improve the quality of client teaching.
   C. define the roles and responsibilities of the advanced practice nurse (APN) in oncology.
   D. describe the client teaching necessary for the client receiving cisplatin chemotherapy.

12. The *scope of oncology nursing practice*
   A. defines the practice of oncology nursing.
   B. describes the role of allied health personnel with oncology clients.
   C. describes oncology nursing practice in a hospital setting only.
   D. delineates the professional responsibilities of the nurse engaged in clinical practice.

ANSWERS

1. *Answer:* C
Rationale: Collaborating with the staff will show that the certified nurse values their views, concerns, and expertise, and therefore this would build cooperation among the staff members. Option A is incorrect because conducting an educational program will only provide the staff with information. Option B is incorrect because evaluating the care of their clients is giving their personal opinion. Option D is incorrect because having a way to contact the nurse is again one-sided. None of Options A, B, or D demonstrates that collaboration has taken place.

2. *Answer:* B
Rationale: By developing a course where interaction would take place, the nurses would be able to gain knowledge and skills to help them become more comfortable with sexuality assessments, leading to better documentation. Option A is incorrect because eliminating the problem is avoidance and will not improve quality of care. Option C is incorrect because the poster may call attention to problems but does not provide the nurse with a means to resolve the problem. Option D is incorrect because nurses may not be familiar with the Annon's PLISSIT sexuality assessment tool. They need some education to help them get over their discomfort with this subject.

3. *Answer:* A
Rationale: Certification's primary concern is to present nurses who have a body of knowledge specific to cancer that would promote their safe practice and therefore protect the public. Option B is incorrect because even though the nursing service may be affected, that would not be the primary purpose. Option C is incorrect because a side benefit of having certified nurses is that they may draw more clients to a facility. Option D is incorrect because a nurse's knowledge will increase from studying for the examination.

4. *Answer:* D
Rationale: Membership in the ONS provides nurses with a wealth of knowledge through publications and local, regional, and national conferences. Programs and scholarships are offered to help members develop as leaders and to promote research and education. Option A is incorrect because ANA serves as a general population of nurses made up of a large number of schools of nursing faculty. Option B is incorrect because HHNA serves nurses caring for a broad base of clients. Option C is incorrect because Sigma Theta Tau is the national honor society for nurses.

5. *Answer:* A
Rationale: Attending an oncology conference provides the nurse with access to content experts who present the latest information on the care of oncology clients and networking opportunities to gain resources from other nurses and vendors. Option B is incorrect because nurses may learn more about medications, but physicians order them. Option C is incorrect because the content may or may not focus on extended care. Option D is incorrect because the content may or may not focus on HMOs.

6. *Answer:* C
Rationale: The nurse is uncomfortable in the situation and can give support, but this client needs someone whose role involves sexuality counseling to help him with his concerns. Option A is incorrect because although it is good to acknowledge the problem, it is not being an advocate. Option B is incorrect because he may have problems with performance. Option D is incorrect because it avoids the problem.

7. *Answer:* B
Rationale: State Nurse Practice Acts are primarily concerned with protecting the public. Two ways they do this are by defining the scope of practice and licensure. They also monitor practice through peer review and apply disciplinary action for nurses violating the standards through hearings. Option A is incorrect because licensing fees usually go to the Board of Nursing Examiners. Option C is

incorrect because the National League for Nursing sets the accreditation standards. Option D is incorrect because mandatory continuing education is not required for relicensure in all states.

8. *Answer:* B
   Rationale: For collaboration to be successful, all parties involved need to be included in the negotiations, and each party's responsibilities need to be specified in the agreement. Option A is incorrect because companies may not be able to provide free expensive equipment and/or supplies for a trial. Option C is incorrect because industry may provide protocols, but they must be approved by the institution's Institutional Review Board (IRB). Option D is incorrect because sites and industry may share in data collection.

9. *Answer:* C
   Rationale: Simplistic advocacy is the act of pleading for the cause of another. Consumer advocacy means that the nurse is required to provide the client with information and let him make the decision. Paternalistic advocacy means that the nurse does something for the client's own good without his consent. Consumer-centric advocacy means that the nurse provides information, then supports the client in his decision.

10. *Answer:* B
    Rationale: Consumer-centric advocacy is the act of a nurse providing a client with information and then supporting the client in his decision. Simplistic advocacy is the act of pleading for the cause of another. Paternalistic advocacy means that the nurse does something for the client's own good without his consent. Consumer advocacy means that the nurse provides information, and the client makes the decision.

11. *Answer:* B
    Rationale: The Oncology Nursing Society believes that oncology nurses have the responsibility of developing, assessing, implementing, and evaluating educational programs for clients, their significant others, and the public. Option A: A generic curriculum is provided in the ONS Publication, *The Master's Degree with a Specialty in Advanced Practice Oncology Nursing* (4th ed.). Option C: Defining the roles and responsibilities of the APN in oncology can be found in the *Statement on the Scope and Standards of Advanced Practice Nursing in Oncology* (3rd ed.). Option D: Patient teaching for the client receiving any oncology treatment is addressed in all the guidelines and recommendations for care published by ONS.

12. *Answer:* A
    Rationale: The scope of oncology nursing practice defines the practice of oncology nursing along the continuum of care and across care delivery settings. Option B: Although standards of care address the role of the oncology nurse in relationship to other ancillary disciplines, the scope of nursing practice specifically addresses the nursing role. Option C: The scope addresses oncology nursing across all care delivery settings. Option D: Standards of professional performance delineate the professional responsibilities of the nurse engaged in clinical practice.

BIBLIOGRAPHY

American Nurses Association. (2001). *Code of ethics for nurses with interpretive statements.* Washington, DC: American Nurses Publishing.

American Nurses Association. (1995). *Nursing: A social policy statement.* Washington, DC: American Nurses Publishing.

Annon, J. (1976). The PLISSIT model: a proposed conceptual scheme for the behavioral treatment of sexual problems, *Journal of Sex Education and Therapy.* 2, 1-15.

Blecher, C.S. (2004). *Standards of oncology education: Patient/significant other and public* (3rd ed.). Pittsburgh: Oncology Nursing Society.

Brandt, J.M., & Wickham, R.S. (Eds.). (2004). *Statement on the scope and standards of oncology nursing practice.* Pittsburgh: Oncology Nursing Society.

Centers for Disease Control. Office of Minority Health. (2003). Retrieved October 29, 2003, from *http://www.cdc.gov/omh/AMH.factsheets/cancer. htm.*

Dadich, K.A., & Yoder-Wise, P.S. (2003) Cancer management: Putting yourself in charge. In P. S. Yoder-Wise (Ed.). *Leading and managing in nursing* (3rd ed.). St. Louis: Mosby, pp. 449-467.

Hewitt, J. (2002). A critical review of the arguments debating the role of the nurse advocate. *Journal of Advanced Nursing* 38(5), 439-445.

Institute of Medicine. (2001). *Crossing the quality chasm: A new health system for the 21st century.* Washington, DC: National Academy Press.

Institute of Medicine. (2003). *Crossing the quality chasm: The IOM health care quality initiative.* Retrieved December 4, 2003, from http://www.ion. edu/ report.asp?id=5432.

Jacobs, L.A. (Ed.).(2003). *Master's degree with a specialty in oncology nursing* (4th ed.). Pittsburgh: Oncology Nursing Society.

Jacobs, L.A. (Ed.). (2003). *Statement on the scope and standards of advanced practice nursing in oncology* (3rd ed.). Pittsburgh: Oncology Nursing Society.

Joint Commission on Accreditation of Healthcare Organizations. (2004). *Comprehensive accreditation manual for hospitals: The official handbook.* Oakbrook Terrace, IL: Joint Commission Resources.

Katz, J. M., & Green, E. (1997). *Managing quality: A guide to system-wide performance management in health care* (2nd ed.). St. Louis, Mosby.

NOTES